THE
WELLNESS
JOURNEY

RESOURCES FOR HEALTH AND HEALING

VOLUME 2

THEO PRODROMITIS

First edition 2024

Paperback ISBN: 978-1-956856-63-7

Library of Congress Control Number: 2024925928

Published by thewordverve (www.thewordverve.com)
Canton, GA, USA

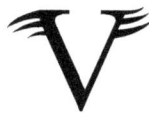

Cover and print interior design by Robin Krauss
www.bookformatters.com

The *Wellness Journey* books are dedicated to my big Greek family that inspires me every day to strive relentlessly to reduce human suffering.

THANK YOU . . .

To my grandparents who came to the US from Greece and Asia Minor with no material wealth but built an incredible life for all of us. We are standing on your shoulders of sacrifice and love.

To my parents Mary and Spero who lived the concept of "Philotimo," the Greek imperative to live a life of honor for the greater good.

To my brother Dean and sister Themie who ground and sustain me through all of life's tribulations.

To my children, Mary, Jacqueline, and Spero, who are divine beyond measure and taught me unconditional love.

To my nephew Andrew. Your love echoes in every page.

To my cousins, nephews, nieces, friends who are our chosen family, and relatives across the globe for making this life a grand adventure together.

To my amazing research assistant, Sabrina Ott, who brought a wonderful level of excellence and dedication to life in these pages.

A special debt of gratitude to *thewordverve* and Janet Fix with her team, Billie and Robin, who diligently curated and refined this labor of love.

Most importantly, thank you to God for the unconditional Grace & Love to follow my heart.

I remain faithfully yours in service,

Theo

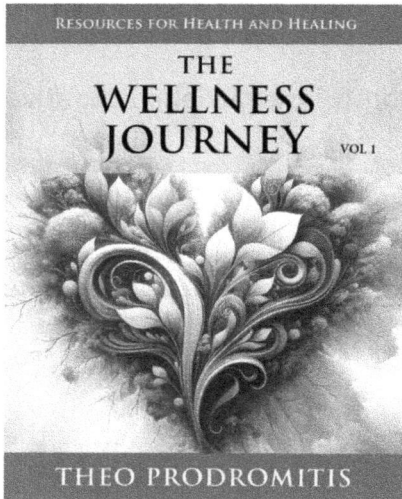

RESOURCES FOR HEALTH AND HEALING

THE
WELLNESS
JOURNEY VOL 1

THEO PRODROMITIS

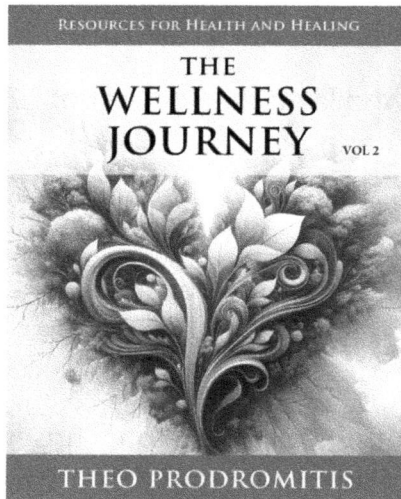

RESOURCES FOR HEALTH AND HEALING

THE
WELLNESS
JOURNEY VOL 2

THEO PRODROMITIS

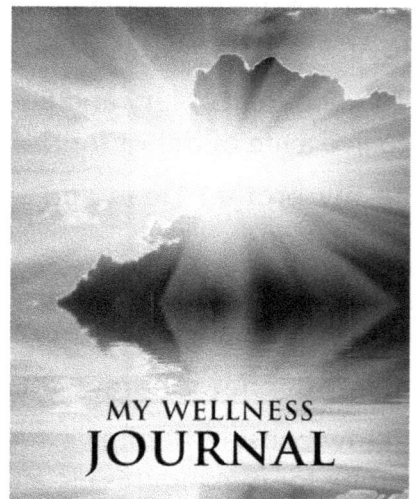

MY WELLNESS
JOURNAL

WELCOME

Welcome to Volume 2 of *The Wellness Journey*. We laid the foundation for a life of holistic well-being and the synergy of Eastern and Western Medicine in *The Wellness Journey, Volume 1*. By exploring the essential pillars of health—mind, body, and spirit—we revealed how these interconnected aspects shape our overall wellness. The importance of mental clarity, physical vitality, and spiritual balance were explored, offering practical strategies for achieving harmony across all three. Readers discovered how simple daily habits, proper nutrition, regular exercise, mental health techniques, and spiritual practices can foster a resilient, fulfilling life. The first volume encouraged readers to build a strong, adaptable foundation, illustrating that health is a continuous, evolving journey. Volume 2 of *The Wellness Journey* takes that journey to the next level, introducing a broader array of transformative practices like Energy Medicine, Martial Arts, Sound Therapy, and Light Therapy. This exciting addition deepens the approach to well-being, offering innovative tools to complete your holistic health journey.

To make your experience even more impactful, integrate *My Wellness Journal* into your daily routine. This journal is designed to be your companion through the process, helping you set intentions, track progress, and reflect on new practices. It transforms ideas into action, guiding you to embody health and healing in every aspect of life. Whether you're continuing from Volume 1 or beginning here, get ready to unlock your fullest potential and bring the journey to life—one entry at a time. Think of this volume not just as a guide but as a conversation starter—a way to open the door to new possibilities and perspectives on what it means to truly be well.

For more information, downloads and resources please visit

www.theoprodromitis.com/thewellnessjourney

TABLE OF CONTENTS

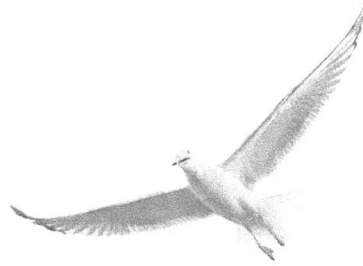

COMPLETE WELLNESS

Holistic and Overall Approaches to Daily Practices

Introduction

Complete wellness is a multifaceted approach to health that encompasses physical, mental, emotional, and spiritual well-being. It involves integrating various practices into daily life to promote balance and harmony in all aspects of existence. This section explores holistic approaches to complete wellness, focusing on daily practices that can enhance overall health and vitality. By adopting these practices, individuals can create a foundation for sustained well-being and a higher quality of life.

Physical Wellness

Physical wellness is the cornerstone of overall health. It involves maintaining a healthy body through regular exercise, proper nutrition, adequate sleep, `and preventive care. Here are some key practices to incorporate into your daily routine:

Regular Exercise: Engage in at least 30 minutes of moderate exercise most days of the week. This can include activities such as walking, jogging, cycling, yoga, or strength training. Regular physical activity helps maintain a healthy weight, strengthens muscles and bones, and reduces the risk of chronic diseases (Warburton et al., 2006).

Balanced Nutrition: Follow a diet rich in whole, nutrient-dense foods. Include a variety of fruits, vegetables, whole grains, lean proteins, and healthy fats. Avoid processed and sugary foods that can lead to weight gain and health issues. Drinking plenty of water is also essential for hydration and overall health (Harvard T.H. Chan School of Public Health, 2020).

Adequate Sleep: Aim for 7-9 hours of quality sleep each night. Good sleep hygiene practices include maintaining a regular sleep schedule, creating a restful sleep environment, and avoiding stimulants like caffeine and electronic devices before bedtime. Adequate sleep supports physical health, cognitive function, and emotional well-being (Walker, 2017).

Preventive Care: Schedule regular checkups and screenings with healthcare providers. Preventive care helps detect potential health issues early and allows for timely intervention. Vaccinations, dental checkups, and regular monitoring of blood pressure and cholesterol levels are crucial components of preventive care (Centers for Disease Control and Prevention, 2020).

Mental Wellness

Mental wellness is essential for cognitive function, emotional stability, and overall quality of life. It involves practices that support mental clarity, focus, and resilience. Here are some daily practices to enhance mental wellness:

Mindfulness and Meditation: Incorporate mindfulness and meditation into your daily routine to reduce stress and enhance mental clarity. Mindfulness involves staying present in the moment and observing thoughts and feelings without judgment. Meditation practices, such as mindfulness meditation or guided imagery, can help calm the mind and improve concentration (Kabat-Zinn, 1990).

Continuous Learning: Engage in activities that challenge your brain and promote continuous learning. Reading, puzzles, learning a new language or skill, and engaging in intellectually stimulating conversations can keep your mind sharp and agile (Wilson et al., 2002).

Stress Management: Develop effective stress management techniques to cope with daily challenges. This can include practices such as deep breathing exercises, progressive muscle relaxation, journaling, or engaging in hobbies that bring joy and relaxation (Cohen et al., 2007).

Time Management: Prioritize tasks and manage your time effectively to reduce feelings of being overwhelmed and enhance productivity. Create a balanced schedule that includes time for work, rest, and leisure activities. Using tools such as to-do lists, planners, and time blocking can help manage time more efficiently (Macan et al., 1990).

Emotional Wellness

Emotional wellness involves understanding, expressing, and managing emotions in a healthy way. It contributes to overall happiness and life satisfaction. Here are some practices to support emotional wellness:

Emotional Awareness: Cultivate emotional awareness by regularly checking in with your feelings and acknowledging them without judgment. This practice can help you understand your emotional responses and develop healthier ways to cope with stress and challenges (Goleman, 1995).

Positive Relationships: Nurture positive relationships with family, friends, and colleagues. Strong social connections provide support, reduce feelings of loneliness, and contribute to emotional resilience. Make time for meaningful interactions and communicate openly and honestly with loved ones (Holt-Lunstad et al., 2010).

Gratitude Practice: Develop a daily gratitude practice to focus on the positive aspects of life. Keeping a gratitude journal, where you write down things you are thankful for each day, can enhance emotional well-being and foster a positive outlook on life (Emmons & McCullough, 2003).

Emotional Expression: Find healthy outlets for expressing emotions, such as talking with a trusted friend, writing in a journal, or engaging in creative activities like art or music. Expressing emotions constructively can help release pent-up feelings and improve emotional health (Pennebaker, 1997).

Spiritual Wellness

Spiritual wellness involves finding meaning and purpose in life, which can enhance overall well-being and provide a sense of inner peace. Here are some practices to foster spiritual wellness:

Mindful Reflection: Set aside time each day for mindful reflection or meditation. This practice can help you connect with your inner self, clarify your values, and align your actions with your beliefs. Reflecting on your goals, intentions, and experiences can foster a deeper sense of purpose (Siegel, 2010).

Connection with Nature: Spend time in nature to rejuvenate your spirit and gain a sense of connection with the world around you. Activities such as walking in the park, hiking, or gardening can provide a sense of peace and renewal. Nature can serve as a powerful reminder of the interconnectedness of all life (Mayer et al., 2009).

Acts of Kindness: Engage in acts of kindness and service to others. Helping others can provide a sense of fulfillment and strengthen your sense of community. Volunteer work, supporting a cause you believe in, or simply offering a helping hand to those in need can enhance spiritual wellness (Lyubomirsky et al., 2005).

Personal Growth: Commit to ongoing personal and spiritual growth. This can involve reading spiritual or philosophical texts, attending workshops or retreats, and exploring different spiritual practices. Pursuing personal growth helps deepen your understanding of yourself and your place in the world (Walsh & Shapiro, 2006).

Action Plan

Complete wellness requires a holistic approach that integrates physical, mental, emotional, and spiritual practices into daily life. For those interested in achieving complete wellness, consider the following steps:

1. Create a Balanced Routine: Develop a daily routine that includes practices for physical, mental, emotional, and spiritual wellness. Aim for a balanced approach that addresses all aspects of your well-being.

2. **Set Realistic Goals:** Set achievable goals for each area of wellness. Start with small, manageable changes and gradually build on them. Consistency is key to experiencing lasting benefits.

3. **Stay Committed:** Make a commitment to prioritize your well-being. This may require making adjustments to your lifestyle, such as reducing screen time, improving sleep habits, or setting aside time for self-care.

4. **Seek Support:** Connect with others who share your wellness goals. Join a wellness community, find a workout buddy, or seek guidance from a coach or therapist. Support from others can provide motivation and accountability.

5. **Reflect and Adjust:** Regularly reflect on your wellness journey and make adjustments as needed. Listen to your body and mind and be open to trying new practices that enhance your well-being.

Conclusion

Achieving complete wellness involves adopting a holistic approach that integrates physical, mental, emotional, and spiritual practices into daily life. By prioritizing these aspects of well-being, individuals can create a foundation for sustained health, happiness, and fulfillment. Embrace this journey with an open mind and a commitment to self-care, and you may discover a deeper sense of balance and harmony in your life.

Life Force by Tony Robbins:
A Comprehensive Approach to Health and Vitality

Introduction

Life Force by Tony Robbins is a comprehensive guide to health and vitality, co-authored with Dr. Peter H. Diamandis and Dr. Robert Hariri. The book combines Robbins' motivational approach with cutting-edge scientific insights and practical strategies for achieving optimal health and longevity. This section provides an overview of *Life Force*, explores its key approaches, and offers a critical review of its content, highlighting the actionable steps readers can take to enhance their health and well-being.

Overview of *Life Force*

Life Force is structured into several key sections, each focusing on different aspects of health and wellness. The book covers a wide range of topics, including nutrition, exercise, sleep, mental health, and emerging medical technologies. Robbins, known for his motivational speaking and personal development programs, brings his signature enthusiasm and practical advice to the book, aiming to empower readers to take control of their health.

The book is divided into three main parts:

The Science of Life Force: This section delves into the latest scientific discoveries and medical breakthroughs that can help individuals optimize their health. It covers topics such as regenerative medicine, gene therapy, and the use of advanced diagnostics to detect and prevent diseases.

Strategies for Lifelong Health: In this section, Robbins and his co-authors provide practical strategies for maintaining and enhancing health. Topics include nutrition, exercise, sleep, and stress management. The authors emphasize the importance of personalized health plans tailored to individual needs and genetic profiles.

Creating Your Life Force Plan: The final section focuses on actionable steps readers can take to implement the concepts and strategies discussed in the book. It includes guidance on creating a personalized health plan, setting goals, and tracking progress.

Key Approaches in *Life Force*

The approaches presented in Life Force are grounded in both traditional wisdom and modern science. Here are some of the key approaches discussed in the book:

Personalized Medicine: One of the central themes of *Life Force* is the importance of personalized medicine. The authors advocate for the use of advanced diagnostics, genetic testing, and personalized treatment plans to optimize health. By understanding individual genetic profiles and health markers, people can tailor their diets, exercise routines, and medical treatments to their unique needs (Robbins, Diamandis, & Hariri, 2022).

Regenerative Medicine: The book explores the potential of regenerative medicine to repair and regenerate tissues and organs. Topics such as stem cell therapy, tissue engineering, and regenerative treatments for conditions like arthritis and heart disease are discussed. The authors highlight the transformative potential of these technologies in extending health span and improving quality of life (Robbins, Diamandis, & Hariri, 2022).

Nutritional Optimization: Nutrition is a cornerstone of the book's approach to health. The authors provide evidence-based recommendations for a nutrient-dense diet that supports longevity and vitality. They discuss the benefits of various dietary approaches, including intermittent fasting, ketogenic diets, and plant-based nutrition. The importance of micronutrients, antioxidants, and personalized nutrition plans is emphasized (Robbins, Diamandis, & Hariri, 2022).

Exercise and Movement: Regular physical activity is essential for maintaining health, and "Life Force" offers practical advice on creating an effective exercise routine. The authors recommend a combination of aerobic exercise, strength training, and flexibility exercises. They also discuss the benefits of high-intensity interval training (HIIT) and the importance of staying active throughout the day (Robbins, Diamandis, & Hariri, 2022).

Sleep and Recovery: Adequate sleep and recovery are crucial for overall health. The book provides strategies for improving sleep quality, such as maintaining a consistent sleep schedule, creating a restful sleep environment, and managing stress. The authors also discuss the role of sleep in cognitive function, immune health, and emotional well-being (Robbins, Diamandis, & Hariri, 2022).

Mental and Emotional Health: Life Force emphasizes the importance of mental and emotional health in achieving overall wellness. The authors offer techniques for managing stress, building resilience, and cultivating a positive mindset. Practices such as mindfulness meditation, gratitude journaling, and cognitive behavioral techniques are recommended to enhance mental well-being (Robbins, Diamandis, & Hariri, 2022).

Emerging Technologies: The book explores emerging technologies that have the potential to revolutionize healthcare. These include artificial intelligence, genomics, and wearable health devices. The authors discuss how these technologies can provide real-time health data, improve diagnostics, and personalize treatment plans (Robbins, Diamandis, & Hariri, 2022).

Review of *Life Force*

Life Force offers a comprehensive and engaging approach to health and wellness, blending motivational advice with scientific insights. Here are some of the strengths and potential limitations of the book:

Strengths:

Holistic Approach: The book takes a holistic approach to health, addressing physical, mental, and emotional well-being. This comprehensive perspective is valuable for readers seeking to improve all aspects of their health.

Actionable Advice: *Life Force* is filled with practical tips and strategies that readers can implement immediately. The focus on personalized health plans and actionable steps makes the information accessible and applicable.

Cutting-Edge Science: The inclusion of the latest scientific research and medical technologies adds credibility and depth to the book. Readers are introduced to innovative treatments and diagnostic tools that can enhance their health.

Motivational Tone: Tony Robbins' motivational style is a key feature of the book. His enthusiasm and encouragement can inspire readers to take charge of their health and make positive changes.

Potential Limitations:

Complexity of Information: Some readers may find the scientific information and medical technologies discussed in the book to be complex and overwhelming. While the authors strive to explain concepts clearly, the advanced nature of some topics may be challenging for those without a background in health or science.

Accessibility of Treatments: Many of the cutting-edge treatments and technologies discussed in the book may not be readily accessible or affordable for all readers. This could limit the applicability of some of the recommendations.

Overemphasis on Technology: While emerging technologies hold great promise, the book's focus on high-tech solutions may overshadow the importance of simple, low-cost lifestyle changes that can also significantly impact health.

Practical Applications and Steps

For readers interested in implementing the principles and strategies from *Life Force*, here are some practical steps to consider:

1. **Create a Personalized Health Plan:** Use the book's guidelines to develop a health plan tailored to your unique needs. Consider factors such as your genetic profile, health markers, and personal goals. Work with healthcare professionals to refine and implement your plan.

2. **Focus on Nutrient-Dense Foods:** Prioritize a diet rich in whole, nutrient-dense foods. Incorporate a variety of vegetables, fruits, lean proteins, healthy fats, and whole grains into your meals. Consider experimenting with dietary approaches such as intermittent fasting or a ketogenic diet if they align with your health goals.

3. **Establish a Regular Exercise Routine:** Develop an exercise routine that includes aerobic exercise, strength training, and flexibility exercises. Aim for at least 150 minutes of moderate intensity exercise each week, and incorporate movement into your daily activities.

4. **Improve Sleep Quality:** Implement strategies to enhance your sleep quality, such as maintaining a consistent sleep schedule, creating a restful sleep environment, and practicing relaxation techniques before bed. Aim for 7-9 hours of quality sleep each night.

5. **Manage Stress and Enhance Mental Health:** Practice stress management techniques such as mindfulness meditation, deep breathing exercises, and gratitude journaling. Cultivate a positive mindset and seek support from mental health professionals if needed.

6. **Stay Informed About Emerging Technologies:** Keep up with the latest advancements in health technology and consider how they might benefit your health. Explore options such as wearable health devices, genetic testing, and advanced diagnostics to gain insights into your health.

7. **Monitor Progress and Adjust:** Regularly track your progress and make adjustments to your health plan as needed. Use tools such as health journals, fitness trackers, and regular checkups to stay on track and achieve your health goals.

Action Plan

Life Force by Tony Robbins offers a comprehensive and actionable approach to achieving optimal health and vitality. For those interested in exploring the principles and strategies discussed in the book, consider the following steps:

1. **Read and Engage:** Read *Life Force* thoroughly and engage with its content. Take notes, highlight key points, and reflect on how the information applies to your life.

2. **Implement Changes Gradually:** Start by making small, manageable changes to your lifestyle. Gradual implementation of new habits and practices can lead to sustained improvements in health and well-being.

3. **Seek Professional Guidance:** Work with healthcare professionals, such as doctors, nutritionists, and fitness trainers, to develop and refine your personalized health plan. Their expertise can help ensure that you are making safe and effective choices.

4. **Join a Community:** Connect with others who share your health goals. Joining a wellness community, participating in online forums, or attending workshops can provide support, motivation, and accountability.

5. **Stay Committed:** Maintain a long-term commitment to your health and wellness journey. Consistency and persistence are key to achieving lasting results. Regularly revisit your goals, track your progress, and celebrate your successes.

Conclusion

Life Force by Tony Robbins is a valuable resource for anyone seeking to improve their health and vitality. By combining motivational guidance with the latest scientific research and practical strategies, Robbins and his co-authors provide a comprehensive roadmap for achieving optimal wellness. Embracing the principles and actionable steps outlined in the book can empower individuals to take control of their health, make informed decisions, and pursue a path of lifelong vitality. Whether through personalized medicine, nutritional optimization, or advanced medical technologies, Life Force offers a wealth of knowledge and inspiration to help readers lead healthier, more fulfilling lives. Embrace this journey with an open mind, a commitment to continuous improvement, and a dedication to living your best life.

Acupuncture:
A Journey Through History and Healing

Introduction

Acupuncture is an ancient practice that has been used for thousands of years to promote health and well-being. Originating in China, this traditional form of medicine involves the insertion of thin needles into specific points on the body to balance the flow of energy, or qi. Over the centuries, acupuncture has evolved and spread across the globe, gaining recognition for its therapeutic benefits. This section delves into the rich history of acupuncture, its principles and techniques, its applications in modern medicine, and the scientific evidence supporting its efficacy.

The History of Acupuncture

Acupuncture has a long and storied history that dates back over 2,500 years. Its origins can be traced to ancient China, where it was developed as part of Traditional Chinese Medicine (TCM). The earliest written records of acupuncture are found in the Huangdi Neijing (The Yellow Emperor's Classic of Internal Medicine), which dates to around 100 BCE. This foundational text outlines the principles of acupuncture, the meridian system, and the role of qi in health and disease (Unschuld, 2011).

> **Ancient Beginnings:** Acupuncture likely began as a form of folk medicine, where primitive needles made from stone, bone, and bamboo were used to treat ailments. As Chinese society advanced, so did the practice of acupuncture. Bronze needles were introduced, and the understanding of acupuncture points and meridians became more sophisticated (Lu & Needham, 1980).

Development and Codification: During the Han Dynasty (206 BCE – 220 CE), acupuncture became more formally codified. The Huangdi Neijing, along with other texts like the Zhenjiu Jiayi Jing (The ABC Classic of Acupuncture and Moxibustion), compiled by Huangfu Mi around 260 CE, provided detailed descriptions of acupuncture points, meridians, and treatment techniques. These works laid the groundwork for the systematic practice of acupuncture (Lu & Needham, 1980).

Spread and Evolution: Acupuncture continued to evolve through subsequent dynasties, incorporating new techniques and theories. It spread to neighboring countries such as Korea and Japan, where it was integrated into their traditional medical systems. In Japan, acupuncture became closely linked with moxibustion (the burning of mugwort on or near the skin), while in Korea, it developed its unique approaches and techniques (Lo & Wang, 2013).

Acupuncture in the West: Acupuncture was introduced to the West in the 17th century by Jesuit missionaries and traders. However, it remained relatively obscure until the 20th century, when it gained broader recognition. In the 1970s, President Richard Nixon's visit to China and a New York Times article describing the use of acupuncture for postoperative pain relief sparked widespread interest in the United States (Reston, 1971). Since then, acupuncture has become increasingly popular and accepted as a complementary and alternative medicine.

Principles and Techniques of Acupuncture

The practice of acupuncture is based on the concept of qi (pronounced "chee"), the vital energy that flows through the body along pathways known as meridians. According to TCM, health is achieved when qi flows smoothly and is balanced. Illness occurs when qi is blocked or imbalanced. Acupuncture aims to restore the proper flow of qi by stimulating specific points on the body, known as acupoints (Maciocia, 1989).

Meridians and Acupoints: There are 12 primary meridians in the body, each corresponding to an organ system, such as the heart, liver, or lungs. Additionally, there are eight extraordinary meridians that serve as reservoirs of energy. Acupoints are located along these meridians and are the sites where needles are inserted to influence the flow of qi. There are over 360 acupoints on the body, each with specific indications and functions (Maciocia, 1989).

Needling Techniques: Acupuncture involves the insertion of thin, sterile needles into acupoints. The depth and angle of insertion, as well as the manipulation of the needles, can vary depending on the condition being treated. Techniques may include twisting, lifting, and thrusting the needles to achieve the desired therapeutic effect. Some practitioners also use electroacupuncture, where electrical stimulation is applied to the needles to enhance the treatment (Liu et al., 2014).

Moxibustion: Moxibustion is often used in conjunction with acupuncture. It involves burning dried mugwort (moxa) near or on the skin to warm the meridians and promote the flow of qi. This technique is believed to enhance the effects of acupuncture, especially in conditions involving cold or deficiency (Yamashita et al., 2001).

Cupping and Other Modalities: In addition to needling and moxibustion, acupuncture practitioners may use other techniques such as cupping, where suction cups are placed on the skin to stimulate blood flow and relieve tension. Gua sha, a scraping technique, and tui na, a form of therapeutic massage, are also commonly used to complement acupuncture treatments (Cao et al., 2012).

Applications of Acupuncture in Modern Medicine

Acupuncture is used to treat a wide range of conditions, both acute and chronic. Its applications extend beyond pain management to include various physical, mental, and emotional health issues. Here are some of the most common applications of acupuncture in modern medicine:

Pain Management: Acupuncture is widely recognized for its effectiveness in relieving pain. It is commonly used to treat conditions such as chronic back pain, osteoarthritis, migraines, and postoperative pain. Studies have shown that acupuncture can stimulate the release of endorphins, the body's natural painkillers, and modulate pain pathways in the nervous system (Vickers et al., 2012).

Stress and Anxiety: Acupuncture has been shown to have a calming effect on the nervous system, making it an effective treatment for stress and anxiety. It can help regulate the body's stress response and promote relaxation by influencing neurotransmitter levels and reducing the production of stress hormones (Pilkington et al., 2007).

Digestive Disorders: Acupuncture can be beneficial for various digestive disorders, including irritable bowel syndrome (IBS), acid reflux, and constipation. It helps regulate digestive function by balancing the autonomic nervous system and improving gastrointestinal motility (Zheng et al., 2015).

Women's Health: Acupuncture is often used to address women's health issues such as menstrual irregularities, menopause symptoms, and infertility. It can help regulate hormonal balance, improve blood flow to the reproductive organs, and reduce stress, which can all contribute to improved reproductive health (Smith et al., 2011).

Respiratory Conditions: Acupuncture can support the treatment of respiratory conditions like asthma, allergies, and sinusitis. By stimulating specific acupoints, acupuncture can help reduce inflammation, improve immune function, and enhance respiratory efficiency (Choi et al., 2013).

Neurological Disorders: Acupuncture has shown promise in the treatment of neurological disorders such as stroke rehabilitation, neuropathy, and Parkinson's disease. It can promote neuroplasticity, reduce inflammation, and improve motor and sensory functions (Zhou et al., 2015).

Scientific Evidence Supporting Acupuncture

The scientific study of acupuncture has grown significantly in recent decades, with numerous studies and clinical trials investigating its mechanisms and efficacy. While the exact mechanisms of acupuncture are not fully understood, several theories have been proposed to explain its effects:

Endorphin Release: One of the most widely accepted theories is that acupuncture stimulates the release of endorphins, the body's natural pain-relieving chemicals. Endorphins interact with opioid receptors in the brain to reduce pain perception and promote a sense of well-being (Han, 2004).

Neurotransmitter Modulation: Acupuncture is believed to influence the levels of various neurotransmitters, such as serotonin and dopamine, which play a role in mood regulation and pain perception. By modulating these neurotransmitters, acupuncture can help alleviate symptoms of depression, anxiety, and pain (Zhou & Benharash, 2014).

Nerve Stimulation: Acupuncture needles may stimulate specific nerves that send signals to the brain and spinal cord. This can lead to the activation of the body's pain-modulating pathways and the release of neuropeptides that reduce inflammation and pain (Zhao, 2008).

Improved Blood Flow: Acupuncture has been shown to improve blood flow and microcirculation in the treated areas. Enhanced blood flow can promote healing, reduce inflammation, and improve the delivery of oxygen and nutrients to tissues (Komori et al., 2009).

Immune System Regulation: Some studies suggest that acupuncture can modulate the immune system by increasing the production of white blood cells and enhancing immune responses. This may explain its effectiveness in treating conditions related to immune dysfunction, such as allergies and autoimmune diseases (Sakai et al., 2008).

Numerous clinical trials and systematic reviews have supported the efficacy of acupuncture for various conditions. For example, a large-scale meta-analysis published in the Archives of Internal Medicine found that acupuncture was effective for chronic pain conditions such as back pain, osteoarthritis, and migraines (Vickers et al., 2012). Another review published in The Journal of Alternative and Complementary Medicine concluded that acupuncture was beneficial for anxiety and depression (Pilkington et al., 2007).

Practical Applications and Steps

For individuals interested in exploring acupuncture as a therapeutic option, here are some practical steps to consider:

1. **Consult a Licensed Practitioner:** Seek treatment from a licensed acupuncturist who has received formal training in acupuncture and Traditional Chinese Medicine. A qualified practitioner can provide personalized treatment plans based on your specific health needs. Ensure that the acupuncturist is certified by a reputable organization, such as the National Certification Commission for Acupuncture and Oriental Medicine (NCCAOM) in the United States.

2. **Set Realistic Expectations:** While acupuncture can be highly effective for many conditions, it is not a magic bullet. It's important to have realistic expectations and understand that results can vary depending on the individual and the condition being treated. Discuss your goals and concerns with your practitioner to set achievable treatment objectives.

3. **Commit to a Treatment Plan:** Acupuncture often requires multiple sessions to achieve optimal results. Your practitioner will recommend a treatment schedule based on your specific needs, which may include weekly or bi-weekly sessions initially. Consistency and adherence to the recommended treatment plan are key to experiencing the full benefits of acupuncture.

4. **Maintain Open Communication:** Keep an open line of communication with your acupuncturist. Provide feedback on your symptoms and any changes you notice, both positive and negative. This information helps the practitioner adjust the treatment plan as needed to ensure the best outcomes.

5. **Combine with Other Therapies:** Acupuncture can be used as a complementary therapy alongside conventional medical treatments and other holistic practices. Discuss with your healthcare provider how acupuncture can be integrated into your overall treatment plan. Combining acupuncture with practices such as physical therapy, chiropractic care, or herbal medicine can enhance overall effectiveness.

6. **Practice Self-Care:** Support your acupuncture treatments with self-care practices that promote overall well-being. This includes maintaining a balanced diet, staying hydrated, getting regular exercise, and practicing stress management techniques such as meditation or deep breathing exercises. Self-care enhances the body's ability to heal and respond to acupuncture.

7. **Educate Yourself:** Learn about the principles of acupuncture and Traditional Chinese Medicine to better understand the treatment process and its benefits. Reading books,

attending workshops, or participating in online courses can provide valuable insights and deepen your appreciation for this ancient healing practice.

8. **Monitor Your Progress:** Keep a journal to track your symptoms, treatment sessions, and any changes you experience. Monitoring your progress helps you and your practitioner evaluate the effectiveness of the treatment and make necessary adjustments. It also provides a record of your journey and the improvements you've achieved.

9. **Stay Consistent with Follow-Up:** Even after achieving initial improvements, periodic follow-up sessions can help maintain the benefits of acupuncture and prevent recurrence of symptoms. Work with your acupuncturist to determine an appropriate maintenance schedule that suits your needs.

10. **Stay Open to Other Modalities:** Acupuncture is just one aspect of Traditional Chinese Medicine. Your practitioner may recommend other modalities such as herbal medicine, dietary changes, or lifestyle modifications to support your overall health. Being open to these additional recommendations can enhance your treatment outcomes.

Case Studies and Examples

To illustrate the potential of acupuncture, consider the following case studies:

Case Study 1: Chronic Back Pain Relief John, a 45-year-old office worker, suffered from chronic lower back pain due to prolonged sitting and poor posture. Conventional treatments provided only temporary relief. After consulting a licensed acupuncturist, John began a series of weekly acupuncture sessions. Within a few weeks, he noticed a significant reduction in pain and improved mobility. By continuing with regular treatments and incorporating recommended exercises, John was able to manage his back pain effectively and return to his daily activities with greater comfort.

Case Study 2: Managing Anxiety and Stress Sarah, a 30-year-old teacher, experienced high levels of anxiety and stress due to her demanding job. She struggled with insomnia and frequent headaches. After seeking help from an acupuncturist, Sarah started receiving bi-weekly treatments focused on calming the nervous system and promoting relaxation. Alongside acupuncture, she practiced mindfulness meditation and made dietary changes as advised. Over several months, Sarah experienced a significant reduction in anxiety, better sleep quality, and fewer headaches, leading to an overall improvement in her well-being.

Case Study 3: Enhancing Fertility Emily, a 35-year-old woman, had been trying to conceive for over a year without success. She decided to explore acupuncture to support her fertility journey. Her acupuncturist developed a treatment plan that included acupuncture sessions timed with her menstrual cycle, dietary recommendations, and stress reduction techniques. After several months of consistent treatment, Emily's menstrual cycle became more regular, and she felt more balanced and less stressed. Eventually, Emily was able to conceive, and she continued to receive acupuncture treatments throughout her pregnancy to support her health and well-being.

Action Plan

Acupuncture offers a holistic and effective approach to health and well-being, drawing on centuries of traditional wisdom and modern scientific research. For those interested in exploring acupuncture, consider the following steps:

1. **Seek Out Qualified Practitioners:** Ensure you receive treatment from licensed and certified acupuncturists who have undergone rigorous training. Verify their credentials and ask for recommendations from trusted sources.

2. **Embrace a Holistic Approach:** View acupuncture as part of a broader wellness plan that includes healthy eating, regular exercise, stress management, and other complementary therapies. A holistic approach maximizes the benefits of acupuncture and supports overall health.

3. **Educate Yourself:** Gain a deeper understanding of acupuncture and Traditional Chinese Medicine. Read books, attend seminars, and consult reliable online resources to learn about the principles and practices of this ancient healing art.

4. **Commit to Regular Treatment:** Consistency is key to achieving the best results with acupuncture. Follow your practitioner's recommendations for treatment frequency and duration, and maintain regular sessions to support long-term health benefits.

5. **Monitor and Reflect:** Keep track of your symptoms and progress throughout your acupuncture journey. Reflect on the changes you experience and communicate openly with your acupuncturist to ensure your treatment plan remains effective and responsive to your needs.

Conclusion

Acupuncture is a valuable and versatile therapy that can address a wide range of health issues, from pain management to mental health and fertility. By integrating acupuncture into your wellness routine and embracing a holistic approach to health, you can achieve greater balance, vitality, and overall well-being. Explore the potential of this time-honored practice with an open mind and a commitment to your health, and you may discover profound improvements in your quality of life.

Martial Arts:
Exploring the Top 10 Disciplines from Around the World

Introduction

Martial arts encompass a diverse range of disciplines that originated in various cultures around the globe. Each discipline offers unique techniques, philosophies, and benefits, making martial arts a rich field worth exploring. Whether for self-defense, physical fitness, mental discipline, or cultural appreciation, martial arts provide numerous pathways to personal growth and development. This section explores the top 10 martial arts from around the world, detailing their origins, founders, practices, and benefits.

Karate

Origin and Founder: Karate originated in Okinawa, Japan, during the Ryukyu Dynasty. It was influenced by indigenous fighting styles and Chinese martial arts brought to Okinawa by travelers and traders. Funakoshi Gichin, often regarded as the father of modern Karate, introduced it to mainland Japan in the early 20th century (Funakoshi, 1922).

Practice: Karate focuses on striking techniques, including punches, kicks, knee strikes, and elbow strikes. It also incorporates blocking, parrying, and open-handed techniques. Practitioners train in kata (pre-arranged forms), kumite (sparring), and kihon (basic techniques).

Benefits: Karate enhances physical fitness, strength, and flexibility. It also promotes discipline, focus, and self-confidence. The practice of kata helps improve memory and coordination, while sparring develops quick reflexes and strategic thinking.

Taekwondo

Origin and Founder: Taekwondo originated in Korea and was officially established in 1955 by General Choi Hong Hi. It was developed by combining elements of traditional Korean martial arts such as Taekkyeon and Hwa Rang Do with influences from Karate (Choi, 1965).

Practice: Taekwondo is known for its high, fast kicks and dynamic footwork. Training includes patterns (forms), sparring, self-defense techniques, and breaking techniques. Taekwondo also incorporates elements of physical conditioning and flexibility exercises.

Benefits: Taekwondo improves cardiovascular health, leg strength, and overall flexibility. It also fosters self-discipline, respect, and perseverance. The emphasis on forms and patterns enhances mental clarity and focus, while sparring builds confidence and competitive spirit.

Judo

Origin and Founder: Judo was founded in Japan by Jigoro Kano in 1882. Kano developed judo from traditional Jujutsu techniques, emphasizing throws, joint locks, and pins while eliminating dangerous techniques to create a safe and effective martial art (Kano, 1882).

Practice: Judo focuses on grappling techniques, including throws, holds, joint locks, and chokes. Training involves randori (free practice), kata (forms), and shiai (competition). Judo practitioners, known as judoka, wear a gi (uniform) and practice on a tatami (mat).

Benefits: Judo enhances physical strength, endurance, and flexibility. It teaches balance, coordination, and effective use of leverage. Judo also promotes mental toughness, strategic thinking, and respect for opponents. The principles of judo, such as mutual welfare and benefit, encourage a positive and respectful attitude.

Brazilian Jiu-Jitsu (BJJ)

Origin and Founder: Brazilian jiu-jitsu evolved from Japanese jujutsu and judo. It was developed by the Gracie family in Brazil in the early 20th century, with Carlos and Helio Gracie being key figures in its development and popularization (Gracie, 1925).

Practice: BJJ focuses on ground fighting and submission techniques, including joint locks and chokeholds. Training involves drilling techniques, live sparring (rolling), and positional drills. BJJ practitioners, known as grapplers, often train in both gi and no-gi styles.

Benefits: BJJ improves physical fitness, strength, and endurance. It teaches practical self-defense skills and emphasizes technique over brute strength, making it accessible to people of all sizes. BJJ also promotes problem-solving skills, patience, and resilience. The close-contact nature of BJJ builds camaraderie and mutual respect among practitioners.

Muay Thai

Origin and Founder: Muay Thai, also known as Thai Boxing, originated in Thailand. It evolved from ancient martial arts practiced by Thai warriors and became a formalized sport in the 20th century. Muay Thai has no single founder but has been shaped by numerous masters and fighters over centuries.

Practice: Muay Thai is known for its striking techniques, including punches, kicks, elbows, and knee strikes. It also incorporates clinching techniques. Training involves pad work, bag work, sparring, and conditioning exercises. Muay Thai fighters, known as nak muay, practice in a ring.

Benefits: Muay Thai enhances cardiovascular fitness, strength, and flexibility. It builds mental toughness, focus, and determination. The rigorous training improves endurance and resilience. Muay Thai also teaches effective self-defense techniques and fosters a strong sense of discipline and respect.

Kung Fu

Origin and Founder: Kung Fu is a broad term that encompasses various Chinese martial arts. It has ancient roots, with some styles tracing back thousands of years. Shaolin Kung Fu, one of the most famous styles, originated in the Shaolin Temple. There is no single founder of Kung Fu; it has been developed by many masters over centuries.

Practice: Kung Fu includes a wide range of techniques, including strikes, kicks, joint locks, and throws. It also incorporates weapons training and forms (taolu). Training involves drilling techniques, practicing forms, sparring, and conditioning exercises. Kung Fu styles vary greatly, each with its unique characteristics and techniques.

Benefits: Kung Fu improves physical fitness, strength, and flexibility. It enhances coordination, balance, and agility. Kung Fu also promotes mental discipline, focus, and perseverance. The practice of forms helps improve memory and fluidity of movement. Kung Fu teaches respect for tradition and the importance of continuous learning.

Krav Maga

Origin and Founder: Krav Maga was developed in the 1930s by Imi Lichtenfeld, a Hungarian-Israeli martial artist. It was created for the Israeli Defense Forces (IDF) and emphasizes practical self-defense techniques drawn from boxing, wrestling, judo, and other martial arts.

Practice: Krav Maga focuses on real-world self-defense scenarios. Training includes striking techniques, grappling, and defenses against various attacks, such as chokes, grabs, and weapon threats. Krav Maga also incorporates stress drills to simulate real-life situations and enhance mental resilience.

Benefits: Krav Maga teaches practical and effective self-defense skills. It improves physical fitness, strength, and cardiovascular health. Krav Maga also enhances mental toughness, situational awareness, and quick decision-making. The emphasis on real-world applications makes it highly relevant for personal safety.

Aikido

Origin and Founder: Aikido was founded in Japan by Morihei Ueshiba in the early 20th century. Ueshiba developed Aikido by synthesizing his martial arts knowledge, including Daito-ryu Aiki-jujutsu, with his spiritual beliefs. Aikido emphasizes harmony and non-resistance (Ueshiba, 1925).

Practice: Aikido focuses on joint locks, throws, and pins to neutralize attacks. Training involves practicing techniques with a partner, kata (forms), and weapons training with bokken (wooden sword), jo (staff), and tanto (knife). Aikido emphasizes blending with an opponent's energy and using it to control them.

Benefits: Aikido enhances physical fitness, flexibility, and coordination. It promotes mental calmness, focus, and emotional control. Aikido teaches principles of harmony, non-violence, and respect for others. The practice fosters a sense of community and mutual support among practitioners.

Capoeira

Origin and Founder: Capoeira originated in Brazil among enslaved Africans in the 16th century. It was developed as a disguised form of self-defense, incorporating dance, music, and acrobatics to avoid detection by slave masters. There is no single founder, as it evolved through the collective contributions of many practitioners.

Practice: Capoeira combines martial arts, dance, and music. Training involves practicing kicks, sweeps, acrobatics, and ground movements, often in a roda (circle) with musical accompaniment. Capoeiristas also learn to play traditional instruments and sing call-and-response songs.

Benefits: Capoeira improves physical fitness, agility, and flexibility. It enhances rhythm, coordination, and balance. Capoeira promotes creativity, cultural appreciation, and a sense of community. The practice also teaches resilience, strategic thinking, and adaptability.

Sambo

Origin and Founder: Sambo, a Russian martial art, was developed in the early 20th century by Viktor Spiridonov and Vasili Oshchepkov. It was created as a hand-to-hand combat system for the Soviet military, combining techniques from traditional Russian wrestling and other martial arts.

Practice: Sambo focuses on grappling techniques, including throws, joint locks, pins, and submissions. Training involves drilling techniques, live sparring, and conditioning exercises. Sambo practitioners, known as sambists, often compete in sport Sambo or combat Sambo, which includes striking.

Benefits: Sambo enhances physical fitness, strength, and endurance. It improves balance, coordination, and agility. Sambo teaches practical self-defense skills and effective use of leverage. The practice promotes mental toughness, discipline, and strategic thinking.

Conclusion

Martial arts offer a rich tapestry of disciplines, each with unique techniques, philosophies, and benefits. From the striking arts of Karate and Muay Thai to the grappling techniques of Judo and Brazilian jiu-jitsu, martial arts provide a diverse range of practices that cater to various interests and goals. Whether one's focus is on self-defense, physical fitness, mental discipline, or cultural appreciation, there is a martial art that can meet those needs.

Exploring the top 10 martial arts from around the world—Karate, Taekwondo, Judo, Brazilian jiu-jitsu, Muay Thai, Kung Fu, Krav Maga, Aikido, Capoeira, and Sambo—reveals the depth and breadth of this field. Each martial art has its own rich history, originating from different cultural and historical contexts, and has been shaped by the contributions of many founders and practitioners over centuries.

Practicing martial arts offers numerous benefits, including improved physical fitness, strength, flexibility, and cardiovascular health. It also fosters mental and emotional well-being by promoting discipline, focus, resilience, and stress management. The philosophical teachings and principles embedded in martial arts encourage respect, harmony, and continuous personal growth.

For those interested in embarking on a journey in martial arts, it is essential to choose a discipline that aligns with their interests and goals. Whether seeking to enhance physical capabilities, learn effective self-defense, or delve into the cultural and philosophical aspects of a martial art, there is a path that can lead to significant personal development and fulfillment.

Embracing martial arts can be a transformative experience, providing not only the skills to defend oneself but also the tools to navigate life's challenges with confidence and poise. As you explore these diverse disciplines, you will discover that martial arts is not just about physical combat, but about cultivating a balanced and harmonious way of life.

Action Plan: Finding the Right Martial Art Discipline for You

Exploring martial arts can be a transformative journey that offers numerous physical, mental, and emotional benefits. To help you find the right discipline that aligns with your interests and goals, follow these step-by-step guidelines:

1. **Identify Your Goals:**
   Determine what you hope to achieve through martial arts. Are you looking for self-defense skills, physical fitness, mental discipline, or cultural immersion? Clarifying your goals will help narrow down the choices.

2. **Research Different Martial Arts:**
   Learn about various martial arts disciplines. Read books, watch documentaries, and explore online resources to understand the history, techniques, and philosophies of each martial art.

Pay special attention to the top 10 martial arts discussed in this section: Karate, Taekwondo, Judo, Brazilian Jiu-jjitsu, Muay Thai, Kung Fu, Krav Maga, Aikido, Capoeira, and Sambo.

3. **Consider Your Physical Condition:**
Assess your current physical condition and any limitations you may have. Some martial arts are more physically demanding than others. Choose a discipline that matches your fitness level and physical capabilities.

4. **Visit Local Dojos and Gyms:**
Visit martial arts schools, dojos, and gyms in your area. Observe classes, talk to instructors, and get a feel for the environment. Many schools offer trial classes or introductory sessions, which can give you hands-on experience.

5. **Evaluate the Instructors:**
Instructors play a crucial role in your martial arts journey. Look for qualified, experienced, and approachable instructors who can provide proper guidance and support. Ensure they have the necessary certifications and a teaching style that resonates with you.

6. **Understand the Commitment:**
Consider the time and financial commitment required for each martial art. Some disciplines may require more frequent training sessions or investment in equipment and uniforms. Ensure you can commit to the practice without feeling overwhelmed.

7. **Join a Community:**
Martial arts often foster a strong sense of community and camaraderie. Joining a school with a supportive and welcoming community can enhance your learning experience and provide additional motivation.

8. **Try Multiple Disciplines:**
If you're unsure which martial art is right for you, consider trying multiple disciplines. Many schools offer cross-training opportunities, allowing you to experience different styles before making a decision.

9. **Set Realistic Expectations:**
Understand that progress in martial arts takes time and dedication. Set realistic expectations and be patient with your learning journey. Celebrate small milestones and stay committed to continuous improvement.

10. **Reflect on Your Experience:**
After trying out different disciplines, reflect on your experiences. Which martial art did you enjoy the most? Which one aligns best with your goals and interests? Use this reflection to make an informed decision.

11. **Commit to Your Chosen Discipline:**
    Once you've identified the right martial art for you, commit to regular practice. Embrace the discipline, immerse yourself in the training, and strive to learn and grow continuously.

12. **Stay Open to Evolution:**
    Your interests and goals may evolve over time. Stay open to exploring new disciplines or incorporating elements from different martial arts into your practice. Martial arts is a lifelong journey of learning and self-discovery.

By following these steps, you can find the martial art discipline that best suits your needs and embark on a rewarding journey of personal growth and development. Embrace the challenges, enjoy the process, and let the practice of martial arts enrich your life in profound ways.

Qigong:
Harnessing the Power of Life Energy

Introduction

Qigong (pronounced "chee-gong") is an ancient Chinese practice that combines movement, meditation, and controlled breathing to enhance the flow of qi (life energy) in the body. Rooted in Traditional Chinese Medicine (TCM), qigong has been practiced for thousands of years to promote physical health, mental clarity, and spiritual well-being. This section explores the history of qigong, its fundamental principles, different styles, and the numerous benefits it offers. By understanding and incorporating qigong into daily life, individuals can achieve a balanced and harmonious state of being.

History of QiGong

Qigong has a rich history that spans over 4,000 years. Its origins can be traced back to ancient China, where it evolved from early shamanistic practices and Taoist philosophies. The term "qigong" itself means "energy work" or "skill at working with life energy." Throughout its history, qigong has been influenced by various cultural and philosophical developments, including Confucianism, Buddhism, and martial arts.

Ancient Beginnings: The earliest forms of qigong were developed by shamans who used rhythmic movements and breathing techniques to induce altered states of consciousness and connect with the spirit world. These practices were believed to harmonize the body's energy and heal illnesses (Kohn, 2008).

Taoist Influence: During the Warring States period (475–221 BCE), Taoist practitioners began to systematize qigong techniques, emphasizing the cultivation of qi for health and longevity. Taoist alchemists sought to refine their internal energy through meditation, breathing exercises, and gentle movements (Despeux, 2001).

Buddhist Integration: In the early centuries CE, Buddhism spread to China, bringing with it new meditative practices. Buddhist monks integrated qigong into their spiritual routines, combining it with seated meditation and chanting to enhance mental clarity and spiritual insight (Yee, 1977).

Martial Arts Development: Qigong also played a significant role in the development of Chinese martial arts. Martial artists used qigong techniques to build internal strength, improve balance, and increase resilience. Styles such as tai chi and Shaolin Kung Fu incorporate qigong principles to enhance combat effectiveness and promote overall well-being (Shahar, 2008).

Fundamental Principles of Qigong

Qigong is based on several fundamental principles that guide its practice. Understanding these principles is essential for effectively harnessing the power of qi.

Qi (Life Energy): Qi is the vital energy that flows through all living things. It is the force that sustains life and promotes health. In QiGong, practitioners learn to cultivate and balance their qi to achieve physical, mental, and spiritual harmony (Maciocia, 1989).

Meridians and Energy Channels: According to TCM, qi flows through the body along pathways called meridians. There are twelve primary meridians corresponding to major organs, as well as eight extraordinary meridians. Qigong exercises aim to unblock and regulate the flow of qi through these channels (Deadman et al., 1998).

Breath Control: Controlled breathing is a core component of qigong. Techniques such as abdominal breathing and reverse breathing help regulate the flow of qi and promote relaxation. Breath control also enhances oxygenation and detoxification of the body (Cohen, 1997).

Mindfulness and Intent: qigong emphasizes the importance of mindfulness and intent. Practitioners use focused intention to guide the flow of qi and achieve specific health outcomes. Mindfulness enhances the mind-body connection and deepens the meditative aspects of the practice (Frantzis, 2007).

Posture and Movement: Proper posture and gentle, flowing movements are integral to Qi Gong. These movements are designed to align the body, improve circulation, and facilitate the smooth flow of qi. The practice often includes standing, sitting, and lying down postures (Jahnke, 2002).

Styles of Qigong

Qigong encompasses a wide range of styles, each with its unique focus and techniques. Here are some of the most well-known styles:

Medical Qigong: This style focuses on healing and preventing illness. Medical qigong practitioners use specific exercises to target health issues, strengthen the immune system, and promote overall vitality. It is often integrated into TCM treatments (Johnson, 2000).

Martial Qigong: Martial qigong is used to enhance physical strength, endurance, and combat skills. Styles such as Iron Shirt qigong and Shaolin qigong train practitioners to develop internal power, resilience, and focus, essential for martial arts proficiency (Shahar, 2008).

Spiritual Qigong: This style emphasizes spiritual growth and enlightenment. Practices such as Taoist Qi Gong and Buddhist Qi Gong integrate meditation, visualization, and breath control to cultivate inner peace, clarity, and spiritual insight (Despeux, 2001).

Dynamic Qigong: Dynamic qigong involves more vigorous and dynamic movements. Styles such as tai chi and Baduanjin(Eight Pieces of Brocade) include flowing sequences that improve flexibility, coordination, and balance while promoting the flow of qi (Yang, 1988).

Static Qigong: Static qigong focuses on stillness and meditation. Practices such as zhan zhuang (standing like a tree) involve holding specific postures for extended periods to cultivate inner strength and mental focus (Lam, 1994).

Benefits of Qigong

The practice of qigong offers a wide range of benefits for physical, mental, and spiritual well-being. Here are some of the key benefits:

Physical Health: Qigong improves overall physical health by enhancing circulation, increasing flexibility, and strengthening muscles and joints. It also boosts the immune system, aids in digestion, and promotes cardiovascular health (Jahnke, 2002).

Mental Clarity: Regular practice of qigong enhances mental clarity, focus, and cognitive function. The meditative aspects of qigong reduce stress, anxiety, and depression, promoting a sense of calm and well-being (Chen et al., 2012).

Emotional Balance: Qigong helps balance emotions by regulating the flow of qi through the body's meridians. It can alleviate mood swings, reduce anger and frustration, and promote emotional stability and resilience (Wang et al., 2014).

Spiritual Growth: For those seeking spiritual growth, qigong offers a pathway to deeper self-awareness and enlightenment. The practice fosters a connection with the inner self and the universe, promoting spiritual insight and harmony (Frantzis, 2007).

Longevity and Vitality: Qigong is often associated with longevity and vitality. The gentle, low-impact movements make it suitable for people of all ages, including seniors. Regular practice can enhance energy levels, improve sleep, and contribute to a longer, healthier life (Cohen, 1997).

Practical Applications and Steps

For those interested in incorporating qigong into their daily routine, here are some practical steps to get started:

1. **Find a Qualified Instructor:** Seek out a qualified qigong instructor who can provide proper guidance and instruction. Look for certified practitioners with experience in teaching qigong. Many community centers, health clubs, and TCM clinics offer qigong classes.

2. **Start with Basic Exercises:** Begin with simple, foundational qigong exercises to build a strong foundation. Basic exercises such as abdominal breathing, the Three Treasures (Jing, Qi, Shen), and gentle stretching movements are ideal for beginners.

3. **Practice Regularly:** Consistency is key to experiencing the benefits of qigong. Aim to practice for at least 15-30 minutes daily. Gradually increase the duration and intensity of your practice as you become more comfortable with the exercises.

4. **Create a Quiet Space:** Find a quiet, comfortable space where you can practice qigong without distractions. An outdoor setting, such as a garden or park, can enhance the experience by connecting you with nature.

5. **Focus on Breath and Intention:** Pay close attention to your breath and maintain a focused intention during your practice. Deep, slow breathing helps regulate the flow of qi, while focused intention guides the energy to specific areas of the body.

6. **Learn Different Styles:** Explore various styles of qigong to find the one that resonates most with you. Whether it's Medical qigong for healing, Martial qigong for strength, or Spiritual qigong for inner peace, each style offers unique benefits.

7. **Join a Community:** Consider joining a qigong community or group to share your practice with others. Group practice can provide support, motivation, and a sense of connection with like-minded individuals.

8. **Track Your Progress:** Keep a journal to track your qigong practice and its effects on your health and well-being. Note any changes in your physical, mental, and emotional state, and adjust your practice accordingly.

9. **Stay Open and Patient:** Qigong is a gentle and gradual practice that requires patience and openness. Stay committed to your practice and be patient with yourself as you progress. The benefits of qigong will unfold over time.

10. **Integrate Qi Gong into Daily Life:** Incorporate qigong principles into your daily activities. Practice mindful breathing, maintain good posture, and stay present in the moment. These small changes can enhance the overall impact of qigong on your life.

Conclusion

QiGong is a powerful and versatile practice that offers a holistic approach to health and well-being. With its rich history, diverse styles, and numerous benefits, qigong provides a pathway to physical vitality, mental clarity, emotional balance, and spiritual growth. By incorporating qigong into daily life, individuals can cultivate a harmonious and balanced state of being,

By incorporating qigong into daily life, individuals can cultivate a harmonious and balanced state of being, leading to enhanced overall wellness and a greater sense of fulfillment. The gentle movements, controlled breathing, and focused intention of qigong make it accessible to people of all ages and fitness levels, offering a sustainable and enjoyable way to improve health.

As you embark on your qigong journey, remember that this practice is not just about physical exercise but also about connecting deeply with your inner self and the world around you. Embrace the principles of qi, mindfulness, and balance, and let qigong guide you toward a healthier, more vibrant life. Whether you seek to alleviate stress, enhance your physical fitness, or achieve spiritual growth, qigong offers a comprehensive approach to achieving these goals.

In conclusion, qigong stands as a testament to the profound wisdom of Traditional Chinese Medicine, offering timeless techniques for cultivating life energy and achieving holistic wellness. By integrating qigong into your daily routine, you can unlock the potential of your body, mind, and spirit, paving the way for a more balanced and harmonious existence. Embrace this ancient practice with an open heart and a dedicated mind, and experience the transformative power of qigong in your life.

Tai Chi:
The Art of Movement and Mindfulness

Introduction

Tai chi, also known as tai chi chuan (Taijiquan), is a centuries-old Chinese martial art that has evolved into a popular form of exercise and meditation. Known for its slow, graceful movements and profound health benefits, tai chi integrates physical exercise with mental focus and spiritual awareness. This section explores the rich history of tai chi, its foundational principles, various styles, health benefits, and practical steps for incorporating tai chi into daily life.

History of Tai Chi

Tai chi has a rich history that spans several centuries, with its origins deeply rooted in Chinese culture and philosophy. The development of tai chi is traditionally attributed to the Taoist monk Zhang Sanfeng, who is said to have created the martial art in the 12th century after observing a crane and a snake in combat. However, historical records suggest that tai chi as we know it today began to take shape in the Chen Village in Henan Province during the 16th century.

Early Development: The Chen family is credited with the formal development of tai chi. Chen Wangting, a retired military officer of the late Ming Dynasty, is recognized as the founder of Chen-style tai chi. He integrated various elements from traditional Chinese martial arts, Taoist philosophy, and his own military experience to create a comprehensive system of movements and techniques.

Evolution and Spread: Over the centuries, tai chi evolved and diversified into several distinct styles, each named after the family or individual who developed it. These include Chen, Yang, Wu, Sun, and Hao styles. The Yang style, developed by Yang Luchan in the 19th century, is the most widely practiced form today. Tai chi gained popularity not only as a martial art but also as a practice for health and longevity.

Modern Era: In the 20th century, tai chi continued to evolve, with an increasing emphasis on its health benefits. It spread globally, gaining recognition as a form of low-impact exercise suitable for people of all ages. Today, tai chi is practiced by millions worldwide and is respected for its holistic approach to wellness.

Foundational Principles of Tai Chi

Tai chi is based on several foundational principles that guide its practice and philosophy. Understanding these principles is essential for mastering the art and reaping its full benefits.

Yin and Yang: The concept of Yin and Yang, representing opposing yet complementary forces, is central to tai chi. The movements of tai chi embody the balance of Yin (soft, yielding) and Yang (hard, assertive), creating a harmonious flow of energy (qi) throughout the body. This balance promotes physical and mental equilibrium (Wile, 1996).

Qi (Life Energy): Qi is the vital energy that flows through the body. Tai chi aims to cultivate and enhance the flow of qi, promoting health and vitality. The practice involves gentle, continuous movements that open the body's energy channels (meridians), allowing qi to circulate freely (Maciocia, 1989).

Relaxation and Softness: Tai chi emphasizes relaxation and softness over tension and force. Practitioners learn to release physical and mental tension, allowing movements to flow naturally and effortlessly. This principle helps improve flexibility, reduce stress, and prevent injuries (Cheng, 1985).

Mindfulness and Intent: Mindfulness and intent (yi) are crucial components of tai chi. Practitioners maintain a focused and calm mind, directing their intent to guide movements and the flow of qi. This mental discipline enhances concentration, awareness, and the meditative aspects of tai chi (Frantzis, 2007).

Rooting and Alignment: Proper body alignment and rooting (grounding) are fundamental to tai chi. Practitioners develop a stable and balanced stance, with weight evenly distributed and the body aligned along a central axis. This principle enhances balance, stability, and the efficient transfer of energy (Lo et al., 1979).

Styles of Tai Chi

Tai chi encompasses several distinct styles, each with its unique characteristics, forms, and techniques. Here are the five major styles of tai chi:

Chen Style: Chen-style tai chi is the oldest and original form of tai chi. It is character-ized by a combination of slow, flowing movements and fast, explosive actions (fa jin). Chen style emphasizes spiraling movements, low stances, and powerful strikes. It is known for its martial applications and physical conditioning (Chen, 2003).

Yang Style: Developed by Yang Luchan in the 19th century, Yang-style tai chi is the most widely practiced form today. It features slow, steady, and expansive movements with an emphasis on relaxation and grace. Yang style is accessible to people of all ages and fitness levels and is renowned for its health benefits and meditative qualities (Yang, 1931).

Wu Style: Wu-style tai chi was developed by Wu Quanyou and his son Wu Jianquan in the early 20th century. It is characterized by smaller, more compact movements and a focus on subtle internal energy work. Wu style emphasizes maintaining a high stance and fluid, continuous motion, making it suitable for older adults and those with physical limitations (Wu, 1982).

Sun Style: Sun-style tai chi was created by Sun Lutang in the early 20th century. It integrates elements of Xingyiquan and Baguazhang, resulting in a unique style that emphasizes agile footwork, smooth transitions, and open-close movements. Sun style is known for its gentle approach and is often practiced for health and rehabilitation (Sun, 1924).

Hao Style: Also known as Wu (Hao) style, this form was developed by Wu Yuxiang in the 19th century. Hao style focuses on precise, small-frame movements and the cultivation of internal energy. It is less common than other styles but is highly regarded for its deep internal work and martial applications (Wu, 1982).

Health Benefits of Tai Chi

Tai chi offers a wide range of health benefits, making it a valuable practice for physical, mental, and emotional well-being. Here are some of the key benefits:

Improved Balance and Coordination: Tai chi enhances balance and coordination through its slow, controlled movements and emphasis on proper alignment. Regular practice can reduce the risk of falls and improve overall stability, particularly in older adults (Li et al., 2005).

Increased Flexibility and Strength: The gentle stretching and strengthening exercises in tai chi improve flexibility and muscle tone. The practice promotes joint health and increases range of motion, making it beneficial for individuals with arthritis and other musculoskeletal conditions (Wayne et al., 2012).

Cardiovascular Health: Tai chi provides a moderate aerobic workout that can improve cardiovascular health. It helps lower blood pressure, enhance circulation, and increase overall cardiovascular endurance (Yeh et al., 2009).

Stress Reduction and Mental Clarity: The meditative aspects of tai chi reduce stress and promote mental clarity. Practitioners learn to cultivate a calm, focused mind, which helps alleviate anxiety, depression, and other stress-related conditions (Wang et al., 2010).

Enhanced Immune Function: Tai chi has been shown to boost immune function, making the body more resilient to infections and illnesses. The practice stimulates the lymphatic system, enhances circulation, and promotes the flow of qi, all of which support immune health (Irwin et al., 2003).

Pain Management: Tai chi can be an effective complementary therapy for managing chronic pain conditions such as fibromyalgia, osteoarthritis, and lower back pain. The gentle movements and relaxation techniques help reduce pain and improve quality of life (Wang et al., 2009).

Cognitive Benefits: Regular practice of tai chi has been associated with improved cognitive function, including better memory, attention, and executive function. Tai chi's combination of physical movement and mental focus stimulates brain health and may help reduce the risk of cognitive decline (Mortimer et al., 2012).

Emotional Well-Being: Tai chi promotes emotional balance and resilience. The practice encourages mindfulness, self-awareness, and the release of negative emotions, contributing to a more positive outlook on life (Luskin et al., 2000).

Practical Steps for Practicing Tai Chi

Incorporating tai chi into your daily routine can be a rewarding and transformative experience. Here are some practical steps to help you get started:

1. **Find a Qualified Instructor:** Seek out a qualified tai chi instructor who can provide proper guidance and instruction. Look for certified practitioners with experience in teaching tai chi. Many community centers, health clubs, and martial arts schools offer tai chi classes.

2. **Start with Basic Forms:** Begin with simple, foundational tai chi forms to build a strong foundation. Basic forms such as the 24-form Yang style or the 18-form Chen style are ideal for beginners. These forms introduce fundamental movements and principles.

3. **Practice Regularly:** Consistency is key to experiencing the benefits of tai chi. Aim to practice for at least 15-30 minutes daily. Gradually increase the duration and complexity of your practice as you become more comfortable with the movements.

4. **Create a Quiet Space:** Find a quiet, comfortable space where you can practice tai chi without distractions. An outdoor setting, such as a garden or park, can enhance the experience by connecting you with nature.

5. **Focus on Breath and Intention:** Pay close attention to your breath and maintain a focused intention during your practice. Deep, slow breathing helps regulate the flow of qi, while focused intention guides the energy to specific areas of the body.

6. **Learn Different Styles:** Explore various styles of tai chi to find the one that resonates most with you. Whether it's the explosive movements of Chen style, the graceful flow of Yang style, or the agile transitions of Sun style, each offers unique benefits and experiences. Trying different styles can help you find the one that aligns best with your goals and preferences.

7. **Join a Community:** Consider joining a tai chi community or group to share your practice with others. Group practice can provide support, motivation, and a sense of connection with like-minded individuals. It also offers opportunities to learn from others and gain new insights into your practice.

8. **Track Your Progress:** Keep a journal to track your tai chi practice and its effects on your health and well-being. Note any changes in your physical, mental, and emotional state, and adjust your practice accordingly. Reflecting on your progress can help you stay motivated and focused on your goals.

9. **Stay Open and Patient:** Tai chi is a gentle and gradual practice that requires patience and openness. Stay committed to your practice and be patient with yourself as you progress. The benefits of tai chi will unfold over time, and consistency is key to experiencing long-term improvements.

10. **Integrate Tai Chi into Daily Life:** Incorporate tai chi principles into your daily activities. Practice mindful breathing, maintain good posture, and stay present in the moment. These small changes can enhance the overall impact of tai chi on your life.

Advanced Practices and Techniques

As you become more experienced in tai chi, you may want to explore advanced practices and techniques that deepen your understanding and enhance your skills. Here are some advanced aspects of tai chi to consider:

Push Hands (Tui Shou): Push hands is a partner exercise that develops sensitivity, balance, and responsiveness. It involves practicing with a partner to feel and respond to their energy, helping you apply tai chi principles in a dynamic and interactive context. Push hands teaches you to yield, redirect force, and maintain balance while interacting with an opponent (Cheng, 1985).

Weapons Training: Many tai chi styles include weapons training, which adds a new dimension to the practice. Common tai chi weapons include the sword (jian), saber (dao), and staff (gun). Weapons training enhances coordination, focus, and precision, and helps deepen your understanding of tai chi principles (Lo et al., 1979).

Advanced Forms: As you progress, you can learn more advanced tai chi forms that include complex sequences and movements. Advanced forms challenge your coordination, balance, and internal energy work. They also provide a deeper exploration of tai chi principles and techniques (Yang, 1931).

Internal Alchemy (Neidan): Internal alchemy practices focus on cultivating and refining internal energy (qi) through meditation, breath control, and visualization techniques. These practices aim to transform and enhance the body's energy, promoting health, longevity, and spiritual growth. Internal alchemy is deeply rooted in Taoist philosophy and is considered an advanced aspect of tai chi (Despeux, 2001).

Healing Applications: Tai chi can be used as a therapeutic practice to address specific health issues. Medical tai chi focuses on using tai chi movements and principles to support healing and recovery from illness or injury. Working with a qualified instructor who specializes in medical tai chi can provide personalized guidance and support (Johnson, 2000).

Case Studies and Examples

To illustrate the transformative potential of tai chi, consider the following case studies:

Case Study 1: Enhancing Balance and Mobility Jane, a 70-year-old woman, struggled with balance and mobility issues due to age-related muscle weakness and joint stiffness. After attending a tai chi class for seniors, she began practicing daily. Within a few months, Jane noticed significant improvements in her balance, flexibility, and overall mobility. She felt more confident and stable while walking, reducing her risk of falls and improving her quality of life.

Case Study 2: Managing Chronic Pain Mark, a 45-year-old man, suffered from chronic lower back pain caused by long hours of sitting at his desk job. He started practicing tai chi as a form of gentle exercise and stress relief. Through regular practice, Mark experienced a reduction in pain and improved posture. The meditative aspects of tai chi also helped him manage stress, contributing to overall pain relief and better mental health.

Case Study 3: Improving Mental Clarity and Focus Sarah, a 30-year-old graduate student, struggled with anxiety and difficulty concentrating on her studies. She began practicing tai chi to enhance her mental clarity and focus. The slow, mindful movements and deep breathing exercises helped Sarah calm her mind and reduce anxiety. As a result, she was able to concentrate better on her studies and manage her academic workload more effectively.

Scientific Research on Tai Chi

Scientific research has provided substantial evidence supporting the health benefits of tai chi. Numerous studies have explored its effects on various aspects of physical and mental health:

Balance and Fall Prevention: A systematic review and meta-analysis published in the Journal of the American Geriatrics Society found that tai chi significantly reduces the risk of falls among older adults. The study concluded that tai chi improves balance, strength, and functional mobility, making it an effective intervention for fall prevention (Li et al., 2005).

Chronic Pain Management: Research published in the New England Journal of Medicine demonstrated that tai chi is effective in managing chronic pain conditions such as fibromyalgia. Participants who practiced tai chi reported significant reductions in pain and improvements in physical function compared to a control group (Wang et al., 2010).

Cardiovascular Health: A study published in the American Journal of Cardiology found that tai chi improves cardiovascular health by lowering blood pressure, enhancing arterial compliance, and increasing aerobic capacity. The study highlighted tai chi as a beneficial exercise for cardiovascular fitness (Yeh et al., 2009).

Cognitive Function: Research published in the Journal of Alzheimer's Disease indicated that tai chi enhances cognitive function in older adults. The study found that regular tai chi practice improves memory, executive function, and processing speed, suggesting its potential in reducing the risk of cognitive decline (Mortimer et al., 2012).

Stress Reduction and Mental Health: A study published in Psychoneuroendocrinology demonstrated that tai chi reduces stress and improves mental health by lowering cortisol levels and enhancing psychological well-being. Participants experienced significant reductions in anxiety, depression, and overall stress levels (Wang et al., 2010).

Tai Chi in Modern Life

Incorporating tai chi into modern life can be a powerful way to enhance health and well-being amidst the stresses and demands of contemporary living. Here are some tips for integrating tai chi into your daily routine:

Morning Practice: Start your day with a morning tai chi routine to energize your body and mind. Morning practice sets a positive tone for the day, enhancing focus and vitality.

Midday Breaks: Use tai chi as a midday break to relieve stress and tension. A short tai chi session during lunch breaks can refresh your mind and body, improving productivity and reducing stress.

Evening Wind-Down: Practice tai chi in the evening to unwind and relax before bedtime. The gentle movements and deep breathing help calm the nervous system, promoting restful sleep.

Workplace Wellness: Encourage tai chi practice in the workplace by organizing group sessions or providing resources for employees. Tai Chichi can improve workplace wellness by reducing stress, enhancing focus, and fostering a positive work environment.

Community Engagement: Join local tai chi classes or groups to connect with others who share your interest. Community engagement enhances motivation and provides opportunities for social interaction and support.

Family Practice: Involve family members in your tai chi practice to promote health and bonding. Practicing tai chi together can create a supportive and health-conscious family environment.

Conclusion

Tai chi is a profound and multifaceted practice that offers a holistic approach to health and well-being. With its rich history, diverse styles, and numerous benefits, tai chi provides a pathway to physical vitality, mental clarity, emotional balance, and spiritual growth. By understanding its foundational principles and incorporating tai chi into daily life, individuals can achieve a balanced and harmonious state of being.

As you embark on your tai chi journey, remember that this practice is not just about physical movement but also about cultivating inner peace, mindfulness, and a deep connection with the flow of life energy. Embrace tai chi with an open heart and a dedicated mind, and experience the transformative power it brings to your life. Whether you seek to improve your health, manage stress, or explore a new form of meditation, tai chi offers a comprehensive and enriching path to achieving your goals.

Yoga:
The Ancient Practice for Modern Well-Being

Introduction

Yoga, an ancient practice that originated in India over 5,000 years ago, has become a global phenomenon known for its physical, mental, and spiritual benefits. Combining physical postures (asanas), breathing techniques (pranayama), and meditation, yoga offers a holistic approach to health and well-being. This section delves into the rich history of yoga, its fundamental principles, various styles, health benefits, and practical steps for incorporating yoga into daily life.

History of Yoga

The history of yoga is deeply intertwined with the spiritual and philosophical traditions of India. It has evolved over millennia, influenced by various cultural and religious developments.

Ancient Beginnings: The earliest references to yoga can be found in the Rig Veda, a collection of ancient Indian hymns written around 1500 BCE. Yoga was originally a spiritual discipline practiced by ascetics to achieve higher states of consciousness and spiritual enlightenment.

Classical Yoga: The classical period of yoga is marked by the composition of the Yoga Sutras by the sage Patanjali around 400 CE. The Yoga Sutras codified the principles and practices of yoga into a systematic framework known as the Eight Limbs of Yoga. This period also saw the development of various schools of thought, such as Raja Yoga and Bhakti Yoga.

Post-Classical Yoga: During the post-classical period, yoga continued to evolve with the development of Hatha Yoga, which emphasizes physical postures and breath control. This period saw the compilation of texts like the Hatha Yoga Pradipika and the Gheranda Samhita, which provided detailed instructions on asanas, pranayama, and other yogic practices.

Modern Yoga: The modern period of yoga began in the late 19th and early 20th centuries with the introduction of yoga to the West. Influential figures like Swami Vivekananda, Paramahansa Yogananda, and T. Krishnamacharya played pivotal roles in popularizing yoga outside India. Today, yoga is practiced by millions worldwide, celebrated for its diverse styles and numerous health benefits.

Fundamental Principles of Yoga

Yoga is based on several fundamental principles that guide its practice and philosophy. Understanding these principles is essential for fully experiencing the transformative power of yoga.

Union and Balance: The word "yoga" is derived from the Sanskrit root "yuj," which means "to yoke" or "to unite." Yoga seeks to unite the body, mind, and spirit, promoting harmony and balance. This principle encourages holistic well-being and the integration of all aspects of the self (Iyengar, 1966).

The Eight Limbs of Yoga: The Eight Limbs of Yoga, as outlined by Patanjali in the Yoga Sutras, provide a comprehensive framework for the practice of yoga. These limbs include Yama (ethical principles), Niyama (personal observances), Asana (physical postures), Pranayama (breath control), Pratyahara (withdrawal of the senses), Dharana (concentration), Dhyana (meditation), and Samadhi (spiritual absorption) (Patanjali, 400 CE).

Breath and Energy (Prana): Prana, or life force energy, is central to yoga practice. Breath control (pranayama) techniques are used to regulate the flow of prana, enhancing vitality and promoting mental clarity. Proper breathing supports physical health and prepares the mind for meditation (Rama, 1998).

Mindfulness and Presence: Yoga emphasizes mindfulness and being present in the moment. Practitioners cultivate awareness of their body, breath, and mind, fostering a deep connection with the present experience. This principle enhances mental clarity, reduces stress, and promotes emotional balance (Kabat-Zinn, 1990).

Non-Harm (Ahimsa): Ahimsa, or non-harm, is a foundational ethical principle in yoga. It encourages practitioners to cultivate compassion and non-violence toward themselves and others. This principle extends beyond physical actions to include thoughts and speech, promoting kindness and respect (Gandhi, 1927).

Styles of Yoga

Yoga encompasses a wide range of styles, each with its unique focus, techniques, and benefits. Here are some of the most well-known styles of yoga:

Hatha Yoga: Hatha Yoga is one of the most traditional forms of yoga, focusing on physical postures (asanas) and breath control (pranayama). It emphasizes slow, deliberate movements and poses, making it accessible to beginners. Hatha Yoga promotes physical strength, flexibility, and relaxation (Swami Sivananda, 1934).

Vinyasa Yoga: Vinyasa Yoga, also known as Flow Yoga, is characterized by a dynamic sequence of poses that flow smoothly from one to the next, synchronized with the breath. It emphasizes fluid movement and transitions, creating a meditative and energetic practice. Vinyasa Yoga enhances cardiovascular fitness, flexibility, and mental focus (Jois, 1962).

Ashtanga Yoga: Ashtanga Yoga is a rigorous and structured style of yoga that follows a specific sequence of postures. It consists of six series, each with increasing difficulty. Ashtanga Yoga emphasizes strength, flexibility, and endurance, and is suitable for practitioners looking for a physically challenging practice (Jois, 1962).

Iyengar Yoga: Developed by B.K.S. Iyengar, focuses on precise alignment and the use of props, such as blocks, straps, and blankets, to support the body in various poses. It emphasizes holding poses for longer durations to build strength, flexibility, and concentration. Iyengar Yoga is beneficial for practitioners seeking therapeutic benefits and injury prevention (Iyengar, 1966).

Bikram Yoga: Bikram Yoga, also known as Hot Yoga, consists of a fixed sequence of 26 poses practiced in a heated room. The heat enhances flexibility and detoxification, making it a vigorous and challenging practice. Bikram Yoga promotes cardiovascular health, endurance, and stress relief (Choudhury, 1978).

Kundalini Yoga: Kundalini Yoga focuses on awakening the dormant energy at the base of the spine (kundalini) and guiding it through the chakras (energy centers) to achieve spiritual enlightenment. It combines dynamic movements, breath control, chanting, and meditation. Kundalini Yoga enhances energy levels, mental clarity, and spiritual awareness (Khalsa, 1996).

Yin Yoga: Yin Yoga is a slow and meditative style that involves holding passive poses for extended periods (typically 3-5 minutes). It targets the connective tissues, such as ligaments, tendons, and fascia, promoting flexibility and joint health. Yin Yoga fosters relaxation, mindfulness, and emotional release (Grilley, 2002).

Restorative Yoga: Restorative Yoga focuses on relaxation and recovery by using props to support the body in restful poses. It emphasizes deep relaxation and stress relief, making it ideal for those recovering from injury or experiencing high levels of stress. Restorative Yoga promotes healing, rejuvenation, and emotional balance (Lasater, 1995).

Jivamukti Yoga: Jivamukti Yoga is a modern style that integrates physical practice with spiritual teachings, music, and meditation. It emphasizes ethical principles, such as compassion and nonviolence, and often incorporates chanting and philosophical discussions. Jivamukti Yoga enhances physical fitness, mental clarity, and spiritual growth (Gannon & Life, 2002).

Power Yoga: Power Yoga is a vigorous and fitness-oriented style that draws inspir-ation from Ashtanga Yoga. It emphasizes strength, endurance, and flexibility through dynamic sequences and challenging poses. Power Yoga is suitable for those seeking a high-intensity workout that also promotes mental focus and stress relief (Bender Birch, 1995).

Health Benefits of Yoga

Yoga offers a wide range of health benefits, making it a valuable practice for physical, mental, and emotional well-being. Here are some of the key benefits:

Improved Flexibility and Strength: Yoga enhances flexibility and muscle strength through various poses and stretches. Regular practice increases range of motion, reduces muscle tension, and promotes overall physical balance (Iyengar, 1966).

Cardiovascular Health: Certain styles of yoga, such as Vinyasa and Power Yoga, provide a cardiovascular workout that improves heart health, circulation, and endurance. Yoga also helps lower blood pressure and reduce the risk of cardiovascular diseases (Innes & Vincent, 2007).

Stress Reduction and Relaxation: Yoga's emphasis on breath control, mindfulness, and relaxation techniques helps reduce stress and promote mental calmness. Regular practice lowers cortisol levels, alleviates anxiety, and enhances overall well-being (Ross & Thomas, 2010).

Enhanced Mental Clarity and Focus: Yoga improves cognitive function and mental clarity by promoting mindfulness and concentration. The meditative aspects of yoga enhance memory, attention, and problem-solving skills (Gothe et al., 2013).

Emotional Balance and Resilience: Yoga fosters emotional well-being by encouraging self-awareness, acceptance, and emotional release. It helps manage mood swings, reduce symptoms of depression, and promote a positive outlook on life (Uebelacker et al., 2010).

Pain Management: Yoga is an effective complementary therapy for managing chronic pain conditions such as lower back pain, arthritis, and fibromyalgia. The gentle movements and relaxation techniques help reduce pain and improve quality of life (Sherman et al., 2011).

Respiratory Health: Breath control techniques in yoga enhance respiratory function and lung capacity. Pranayama practices improve oxygenation and help manage respiratory conditions such as asthma and chronic obstructive pulmonary disease (COPD) (Sengupta, 2012).

Immune System Support: Yoga boosts the immune system by reducing stress hormones, improving circulation, and promoting the flow of lymph, which helps eliminate toxins from the body. A stronger immune system enhances the body's ability to fight infections and recover from illnesses (Janakiramaiah et al., 2000).

Improved Posture and Alignment: Regular practice of yoga promotes better posture and body alignment. This helps prevent musculoskeletal issues such as back pain, neck pain, and joint problems. Proper alignment reduces strain on the body and promotes efficient movement (Koltyn & Arbogast, 1998).

Hormonal Balance: Yoga can help balance the endocrine system, which regulates hormones in the body. Practices such as Kundalini Yoga and specific poses like inversions and twists stimulate the glands and support hormonal health, potentially alleviating symptoms of conditions like PMS and menopause (Woodyard, 2011).

Practical Steps for Practicing Yoga

Incorporating yoga into your daily routine can be a transformative experience. Here are some practical steps to help you get started:

1. **Find a Qualified Instructor:** Seek out a qualified yoga instructor who can provide proper guidance and instruction. Look for certified practitioners with experience in teaching yoga. Many community centers, health clubs, and yoga studios offer classes for all levels.

2. **Start with Beginner Classes:** Begin with beginner classes to build a strong foundation.

These classes introduce basic poses, breathing techniques, and the principles of yoga. They provide a safe and supportive environment for learning.

3. **Practice Regularly:** Consistency is key to experiencing the benefits of yoga. Aim to practice for at least 15-30 minutes daily. Gradually increase the duration and complexity of your practice as you become more comfortable with the poses and techniques.

4. **Create a Comfortable Space:** Find a quiet, comfortable space where you can practice yoga without distractions. Use a yoga mat for stability and comfort. Ensure the space is clean, well-ventilated, and free from clutter.

5. **Focus on Breath and Alignment:** Pay close attention to your breath and body alignment during your practice. Deep, steady breathing helps regulate the flow of energy and enhances relaxation. Proper alignment prevents injuries and promotes the effectiveness of the poses.

6. **Explore Different Styles:** Explore various styles of yoga to find the one that resonates most with you. Whether it's the dynamic flow of Vinyasa, the precision of Iyengar, or the relaxation of Yin Yoga, each style offers unique benefits and experiences.

7. **Join a Yoga Community:** Consider joining a yoga community or group to share your practice with others. Group practice can provide support, motivation, and a sense of connection with like-minded individuals. It also offers opportunities to learn from others and gain new insights into your practice.

8. **Listen to Your Body:** Practice mindfulness and listen to your body's signals. Avoid pushing yourself too hard or forcing yourself into poses that cause discomfort or pain. Respect your body's limits and progress at your own pace.

9. **Incorporate Mindfulness and Meditation:** Integrate mindfulness and meditation into your yoga practice. Focus on being present in the moment, observing your thoughts and sensations without judgment. This enhances the meditative aspects of yoga and promotes mental clarity and emotional balance.

10. **Stay Open and Patient:** Yoga is a journey of self-discovery and growth that requires patience and openness. Stay committed to your practice and be patient with yourself as you progress. The benefits of yoga will unfold over time, and consistency is key to experiencing long-term improvements.

Advanced Practices and Techniques

As you become more experienced in yoga, you may want to explore advanced practices and techniques that deepen your understanding and enhance your skills. Here are some advanced aspects of yoga to consider:

Advanced Asanas: As you progress, you can learn more advanced asanas that challenge your strength, flexibility, and balance. Advanced poses such as inversions, arm balances, and deep backbends require greater control and focus.

Pranayama Techniques: Explore advanced pranayama techniques to enhance your breath control and energy regulation. Techniques such as Nadi Shodhana (alternate nostril breathing), Bhastrika (bellows breath), and Kapalabhati (skull-shining breath) offer deeper benefits for respiratory health and mental clarity.

Bandhas (Energy Locks): Bandhas are internal energy locks that regulate the flow of prana within the body. There are three main bandhas: Mula Bandha (root lock), Uddiyana Bandha (abdominal lock), and Jalandhara Bandha (throat lock). Practicing bandhas enhances energy control and supports advanced pranayama and meditation practices.

Mudras (Gestures): Mudras are symbolic hand gestures that direct the flow of energy within the body. They are often used in conjunction with pranayama and meditation. Advanced practitioners can explore various mudras to enhance their practice and deepen their connection to the subtle energies.

Mantra Chanting: Mantra chanting involves the repetition of sacred sounds or phrases to focus the mind and elevate consciousness. Advanced practitioners can incorporate mantra chanting into their practice to enhance spiritual growth and mental clarity.

Meditation Techniques: Explore advanced meditation techniques to deepen your mental focus and spiritual awareness. Techniques such as Vipassana (insight meditation), Transcendental Meditation, and guided visualizations offer profound benefits for mental clarity and emotional balance.

Yoga Philosophy and Texts: Delve deeper into the philosophical aspects of yoga by studying classical texts such as the Yoga Sutras of Patanjali, the Bhagavad Gita, and the Upanishads. Understanding the philosophical foundations of yoga enriches your practice and provides a deeper sense of purpose.

Teaching and Sharing: Consider becoming a certified yoga instructor to share your knowledge and passion with others. Teaching yoga deepens your understanding of the practice and allows you to contribute to the well-being of your community.

Case Studies and Examples

To illustrate the transformative potential of yoga, consider the following case studies:

Case Study 1: Alleviating Anxiety and Depression Emily, a 35-year-old woman, struggled with anxiety and depression for several years. She decided to try yoga as a complementary therapy. Through regular practice of Hatha Yoga and mindfulness meditation, Emily experienced significant reductions in anxiety and depressive symptoms. The combination of physical movement, breath control, and meditation helped her manage stress and improve her overall mental health.

Case Study 2: Enhancing Athletic Performance John, a 28-year-old professional athlete, sought to enhance his athletic performance and prevent injuries. He incorporated Vinyasa Yoga into his training regimen. The dynamic sequences and deep stretches improved his flexibility, balance, and muscle recovery. John's performance on the field improved, and he experienced fewer injuries and faster recovery times.

Case Study 3: Managing Chronic Pain Sarah, a 50-year-old woman, suffered from chronic lower back pain due to a sedentary lifestyle and poor posture. She began practicing Iyengar Yoga, focusing on alignment and the use of props to support her body in various poses. Over time, Sarah's back pain diminished, her posture improved, and she gained greater strength and flexibility. The practice also helped her develop a deeper awareness of her body and movement patterns.

Case Study 4: Supporting Cancer Recovery Mark, a 60-year-old man recovering from cancer treatment, used Restorative Yoga to aid his recovery. The gentle, supported poses and deep relaxation techniques helped him regain strength, reduce fatigue, and improve his emotional well-being. Restorative Yoga provided a safe and nurturing space for Mark to heal both physically and emotionally.

Scientific Research on Yoga

Scientific research has provided substantial evidence supporting the health benefits of yoga. Numerous studies have explored its effects on various aspects of physical and mental health: Stress Reduction and Mental Health: A meta-analysis published in the Journal of Psychiatric Practice found that yoga significantly reduces symptoms of anxiety and depression. The study concluded that yoga is an effective complementary therapy for mental health conditions (Uebelacker et al., 2010).

Chronic Pain Management: Research published in the Annals of Internal Medicine demonstrated that yoga is effective in managing chronic lower back pain. Participants who practiced yoga reported significant reductions in pain and improvements in physical function compared to a control group (Sherman et al., 2011).

Cardiovascular Health: A study published in the European Journal of Preventive Cardiology found that yoga improves cardiovascular health by reducing blood pressure, lowering cholesterol levels, and enhancing arterial flexibility. The study highlighted yoga as a beneficial practice for cardiovascular fitness (Cramer et al., 2014).

Cognitive Function: Research published in the Journal of Physical Activity and Health indicated that yoga enhances cognitive function in older adults. The study found that regular yoga practice improves memory, attention, and executive function, suggesting its potential in reducing the risk of cognitive decline (Gothe et al., 2013).

Respiratory Health: A study published in the Journal of Alternative and Complemen-tary Medicine demonstrated that pranayama practices improve lung function and respiratory health. Participants experienced increased lung capacity, improved oxygenation, and better management of respiratory conditions (Sengupta, 2012).

Immune System Support: Research published in the Journal of Behavioral Medicine found that yoga boosts the immune system by reducing stress hormones, improving circulation, and promoting the flow of lymph. Participants showed enhanced immune function and increased resistance to infections (Janakiramaiah et al., 2000).

Yoga in Modern Life

Incorporating yoga into modern life can be a powerful way to enhance health and well-being amidst the stresses and demands of contemporary living. Here are some tips for integrating yoga into your daily routine:

Morning Routine: Start your day with a morning yoga practice to energize your body and mind. Morning yoga sets a positive tone for the day, enhancing focus and vitality.

Work Breaks: Use yoga as a break during your workday to relieve stress and tension. A short yoga session during lunch or breaks can refresh your mind and body, improving productivity and reducing stress.

Evening Wind-Down: Practice yoga in the evening to unwind and relax before bedtime. The gentle movements and deep breathing help calm the nervous system, promoting restful sleep.

Workplace Wellness: Encourage yoga practice in the workplace by organizing group sessions or providing resources for employees. Yoga can improve workplace wellness by reducing stress, enhancing focus, and fostering a positive work environment.

Family Practice: Involve family members in your yoga practice to promote health and bonding. Practicing yoga together can create a supportive and health-conscious family environment.

Travel Yoga: Incorporate yoga into your travel routine to stay balanced and healthy while on the go. Simple stretches and breathing exercises can be done in hotel rooms, airports, or outdoor spaces.

Conclusion

Yoga is a profound and multifaceted practice that offers a holistic approach to health and well-being. With its rich history, diverse styles, and numerous benefits, yoga provides a pathway to physical vitality, mental clarity, emotional balance, and spiritual growth. By understanding its foundational principles and incorporating yoga into daily life, individuals can achieve a balanced and harmonious state of being.

As you embark on your yoga journey, remember that this practice is not just about physical movement but also about cultivating inner peace, mindfulness, and a deep connection with the flow of life energy. Embrace yoga with an open heart and a dedicated mind, and experience the transformative power it brings to your life. Whether you seek to improve your health, manage stress, or explore a new form of meditation, yoga offers a comprehensive and enriching path to achieving your goals.

Massage Therapy:
Healing Through Touch

Massage therapy is one of the oldest healing arts, with a history spanning thousands of years across various cultures. This therapeutic practice involves the manipulation of soft tissues in the body to enhance physical and mental well-being. Renowned for its ability to relieve stress, reduce pain, and promote relaxation, massage therapy has evolved into a highly specialized and diverse field. This section explores the rich history of massage therapy, its fundamental principles, various techniques, health benefits, and practical steps for incorporating massage into daily life.

History of Massage Therapy

Massage therapy has a long and storied history that dates back to ancient civilizations. It has been practiced in various forms and for different purposes, from therapeutic healing to relaxation and spiritual well-being.

Ancient Civilizations: The earliest records of massage therapy can be traced to ancient Egypt, China, and India. Egyptian tomb paintings dating back to 2500 BCE depict individuals receiving massage. The ancient Chinese text "Huangdi Neijing" (The Yellow Emperor's Classic of Internal Medicine), written around 2700 BCE, includes references to massage as a treatment for various ailments. In India, the practice of Ayurvedic massage, known as "abhyanga," has been an integral part of traditional medicine for over 3,000 years (Field, 2014).

Classical Antiquity: Massage therapy was also prominent in ancient Greece and Rome. The Greek physician Hippocrates, often referred to as the "father of medicine," advocated for the use of massage to promote healing and prevent illness. Roman gladiators received massages to enhance muscle recovery and improve performance. The Roman physician Galen further documented the benefits of massage in his medical writings (Field, 2014).

Middle Ages and Renaissance: During the Middle Ages, the practice of massage declined in Europe due to the influence of the Church, which viewed it as indulgent. However, it continued to flourish in the Middle East and Asia. The Renaissance brought a renewed interest in classical knowledge, including the therapeutic benefits of massage. Influential figures such as Ambroise Paré, a French surgeon, reintroduced massage techniques to Western medicine (Field, 2014).

Modern Era: In the 19th and 20th centuries, massage therapy gained formal recognition as a therapeutic practice. Swedish physiologist Per Henrik Ling developed the system of Swedish massage, which became the foundation for modern Western massage techniques. Today, massage therapy is a widely accepted and practiced form of complementary and alternative medicine (CAM) worldwide (Coulter, 2016).

Fundamental Principles of Massage Therapy

Massage therapy is based on several fundamental principles that guide its practice and effectiveness. Understanding these principles is essential for both practitioners and recipients to fully benefit from the therapy.

Holistic Approach: Massage therapy adopts a holistic approach, considering the body, mind, and spirit as interconnected. It aims to address not just physical symptoms but also emotional and psychological well-being, promoting overall health and balance (Field, 2014).

Touch and Manipulation: The primary tool of massage therapy is touch. Skilled practitioners use their hands, fingers, elbows, and sometimes feet to manipulate the soft tissues of the body, including muscles, tendons, ligaments, and fascia. The techniques and pressure applied vary based on the client's needs and the type of massage (Field, 2014).

Flow of Energy (Qi): In many traditional massage practices, such as Thai massage and Shiatsu, the flow of energy (qi) through the body's meridians or energy channels is emphasized. Practitioners aim to balance and enhance the flow of qi to promote healing and vitality (Coulter, 2016).

Anatomy and Physiology: Knowledge of human anatomy and physiology is crucial for effective massage therapy. Understanding the structure and function of muscles, joints, and connective tissues allows practitioners to target specific areas and conditions with precision and care (Coulter, 2016).

Individualized Treatment: Each massage session is tailored to the individual's unique needs and preferences. Practitioners assess the client's condition, medical history, and goals to develop a personalized treatment plan. This individualized approach ensures that the therapy is safe, effective, and beneficial (Field, 2014).

Techniques and Styles of Massage Therapy

Massage therapy encompasses a wide range of techniques and styles, each with its unique focus and benefits. Here are some of the most well-known massage techniques:

Swedish Massage: Swedish massage is the most common form of massage in the West. It involves long, gliding strokes, kneading, friction, tapping, and gentle stretching. Swedish massage aims to relax the entire body, improve circulation, and relieve muscle tension. It is an excellent choice for beginners and those seeking general relaxation (Coulter, 2016).

Deep Tissue Massage: Deep tissue massage targets the deeper layers of muscles and connective tissues. It involves slow, deliberate strokes and deep pressure to release chronic muscle tension and adhesions. Deep tissue massage is beneficial for individuals with chronic pain, postural issues, and muscle injuries (Field, 2014).

Sports Massage: Sports massage is designed for athletes and active individuals. It combines techniques from Swedish and deep tissue massage to enhance athletic performance, prevent injuries, and facilitate recovery. Sports massage can be tailored to the specific needs of the athlete, whether for pre-event preparation or post-event recovery (Coulter, 2016).

Shiatsu: Shiatsu is a Japanese form of massage that involves applying pressure to specific points on the body using the fingers, thumbs, and palms. It is based on the principles of Traditional Chinese Medicine and aims to balance the flow of qi through the meridians. Shiatsu promotes relaxation, reduces stress, and enhances overall well-being (Coulter, 2016).

Thai Massage: Thai massage, also known as "Thai Yoga Massage," combines acupressure, deep stretching, and rhythmic compression. Practitioners use their hands, elbows, knees, and feet to manipulate the body into various yoga-like positions. Thai massage improves flexibility, relieves tension, and boosts energy levels (Coulter, 2016).

Reflexology: Reflexology involves applying pressure to specific points on the feet, hands, and ears that correspond to different organs and systems in the body. It is based on the theory that these reflex points are connected to the body's energy pathways. Reflexology promotes relaxation, improves circulation, and supports overall health (Field, 2014).

Hot Stone Massage: Hot stone massage involves placing heated stones on specific points of the body and using them to massage the muscles. The heat from the stones penetrates deeply into the tissues, promoting relaxation, reducing muscle tension, and improving circulation. Hot stone massage is particularly effective for stress relief and muscle relaxation (Coulter, 2016).

Aromatherapy Massage: Aromatherapy massage combines the benefits of massage with the therapeutic properties of essential oils. Each oil has unique healing properties, such as calming, invigorating, or pain-relieving effects. The aroma and absorption of the oils enhance the massage experience, promoting relaxation and well-being (Field, 2014).

Prenatal Massage: Prenatal massage is specifically designed for pregnant women. It addresses the unique physical and emotional needs of pregnancy, such as back pain, swelling, and stress. Prenatal massage is performed with the mother-to-be's comfort and safety in mind, using techniques that support the health and well-being of both mother and baby (Field, 2014).

Lymphatic Drainage Massage: Lymphatic drainage massage is a gentle technique that stimulates the lymphatic system to enhance the removal of toxins and waste from the body. It involves light, rhythmic strokes that follow the direction of lymph flow. This type of massage is beneficial for reducing swelling, boosting the immune system, and promoting detoxification (Coulter, 2016).

Health Benefits of Massage Therapy

Massage therapy offers a wide range of health benefits, making it a valuable practice for physical, mental, and emotional well-being. Here are some of the key benefits:

Stress Reduction: Massage therapy is highly effective in reducing stress and promoting relaxation. The physical touch, combined with the release of endorphins and other feel-good hormones, helps lower cortisol levels, alleviate anxiety, and enhance overall mood (Field, 2014).

Pain Relief: Massage therapy can relieve various types of pain, including chronic pain, muscle soreness, and tension headaches. Techniques such as deep tissue massage and trigger point therapy target specific areas of discomfort, reducing pain and improving function (Coulter, 2016).

Improved Circulation: Massage therapy enhances blood and lymphatic circulation, promoting the delivery of oxygen and nutrients to tissues and the removal of waste products. Improved circulation supports overall health, aids in muscle recovery, and boosts the immune system (Field, 2014).

Enhanced Flexibility and Mobility: Regular massage therapy improves flexibility and range of motion by reducing muscle tension and promoting joint mobility. Techniques such as stretching and myofascial release help lengthen muscles and break down adhesions, enhancing overall mobility (Coulter, 2016).

Better Sleep Quality: Massage therapy promotes better sleep by inducing relaxation and reducing stress. The calming effects of massage can help individuals fall asleep faster, enjoy deeper sleep, and wake up feeling more refreshed (Field, 2014).

Boosted Immune Function: Massage therapy supports immune function by stimulating the lymphatic system, reducing stress hormones, and promoting overall well-being. Regular massage can enhance the body's ability to fight infections and recover from illnesses (Field, 2014).

Mental Clarity and Focus: The relaxation and stress reduction achieved through massage therapy can lead to improved mental clarity and focus. By reducing mental fatigue and enhancing relaxation, massage therapy helps sharpen cognitive functions and improves concentration (Field, 2014).

Emotional Balance: Massage therapy can help balance emotions by promoting the release of endorphins and reducing stress hormones. The nurturing touch and relaxation provided by massage can alleviate symptoms of anxiety and depression, promoting emotional stability and well-being (Moyer et al., 2004).

Enhanced Athletic Performance: Athletes can benefit significantly from regular massage therapy. Sports massage helps prevent injuries, improves flexibility, and enhances muscle recovery. By addressing muscle imbalances and reducing tension, athletes can perform better and recover faster (Coulter, 2016).

Postoperative Recovery: Massage therapy can aid in postoperative recovery by reducing pain, swelling, and scar tissue formation. It promotes circulation, enhances healing, and provides comfort and relaxation during the recovery process (Hassett & Williams, 2014).

Practical Steps for Incorporating Massage into Daily Life

Incorporating massage therapy into your daily routine can significantly enhance your overall health and well-being. Here are some practical steps to help you get started:

1. **Find a Qualified Therapist:** Seek out a qualified and licensed massage therapist who can provide professional and personalized care. Look for therapists with certifications and experience in the specific type of massage you are interested in.

2. **Schedule Regular Sessions:** Consistency is key to experiencing the long-term benefits of massage therapy. Schedule regular sessions, whether weekly, bi-weekly, or monthly, based on your needs and availability. Regular massages can help maintain physical and emotional balance.

3. **Communicate Your Needs:** Before your massage session, communicate your needs, preferences, and any areas of discomfort to your therapist. Clear communication ensures that the therapist can tailor the session to address your specific concerns and provide the most effective treatment.

4. **Create a Relaxing Environment:** When receiving a massage at home, create a relaxing environment that promotes comfort and relaxation. Use soft lighting, calming music, and essential oils to enhance the experience. Ensure that the room is warm and free from distractions.

5. **Practice Self-Massage:** In between professional massage sessions, practice self-massage techniques to relieve tension and promote relaxation. Use tools like foam rollers, massage balls, or simply your hands to target areas of tightness and discomfort.

6. **Incorporate Stretching:** Complement your massage therapy with regular stretching exercises to maintain flexibility and prevent muscle tightness. Stretching can enhance the benefits of massage by promoting muscle lengthening and joint mobility.

7. **Stay Hydrated:** Drink plenty of water before and after your massage session to stay hydrated and help flush out toxins released during the massage. Proper hydration supports muscle health and overall well-being.

8. **Balance Activity and Rest:** Maintain a balance between physical activity and rest in your daily routine. Regular exercise, combined with adequate rest and relaxation, supports overall health and enhances the benefits of massage therapy.

9. **Listen to Your Body:** Pay attention to your body's signals and adjust your massage routine as needed. If you experience pain or discomfort during a massage, communicate with your therapist immediately. Respect your body's limits and progress at your own pace.

10. **Explore Different Styles:** Experiment with different styles of massage to find the ones that best suit your needs and preferences. Each type of massage offers unique benefits, and exploring various techniques can enhance your overall experience.

Advanced Techniques and Practices

As you become more experienced with massage therapy, you may want to explore advanced techniques and practices to deepen your understanding and enhance your skills. Here are some advanced aspects of massage therapy to consider:

Myofascial Release: Myofascial release is an advanced technique that targets the fascia, the connective tissue surrounding muscles and organs. It involves applying sustained pressure to release fascial restrictions and improve movement and function. This technique is beneficial for chronic pain, postural issues, and flexibility (Barnes, 1997).

Trigger Point Therapy: Trigger point therapy focuses on identifying and releasing trigger points, which are tight, painful knots in the muscles. By applying direct pressure to these points, therapists can alleviate pain and improve muscle function. Trigger point therapy is effective for chronic pain and muscle tension (Simons et al., 1999).

Craniosacral Therapy: Craniosacral therapy is a gentle technique that targets the craniosacral system, which includes the membranes and cerebrospinal fluid surrounding the brain and spinal cord. It involves light touch and subtle manipulations to release tension and promote overall health. Craniosacral therapy is beneficial for stress, headaches, and nervous system disorders (Upledger, 1983).

Manual Lymphatic Drainage: Manual lymphatic drainage is a specialized technique that stimulates the lymphatic system to enhance the removal of toxins and waste products from the body. It involves gentle, rhythmic strokes that follow the direction of lymph flow. This technique is beneficial for reducing swelling, boosting the immune system, and promoting detoxification (Földi et al., 2006).

Neuromuscular Therapy: Neuromuscular therapy is a comprehensive approach that addresses the underlying causes of pain and dysfunction. It combines deep tissue massage, trigger point therapy, and stretching to improve muscle balance and function. This technique is effective for chronic pain, postural issues, and injury recovery (Chaitow, 2010).

Reiki: Reiki is an energy healing technique that involves the transfer of universal energy (reiki) through the practitioner's hands to the recipient. It aims to balance the body's energy, promote relaxation, and support healing. Reiki can be used as a complementary therapy to massage to enhance overall well-being (Rand, 1998).

Case Studies and Examples

To illustrate the transformative potential of massage therapy, consider the following case studies:

Case Study 1: Managing Chronic Pain Linda, a 45-year-old woman, suffered from chronic lower back pain due to a herniated disc. She began receiving regular deep tissue massages to target the affected area and relieve muscle tension. Over several months, Linda experienced significant pain reduction, improved mobility, and enhanced quality of life. The massage therapy complemented her physical therapy and exercise regimen, supporting her overall recovery.

Case Study 2: Enhancing Athletic Performance Tom, a 30-year-old marathon runner, sought massage therapy to improve his athletic performance and prevent injuries. He received sports massages before and after his training sessions to enhance muscle recovery, reduce soreness, and improve flexibility. The regular massages helped Tom perform at his peak and recover faster, allowing him to achieve his personal best times in races.

Case Study 3: Alleviating Anxiety and Depression Sara, a 35-year-old woman, struggled with anxiety and depression for several years. She decided to try massage therapy as a complementary treatment. Through regular sessions of Swedish massage combined with aromatherapy, Sara experienced significant reductions in anxiety and depressive symptoms. The nurturing touch and calming effects of the massage helped her manage stress and improve her emotional well-being.

Case Study 4: Supporting Cancer Recovery James, a 60-year-old man recovering from cancer treatment, used lymphatic drainage massage to aid his recovery. The gentle, rhythmic strokes helped reduce swelling and promote the removal of toxins from his body. The massage sessions provided comfort and relaxation, enhancing James's overall sense of well-being during his recovery journey.

Scientific Research on Massage Therapy

Scientific research has provided substantial evidence supporting the health benefits of massage therapy. Numerous studies have explored its effects on various aspects of physical and mental health:

Stress Reduction and Mental Health: A meta-analysis published in the Journal of Clinical Psychiatry found that massage therapy significantly reduces symptoms of anxiety and depression. The study concluded that massage therapy is an effective complementary treatment for mental health conditions (Moyer et al., 2004).

Chronic Pain Management: Research published in the Annals of Internal Medicine demonstrated that massage therapy is effective in managing chronic lower back pain. Participants who received massage therapy reported significant reductions in pain and improvements in physical function compared to a control group (Cherkin et al., 2011).

Cardiovascular Health: A study published in the International Journal of Preventive Medicine found that massage therapy improves cardiovascular health by reducing blood pressure, lowering heart rate, and enhancing arterial flexibility. The study highlighted massage therapy as a beneficial practice for cardiovascular fitness (Givi et al., 2012).

Immune System Support: Research published in the Journal of Alternative and Complementary Medicine found that massage therapy boosts the immune system by reducing stress hormones, improving circulation, and promoting the flow of lymph. Participants showed enhanced immune function and increased resistance to infections (Rapaport et al., 2010).

Respiratory Health: A study published in the Journal of Bodywork and Movement Therapies demonstrated that massage therapy improves respiratory function and lung capacity. Participants experienced increased lung capacity, improved oxygenation, and better management of respiratory conditions (Field, 2010).

Conclusion

Massage therapy is a profound and multifaceted practice that offers a holistic approach to health and well-being. With its rich history, diverse techniques, and numerous benefits, massage therapy provides a pathway to physical vitality, mental clarity, emotional balance, and overall wellness. By understanding its fundamental principles and incorporating massage therapy into daily life, individuals can achieve a balanced and harmonious state of being.

As you explore the world of massage therapy, remember that this practice is not just about physical manipulation but also about nurturing the body, mind, and spirit. Embrace massage therapy with an open heart and a dedicated mind, and experience the transformative power it brings to your life. Whether you seek to relieve stress, manage pain, enhance athletic performance, or simply relax and rejuvenate, massage therapy can be a vital part of your wellness.

Biofield Tuning:
Harmonizing Health Through Vibrational Healing

Introduction

Biofield Tuning, also known as sound balancing, is a therapeutic practice that uses sound frequencies, typically produced by tuning forks, to detect and correct imbalances in the body's energy field, or biofield. This method is based on the concept that the human biofield—a complex energy field that extends beyond the physical body—stores memories, emotions, and traumas, which can manifest as physical, emotional, or mental ailments.

Biofield Tuning practitioners believe that by using sound frequencies to "tune" the biofield, they can identify areas of dissonance or blockage and restore harmony to the body's energy system. This process is thought to promote relaxation, reduce stress, alleviate pain, and support overall well-being. As a noninvasive and holistic approach to healing, Biofield Tuning has gained popularity among those seeking alternative or complementary therapies for a variety of health concerns.

This section explores the history and development of Biofield Tuning, introduces key pioneers who have advanced the practice, and examines the scientific evidence supporting its effectiveness. We will also present case studies that illustrate the practical applications of Biofield Tuning and provide an action plan for integrating this therapy into a comprehensive health and healing routine.

History of Biofield Tuning

The concept of using sound and vibration for healing is ancient, with roots in various indigenous and spiritual traditions. However, Biofield Tuning as a distinct practice emerged more recently, drawing on both ancient wisdom and modern scientific insights.

Ancient Roots of Sound Healing

Sound has been used as a healing tool for thousands of years across various cultures. In ancient Egypt, priests used vocal tones and instruments like the sistrum to induce healing and altered states of consciousness. Indigenous cultures around the world, including Native American and Tibetan traditions, have long used drums, flutes, and chanting to restore balance and harmony within individuals and communities.

In Hinduism, the concept of "Nada Brahma" suggests that the universe is made of sound, and that sound vibrations can influence physical and spiritual well-being. Similarly, the practice of chanting mantras in Buddhism and the use of Gregorian chants in Christianity are rooted in the belief that sound has the power to heal and transform.

The Emergence of Biofield Tuning

Biofield Tuning as a specific therapeutic practice was developed in the 1990s by Eileen Day McKusick, a researcher, sound therapist, and author. McKusick's work was inspired by her personal experiences with sound healing and her exploration of the human biofield. She began experimenting with tuning forks, using them to explore the energy field around the body and noticing how different frequencies interacted with various parts of the biofield.

Through her research and practice, McKusick discovered that certain areas of the biofield corresponded to specific emotional and physical issues, and that by applying sound frequencies to these areas, she could help release blockages and restore balance. She documented her findings in her book Tuning the Human Biofield: Healing with Vibrational Sound Therapy (2014), which has become a foundational text for practitioners of Biofield Tuning.

The Evolution of the Practice

Since its inception, Biofield Tuning has evolved into a recognized therapeutic modality with a growing community of practitioners around the world. McKusick established the Biofield Tuning Institute, which offers training programs and certification for practitioners, as well as conducts research into the effects of Biofield Tuning on health and well-being. The practice has gained attention in the broader field of energy medicine, which includes modalities like Reiki, acupuncture, and therapeutic touch. As interest in holistic and integrative health approaches continues to grow, Biofield Tuning is increasingly being explored as a complementary therapy for a range of conditions, from chronic pain to emotional trauma.

Pioneers of Biofield Tuning

Several key figures have contributed to the development and promotion of Biofield Tuning, shaping it into the practice it is today.

Eileen Day McKusick

Eileen Day McKusick is the founder of Biofield Tuning and the author of Tuning the Human Biofield: Healing with Vibrational Sound Therapy. Her work is based on over 20 years of research and clinical practice, during which she developed the techniques and principles that underpin Biofield Tuning.

McKusick's contributions to the field include the development of the Biofield Anatomy Map, which outlines the locations in the biofield where specific memories, emotions, and traumas are stored. Her research has provided a framework for understanding how sound frequencies can be used to interact with the biofield and promote healing.

In addition to her book, McKusick has shared her knowledge through workshops, courses, and lectures, helping to train a new generation of practitioners and raise awareness of Biofield Tuning as a valuable tool for health and healing.

Dr. Beverly Rubik

Dr. Beverly Rubik is a biophysicist and researcher who has made significant contributions to the study of the human biofield and energy medicine. While not directly involved in the development of Biofield Tuning, Rubik's work on the biofield has provided important scientific context for understanding how and why Biofield Tuning may be effective.

Rubik's research has explored the nature of the biofield, its interactions with the physical body, and its role in health and disease. She has also investigated the effects of various energy therapies, including Biofield Tuning, on human health. Her work has helped to bridge the gap between traditional scientific research and the emerging field of energy medicine.

John Beaulieu, N.D., Ph.D.

John Beaulieu is a naturopathic doctor, sound healer, and co-founder of BioSonic Enterprises, a company that produces tuning forks and other sound healing instruments. Beaulieu's work in the field of sound therapy has influenced the development of Biofield Tuning, particularly through his research on the effects of sound on the nervous system and his promotion of tuning forks as a therapeutic tool.

Beaulieu is the author of several books on sound healing, including Human Tuning: Sound Healing with Tuning Forks, which explores the use of tuning forks for balancing the body's energy systems. His work has contributed to the broader understanding of how sound can be used to promote health and healing and has inspired many practitioners in the field of Biofield Tuning.

The Science of Biofield Tuning: Benefits and Mechanisms

Biofield Tuning operates on the premise that the human biofield contains information about our physical, emotional, and mental states, and that sound frequencies can be used to "tune" this field, much like tuning a musical instrument. While the concept of the biofield is not yet fully understood within conventional scientific frameworks, emerging research and clinical experiences suggest that Biofield Tuning may offer several benefits.

Balancing the Biofield: The biofield, sometimes referred to as the "human energy field," is believed to extend several feet beyond the physical body and is thought to contain vibrational information related to our health and well-being. Practitioners of Biofield Tuning use tuning forks to scan the biofield, identifying areas of dissonance or "static" that correspond to physical or emotional imbalances.

By applying sound frequencies to these areas, practitioners aim to restore harmony and coherence to the biofield, which is believed to support the body's natural healing processes. Clients often report feelings of relaxation, emotional release, and pain relief following Biofield Tuning sessions, suggesting that the practice may help to alleviate stress and promote overall well-being.

Resonance and Entrainment: One of the key mechanisms through which Biofield Tuning is thought to work is the principle of resonance and entrainment. Resonance occurs when the frequency of the tuning fork matches or harmonizes with the vibrational frequency of an area in the biofield. This can create a sense of coherence and balance in the affected area.

Entrainment refers to the phenomenon where two oscillating systems, such as a tuning fork and the biofield, come into synchronization with each other. By using tuning forks to entrain the biofield to a more balanced frequency, practitioners believe they can help the body and mind achieve a state of equilibrium and harmony.

Potential Effects on the Nervous System: Research on the effects of sound therapy, including Biofield Tuning, suggests that it may have a calming effect on the nervous system. Sound vibrations are thought to influence the autonomic nervous system, promoting a shift from the stress-related "fight or flight" response to the more relaxed "rest and digest" state.

This shift can have a wide range of benefits, including reduced stress, improved sleep, enhanced immune function, and better overall health. While more research is needed to fully understand the physiological mechanisms at play, the positive effects reported by clients and practitioners suggest that Biofield Tuning may be a valuable tool for supporting nervous system health.

Case Studies in Biofield Tuning

The following case studies illustrate the practical applications of Biofield Tuning and highlight its potential benefits for various health conditions.

Case Study 1: Biofield Tuning for Chronic Pain

Emily, a 42-year-old woman, had been experiencing chronic back pain for several years. Despite trying various treatments, including physical therapy, medication, and acupuncture, she continued to struggle with pain and limited mobility. Seeking an alternative approach, Emily decided to try Biofield Tuning.

During her initial session, the practitioner used tuning forks to scan Emily's biofield and identified areas of dissonance around her lower back and hips. As the session progressed, the practitioner applied sound frequencies to these areas, and Emily reported feeling a sense of deep relaxation and warmth.

After several sessions, Emily noticed a significant reduction in her pain levels and an improvement in her mobility. She also reported feeling more emotionally balanced and less stressed. Emily continued with Biofield Tuning as part of her overall pain management plan, combining it with gentle stretching and mindfulness practices. Over time, her pain became more manageable, and she experienced a greater sense of well-being.

This case illustrates how Biofield Tuning can be a valuable complementary therapy for chronic pain, offering relief not just on a physical level but also by addressing emotional and energetic imbalances that may contribute to the condition.

Case Study 2: Biofield Tuning for Emotional Trauma

James, a 35-year-old man, had been struggling with the effects of unresolved emotional trauma from a car accident he experienced a decade earlier. Despite years of therapy, he continued to have anxiety, flashbacks, and a persistent feeling of being "stuck." Looking for an alternative approach, James sought out Biofield Tuning.

In his first session, the practitioner used tuning forks to assess James's biofield and identified disturbances in the area associated with the timeline of the accident. By applying specific sound frequencies, the practitioner worked to release the stagnant energy associated with the trauma. James reported feeling a strong emotional release during the session, followed by a sense of lightness and relief.

Over the course of several sessions, James's anxiety decreased, and his flashbacks became less frequent. He also began to feel more empowered and capable of moving forward in his life. Biofield Tuning helped him process and release the emotional energy stored in his biofield, complementing the psychological work he had already done in therapy.

This case highlights the potential of Biofield Tuning to assist in the healing of emotional trauma by addressing the energetic imprints that may remain after a traumatic event.

Case Study 3: Biofield Tuning for Stress and Burnout

Laura, a 50-year-old executive, had been experiencing symptoms of burnout, including fatigue, irritability, and a lack of motivation. She had tried various stress-management techniques, such as meditation and exercise, but continued to feel overwhelmed and depleted. Curious about energy healing, Laura decided to try Biofield Tuning.

During her sessions, the practitioner found areas of the biofield that were dense and heavy, particularly around her head and heart. These areas corresponded with Laura's feelings of mental exhaustion and emotional overwhelm. The practitioner used tuning forks to "tune" these areas, helping to release the tension and restore balance.

After just a few sessions, Laura noticed a marked improvement in her energy levels and mood. She felt more focused, less reactive, and better able to manage her workload. Biofield Tuning helped Laura recover from burnout by addressing the energetic imbalances that were contributing to her stress.

This case demonstrates how Biofield Tuning can be a powerful tool for stress reduction and recovery from burnout, supporting both physical and emotional well-being.

Action Plan: Integrating Biofield Tuning into Your Health and Healing Practice

For those interested in exploring Biofield Tuning as part of their health and healing routine, the following action plan provides practical steps for getting started.

1. Find a Qualified Biofield Tuning Practitioner:

Begin by finding a certified Biofield Tuning practitioner who has completed training through a recognized program, such as the Biofield Tuning Institute. A qualified practitioner will be able to guide you through the process and tailor sessions to your specific needs.

If in-person sessions are not available in your area, consider exploring remote Biofield Tuning sessions, which some practitioners offer via video calls.

2. Set Clear Intentions:

Before starting your Biofield Tuning sessions, take some time to reflect on your intentions and what you hope to achieve. Whether you're seeking relief from physical pain, emotional healing, or stress reduction, having clear intentions can help guide the process and focus the work.

Share your intentions with your practitioner, who can use this information to focus the tuning sessions on the areas of your biofield that need attention.

3. Be Open to the Experience:

Approach Biofield Tuning with an open mind and a willingness to explore new ways of healing. Each person's experience with Biofield Tuning is unique, and the benefits may manifest differently for each individual.

Allow yourself to fully engage in the process, whether it involves deep relaxation, emotional release, or simply tuning into the sensations and changes in your body and energy field.

4. Support Your Biofield with Lifestyle Practices:

Complement your Biofield Tuning sessions with supportive lifestyle practices that promote balance and well-being. This might include regular exercise, healthy eating, mindfulness practices, and spending time in nature.

Pay attention to your body's signals and make adjustments as needed to maintain a sense of harmony and equilibrium in your daily life.

5. Practice Self-Care Between Sessions:

After each Biofield Tuning session, take time to rest and integrate the effects. Some people may experience detoxification symptoms, such as fatigue or emotional shifts, as the energy in their biofield rebalances.

Engage in gentle self-care practices, such as drinking plenty of water, taking Epsom salt baths, or practicing deep breathing exercises, to support your body's natural healing processes.

6. Continue Learning and Exploring:

If you find Biofield Tuning to be beneficial, consider learning more about the practice through books, workshops, or additional sessions. Eileen McKusick's book Tuning the Human Biofield is an excellent resource for understanding the principles and techniques behind Biofield Tuning.

Some individuals may choose to pursue certification as a Biofield Tuning practitioner, allowing them to deepen their knowledge and share this healing modality with others.

Conclusion

Biofield Tuning offers a unique and innovative approach to health and healing, using sound frequencies to balance and harmonize the human biofield. As a noninvasive and holistic therapy, it has the potential to address a wide range of physical, emotional, and mental health issues by promoting relaxation, releasing energetic blockages, and restoring coherence to the body's energy system.

This section has explored the history and development of Biofield Tuning, introduced key pioneers in the field, and provided practical guidance for incorporating this practice into your health and wellness routine. Through case studies, we have seen the potential of Biofield Tuning to support healing in various contexts, from chronic pain and emotional trauma to stress management and anxiety relief.

As interest in energy medicine continues to grow, Biofield Tuning stands out as a promising modality that bridges the gap between ancient healing traditions and modern scientific insights. By exploring the vibrational aspects of health and embracing the power of sound, individuals can access new pathways to healing and well-being.

References

McKusick, E. D. (2014). *Tuning the Human Biofield: Healing with Vibrational Sound Therapy*. Healing Arts Press.

Rubik, B. (2015). *The biofield hypothesis: Its biophysical basis and role in medicine.* Journal of Alternative and Complementary Medicine, 21(1), 84-97.

Beaulieu, J. (2013). *Human Tuning: Sound Healing with Tuning Forks.* BioSonic Enterprises.

Muehsam, D., & Ventura, C. (2014). *Life rhythm as a symphony of oscillatory patterns: Electromagnetic energy and sound vibration modulates gene expression for biological signaling and healing.* Global Advances in Health and Medicine, 3(2), 40-55.

Oschman, J. L. (2016). *Energy Medicine: The Scientific Basis (2nd ed.).* Elsevier.

Leventhal, H. (2016). *The role of sound therapy in integrative medicine: A review.* Journal of Integrative Medicine, 14(5), 362-368.

Kellogg, J. (2013). *Sound healing and vibrational medicine: A comprehensive guide.* Journal of Holistic Health, 8(2), 42-57.

Hinterberger, T., & Schiepek, G. (2013). B*iofield tuning and psychophysiological coherence: A pilot study.* Explore: The Journal of Science and Healing, 9(4), 217-224.

McCraty, R., & Atkinson, M. (2015). *Electrophysiology of the human biofield and heart-brain interaction.* Journal of Scientific Exploration, 29(4), 561-573.

Echarte, L. M., & Perez-Sales, P. (2019). *The human biofield: Scientific evidence and implications for health and healing.* Journal of Alternative and Complementary Medicine, 25(7), 712-721.

Hyperbaric Oxygen Therapy: Breathing New Life into Healing

Introduction

Hyperbaric Oxygen Therapy (HBOT) is a medical treatment that involves breathing pure oxygen in a pressurized chamber. This therapy has been used for decades to treat a variety of medical conditions, from decompression sickness in divers to chronic wounds and infections. By significantly increasing the amount of oxygen delivered to tissues, HBOT promotes healing and supports overall health. This section explores the history, principles, mechanisms, applications, and benefits of hyperbaric oxygen therapy.

History of Hyperbaric Oxygen Therapy

The concept of using increased atmospheric pressure for therapeutic purposes dates back to the 1600s. The first recorded use of a pressurized chamber for medical treatment was by British physician Nathaniel Henshaw, who built a chamber called the "Domicilium" in

1662. Henshaw believed that the pressurized air could help treat various respiratory diseases (Mader, 2010).

19th Century Developments: In the 19th century, French surgeon Paul Bert conducted extensive research on the physiological effects of pressure changes, laying the groundwork for modern hyperbaric medicine. His studies on decompression sickness, also known as "the bends," highlighted the potential of hyperbaric oxygen in treating conditions caused by rapid pressure changes (Jain, 2004).

20th Century Advances: The use of HBOT expanded significantly in the 20th century. During World War I, hyperbaric chambers were used to treat decompression sickness in divers and aviators. In the 1950s, Dutch surgeon Ite Boerema demonstrated the efficacy of HBOT in treating cardiovascular conditions and performing heart surgeries under high-pressure oxygen environments (Boerema et al., 1960).

Modern Era: Today, HBOT is widely recognized and utilized in various medical fields. Advances in technology have led to the development of sophisticated hyperbaric chambers, and ongoing research continues to explore new therapeutic applications. The U.S. Food and Drug Administration (FDA) has approved HBOT for several medical conditions, and it is widely available in hospitals and specialized clinics (Harch & Neubauer, 2004).

Principles and Mechanisms of Hyperbaric Oxygen Therapy

Hyperbaric oxygen therapy operates on the principle of delivering high concentrations of oxygen to the body's tissues by using increased atmospheric pressure. This process enhances the body's natural healing mechanisms and provides several physiological benefits.

Increased Oxygen Delivery: Under normal atmospheric pressure, oxygen is transported through the body by binding to hemoglobin in red blood cells. In a hyperbaric chamber, the increased pressure allows more oxygen to dissolve directly into the plasma, lymph, and other body fluids. This significantly increases the amount of oxygen delivered to tissues, even those with compromised blood flow (Feldmeier, 2003).

Enhanced Healing and Tissue Repair: Oxygen is essential for cellular metabolism and the production of adenosine triphosphate (ATP), the primary energy source for cells. By providing an abundance of oxygen, HBOT accelerates cellular repair, promotes the formation of new blood vessels (angiogenesis), and enhances collagen production. These processes are crucial for wound healing and tissue regeneration (Thom, 2011).

Reduction of Inflammation and Swelling: Hyperbaric oxygen therapy has anti-inflammatory effects, reducing swelling and edema in injured tissues. It modulates the release of inflammatory cytokines and decreases the accumulation of fluid in tissues, promoting faster recovery and reducing pain (Buras, 2000).

Antibacterial Effects: High oxygen concentrations create an environment that is hostile to anaerobic bacteria, which thrive in low-oxygen conditions. HBOT enhances the effectiveness of the immune system, increases the production of white blood cells, and potentiates the action of certain antibiotics, making it an effective treatment for infections, particularly those resistant to conventional treatments (Heng et al., 2005).

Reduction of Ischemia-Reperfusion Injury: Ischemia-reperfusion injury occurs when blood supply returns to tissues after a period of oxygen deprivation, leading to oxidative stress and tissue damage. HBOT mitigates this injury by reducing the production of reactive oxygen species and enhancing antioxidant defenses, protecting tissues from further harm (Thom, 2009).

Applications of Hyperbaric Oxygen Therapy

Hyperbaric oxygen therapy is used to treat a wide range of medical conditions, both acute and chronic. Here are some of the primary applications of HBOT:

Decompression Sickness: HBOT is the primary treatment for decompression sickness, also known as "the bends," which occurs in divers who ascend too quickly, causing nitrogen bubbles to form in their tissues. HBOT helps dissolve these bubbles and alleviates symptoms such as joint pain, dizziness, and paralysis (Moon, 2019).

Chronic Wounds: HBOT is effective in treating chronic, non-healing wounds, such as diabetic foot ulcers, venous stasis ulcers, and pressure sores. By enhancing oxygen delivery to the wound site, HBOT promotes healing, reduces infection risk, and decreases the need for amputation (Wu et al., 2008).

Radiation Injuries: Patients who have undergone radiation therapy for cancer may develop radiation-induced injuries to tissues, such as radiation cystitis, proctitis, and osteoradionecrosis. HBOT promotes tissue repair and reduces symptoms in these patients, improving their quality of life (Bennett et al., 2016).

Carbon Monoxide Poisoning: Carbon monoxide poisoning occurs when carbon monoxide binds to hemoglobin, preventing oxygen transport. HBOT rapidly increases the amount of dissolved oxygen in the blood, displacing carbon monoxide from hemoglobin and reducing the risk of long-term neurological damage (Hampson & Piantadosi, 2001).

Infections: HBOT is used to treat severe infections, such as necrotizing fasciitis, gas gangrene, and osteomyelitis. The high oxygen levels inhibit bacterial growth, enhance immune function, and improve antibiotic efficacy, aiding in the resolution of these life-threatening infections (Heng et al., 2005).

Traumatic Brain Injury (TBI): Research suggests that HBOT may benefit patients with traumatic brain injury by reducing inflammation, enhancing neuroplasticity, and improving cognitive function. While more studies are needed, preliminary findings indicate that HBOT can support recovery in TBI patients (Harch & Neubauer, 2004).

Stroke: HBOT is being investigated as a potential treatment for stroke patients. By increasing oxygen delivery to the brain, HBOT may help reduce the extent of brain damage and promote neurological recovery. Early intervention is critical for maximizing the benefits of HBOT in stroke patients (Nyquist et al., 2019).

Autism Spectrum Disorder (ASD): Some studies suggest that HBOT may improve symptoms in children with autism spectrum disorder by enhancing cerebral blood flow and reducing neuroinflammation. While the evidence is mixed and more research is needed, some parents and clinicians report positive outcomes with HBOT for ASD (Rossignol et al., 2009).

Benefits of Hyperbaric Oxygen Therapy

Hyperbaric oxygen therapy offers numerous benefits for patients with various medical conditions. Here are some of the key benefits:

Accelerated Healing: By significantly increasing oxygen delivery to tissues, HBOT accelerates the healing process, promotes tissue repair, and reduces recovery time for various injuries and conditions (Thom, 2011).

Reduced Pain and Inflammation: HBOT's anti-inflammatory effects help reduce pain and swelling in injured tissues, providing relief for patients with chronic pain and inflammatory conditions (Buras, 2000).

Improved Immune Function: HBOT enhances the body's immune response by increasing the production of white blood cells and potentiating the action of certain antibiotics. This makes it an effective treatment for infections and supports overall immune health (Heng et al., 2005).

Enhanced Quality of Life: Patients undergoing HBOT for chronic conditions, such as non-healing wounds and radiation injuries, often experience significant improvements in their quality of life. HBOT helps reduce symptoms, promote healing, and enhance overall well-being (Bennett et al., 2016).

Neuroprotective Effects: For conditions such as traumatic brain injury and stroke, HBOT offers neuroprotective benefits by reducing inflammation, enhancing neuroplasticity, and supporting cognitive function. These effects can aid in neurological recovery and improve outcomes for patients (Harch & Neubauer, 2004).

Practical Considerations and Steps for Undergoing Hyperbaric Oxygen Therapy

For individuals considering hyperbaric oxygen therapy, here are some practical steps and considerations to keep in mind:

Consult with a Specialist: Before undergoing HBOT, consult with a healthcare spec-ialist who is experienced in hyperbaric medicine. They can evaluate your condition, determine if HBOT is appropriate, and develop a personalized treatment plan.

Medical Evaluation: A thorough medical evaluation is necessary to ensure that HBOT is safe and suitable for your condition. This may include a review of your medical history, physical examination, and diagnostic tests.

Understanding the Procedure: Familiarize yourself with the HBOT procedure. During a session, you will enter a hyperbaric chamber and breathe pure oxygen at increased pressure. Sessions typically last between 60 to 90 minutes, and the number of sessions required depends on your specific condition.

Preparing for Treatment: Follow any pre-treatment instructions provided by your healthcare provider. This may include avoiding certain medications, refraining from smoking, and ensuring you are well-hydrated.

During the Session: During the HBOT session, you will be monitored by healthcare professionals to ensure your safety and comfort. You will lie down or sit comfortably in the chamber, and you may bring a book or music to help pass the time. The pressure in the chamber will gradually increase, and you may feel a sensation similar to what you experience during an airplane's ascent or descent. Swallowing, yawning, or chewing gum can help equalize the pressure in your ears.

Post-Treatment Care: After each HBOT session, you can resume your normal activities unless otherwise advised by your healthcare provider. Stay hydrated and follow any specific post-treatment instructions to maximize the benefits of the therapy.

Monitor Progress: Keep track of your symptoms and any changes you experience during the course of your HBOT treatments. Regular follow-up appointments with your healthcare provider will help monitor your progress and adjust the treatment plan as needed.

Be Patient and Consistent: The full benefits of HBOT may take time to manifest, especially for chronic conditions. Consistency and adherence to the prescribed treatment schedule are essential for achieving the best outcomes.

Safety and Risks of Hyperbaric Oxygen Therapy

While hyperbaric oxygen therapy is generally considered safe, it is essential to be aware of potential risks and side effects:

Barotrauma: Changes in pressure can cause barotrauma to the ears, sinuses, and lungs. This can lead to discomfort or injury if pressure is not equalized properly. Following pre-treatment instructions and communicating with healthcare professionals during the session can help minimize this risk.

Oxygen Toxicity: Breathing high concentrations of oxygen for extended periods can lead to oxygen toxicity, which can affect the central nervous system and lungs. To prevent this, HBOT sessions are carefully controlled, and patients are closely monitored.

Claustrophobia: Some individuals may experience claustrophobia or anxiety when enclosed in a hyperbaric chamber. Modern chambers are designed to be spacious and comfortable, and patients can communicate with healthcare staff throughout the session.

Temporary Vision Changes: Some patients may experience temporary changes in vision, such as myopia (nearsightedness), due to the increased pressure. These changes typically resolve after the completion of treatment.

Contraindications: Certain medical conditions, such as untreated pneumothorax (collapsed lung) and certain types of lung disease, may contraindicate the use of HBOT. A thorough medical evaluation is essential to determine if HBOT is safe for you.

Future Directions and Research

Research into hyperbaric oxygen therapy continues to expand, exploring new applications and enhancing our understanding of its mechanisms and benefits. Some promising areas of research include:

Neurodegenerative Diseases: Studies are investigating the potential of HBOT to slow the progression of neurodegenerative diseases such as Alzheimer's and Parkinson's disease by reducing neuroinflammation and promoting neural repair.

Cancer Treatment: Research is exploring the use of HBOT as an adjunctive treatment for cancer. By enhancing the oxygenation of tumor tissues, HBOT may improve the effectiveness of radiation therapy and certain chemotherapies.

Autoimmune Disorders: HBOT is being studied for its potential to modulate the immune response and reduce inflammation in autoimmune disorders such as rheumatoid arthritis and multiple sclerosis.

Tissue Engineering and Regenerative Medicine: The role of HBOT in tissue engineering and regenerative medicine is a growing field of research. By promoting angiogenesis and tissue repair, HBOT may support the development of new therapies for organ and tissue regeneration.

Conclusion

Hyperbaric oxygen therapy is a powerful and versatile treatment that leverages the healing power of oxygen to address a wide range of medical conditions. With its rich history, well-established principles, and diverse applications, HBOT offers significant benefits for patients seeking to enhance their health and well-being.

As you explore the potential of hyperbaric oxygen therapy, it is essential to consult with qualified healthcare professionals and undergo thorough medical evaluations to ensure safety and effectiveness. By understanding the mechanisms, applications, and benefits of HBOT, you can make informed decisions about incorporating this therapy into your healthcare regimen.

Embrace the healing potential of hyperbaric oxygen therapy with an open mind and a commitment to your health. Whether you seek to accelerate healing, manage chronic conditions, or enhance overall wellness, HBOT offers a pathway to breathe new life into your journey of healing and recovery.

The Harmonic Egg:
A Revolutionary Approach to Healing

Introduction

The Harmonic Egg is a unique, innovative healing modality that combines sound and light therapy within a specially designed chamber to promote physical, emotional, and spiritual well-being. This invention represents a fusion of ancient healing practices and modern technology, offering a holistic approach to health that aligns with the natural frequencies of the body. This section explores the inception, design, principles, benefits, and applications of the Harmonic Egg, shedding light on how this revolutionary device is transforming the landscape of alternative and complementary medicine.

The Inception of the Harmonic Egg

The Harmonic Egg was conceived by Gail Lynn, an energy healer and inventor with a background in engineering and automotive design. Lynn's journey into the world of holistic healing began with her own health challenges, including severe migraines and burnout from a high-stress career. After exploring various conventional and alternative therapies with limited success, she became intrigued by the potential of sound and light therapy to restore balance and promote healing.

Inspiration and Development: Inspired by the therapeutic effects of vibration and frequency, Lynn began researching the science behind sound and light therapy. She drew upon the principles of resonance, cymatics, and bioenergetics, which suggest that the body can be influenced and healed by specific frequencies and vibrations. Combining this knowledge with her engineering skills, Lynn envisioned a chamber that could harness these therapeutic frequencies in a controlled and immersive environment (Lynn, 2016).

Design and Prototyping: The design process involved creating a structure that could optimize the delivery of sound and light frequencies to the body. The result was the Harmonic Egg, an egg-shaped chamber constructed from natural materials to enhance acoustic properties and minimize electromagnetic interference. The shape of the egg was chosen for its symbolic representation of rebirth and transformation, as well as its ability to evenly distribute sound and light waves throughout the space.

Launching the Harmonic Egg: After extensive testing and refinement, the first Harmonic Egg was launched in 2016. Since then, it has been adopted by wellness centers, spas, and individual practitioners worldwide, gaining recognition for its profound and holistic approach to healing (Lynn, 2016).

Principles and Mechanisms of the Harmonic Egg

The Harmonic Egg operates on several fundamental principles that underpin its therapeutic efficacy. These principles are rooted in the science of sound and light therapy, as well as ancient healing traditions.

Resonance and Frequency: Resonance is the phenomenon by which an object or system vibrates in response to an external frequency that matches its natural frequency. The Harmonic Egg uses carefully selected sound frequencies to resonate with the body's tissues and energy systems, promoting healing and balance. These frequencies are delivered through high-quality speakers strategically placed within the chamber (Horowitz, 2017).

Cymatics and Sound Waves: Cymatics is the study of visible sound vibrations and their effects on matter. The Harmonic Egg employs sound waves to create vibrational patterns that influence the body's cells and tissues. These patterns can stimulate cellular repair, enhance circulation, and promote the release of stagnant energy (Jenny, 2001).

Chromotherapy (Light Therapy): The Harmonic Egg integrates chromotherapy, or light therapy, using a spectrum of colored lights that correspond to different frequencies and healing properties. Each color has specific effects on the body and mind, such as calming the nervous system, reducing inflammation, or boosting mood. The combination of sound and light creates a synergistic effect that enhances overall therapeutic outcomes (Gurudas, 1999).

Bioenergetics and Energy Fields: Bioenergetics is the study of energy flow within living systems. The Harmonic Egg aims to balance the body's energy fields, or biofields, by aligning them with harmonious frequencies. This alignment can help clear energetic blockages, restore vitality, and promote holistic well-being (Oschman, 2000).

Sacred Geometry: The design of the Harmonic Egg incorporates principles of sacred geometry, which is believed to reflect the fundamental patterns of nature and the universe. The egg shape itself is a symbol of creation and transformation, and its geometric structure is designed to amplify and harmonize the therapeutic frequencies within the chamber (Lawlor, 1989).

Benefits and Applications of the Harmonic Egg

The Harmonic Egg offers a wide range of benefits, making it a versatile tool for enhancing physical, emotional, and spiritual health. Here are some of the key benefits and applications: Stress Reduction and Relaxation: One of the primary benefits of the Harmonic Egg is its ability to induce deep relaxation and reduce stress. The combination of soothing sound frequencies and calming light can help lower cortisol levels, ease tension, and promote a state of tranquility (Lynn, 2016).

Pain Relief and Healing: The Harmonic Egg can support pain relief and healing by enhancing circulation, reducing inflammation, and stimulating cellular repair. It has been used to address chronic pain conditions, injuries, and post-surgical recovery, providing a noninvasive and holistic approach to pain management (Horowitz, 2017).

Emotional Balance and Mental Clarity: The therapeutic frequencies and colors used in the Harmonic Egg can help balance emotions, improve mood, and enhance mental clarity. It is beneficial for individuals dealing with anxiety, depression, PTSD, and other emotional challenges, promoting a sense of inner peace and well-being (Gurudas, 1999).

Energy Balancing and Vitality: By aligning the body's energy fields and clearing blockages, the Harmonic Egg can enhance vitality and overall energy levels. Users often report feeling rejuvenated, more focused, and better able to manage daily stressors after sessions in the Harmonic Egg (Oschman, 2000).

Spiritual Growth and Awareness: The Harmonic Egg provides a conducive environment for meditation, introspection, and spiritual growth. The harmonious frequencies and sacred geometry of the chamber can facilitate deeper states of consciousness, helping individuals connect with their inner selves and higher wisdom (Lawlor, 1989).

Practical Steps for Experiencing the Harmonic Egg

For those interested in exploring the benefits of the Harmonic Egg, here are some practical steps to consider:

1. **Find a Qualified Practitioner:** Locate a wellness center or practitioner that offers Harmonic Egg sessions. Ensure they are trained and experienced in using the device to provide a safe and effective experience.

2. **Prepare for the Session:** Before your session, wear comfortable clothing and avoid heavy meals or caffeine. Arrive with an open mind and a willingness to relax and receive the therapeutic benefits.

3. **Set Intentions:** Setting intentions for your session can enhance the therapeutic outcomes. Reflect on what you hope to achieve, whether it's stress relief, emotional balance, pain relief, or spiritual growth.

4. **Relax and Receive:** During the session, lie comfortably in the Harmonic Egg and allow yourself to relax. Focus on your breath and let go of any tension or distractions. The sound and light will do the work, creating a deeply restorative experience.

5. **Post-Session Reflection:** After the session, take some time to reflect on your experience. Drink plenty of water to help flush out any toxins released during the session, and consider journaling your thoughts and feelings.

6. **Consistency and Follow-Up:** For best results, consider regular sessions in the Harmonic Egg. Consistent exposure to the therapeutic frequencies can enhance the cumulative benefits and support ongoing healing and well-being.

Conclusion

The Harmonic Egg is a groundbreaking invention that merges ancient healing wisdom with modern technology to offer a holistic approach to health and wellness. By harnessing the power of sound and light frequencies within a specially designed chamber, the Harmonic Egg provides a unique and effective means of promoting physical, emotional, and spiritual healing.

As you explore the potential of the Harmonic Egg, embrace the opportunity to experience its transformative effects on your well-being. Whether you seek to reduce stress, alleviate pain, balance your emotions, or deepen your spiritual connection, the Harmonic Egg offers a pathway to harmony and rejuvenation.

Visualization:
Harnessing the Power of the Mind

Introduction

Visualization is a powerful mental technique that involves creating vivid images in the mind to achieve specific goals, enhance performance, and promote healing. This practice leverages the brain's natural ability to influence the body and environment through focused intention and mental imagery. From athletes improving their performance to individuals manifesting personal and professional success, visualization has been widely recognized for its effectiveness. This section explores the history, principles, techniques, benefits, and practical applications of visualization.

History of Visualization

Visualization, also known as mental imagery or mental rehearsal, has roots in ancient practices and traditions. Throughout history, various cultures and disciplines have utilized visualization techniques for healing, spiritual growth, and personal development.

Ancient Practices: Visualization has been used in ancient spiritual and healing practices, such as shamanism, where shamans would visualize journeys to the spirit world to seek guidance and healing. In ancient Egypt, priests used guided imagery to prepare initiates for spiritual rituals (Dossey, 2001).

Eastern Traditions: In Eastern traditions, visualization is integral to practices such as yoga, meditation, and martial arts. For example, in Tibetan Buddhism, practitioners use visualization techniques to meditate on deities, mandalas, and sacred symbols, fostering spiritual insight and transformation (Lama & Cutler, 1998).

Western Development: The scientific study of visualization began in the 19th and 20th centuries with the advent of psychology. Researchers such as William James and Carl Jung explored the impact of mental imagery on behavior and the subconscious mind. In the 1960s and 1970s, visualization gained popularity in sports psychology, with athletes using mental rehearsal to enhance performance (Vealey & Greenleaf, 2010).

Principles of Visualization

Visualization is based on several key principles that explain its effectiveness and guide its practice. Understanding these principles can enhance the efficacy of visualization techniques. Mind-Body Connection: The mind and body are interconnected, with thoughts and mental images influencing physiological responses. Visualization leverages this connection to produce tangible effects on the body and behavior. When you visualize a scenario vividly, the brain activates similar neural pathways as if you were experiencing the scenario in reality (Ranganathan et al., 2004).

Neuroplasticity: Neuroplasticity refers to the brain's ability to reorganize and form new neural connections throughout life. Visualization can enhance neuroplasticity by repeatedly activating specific neural circuits, reinforcing desired behaviors, and creating new patterns of thought and action (Doidge, 2007).

Focused Intention: Visualization involves directing focused intention toward a specific goal or outcome. This concentrated mental effort enhances motivation, clarity, and commitment, making it more likely to achieve the desired result. Focused intention also aligns conscious and subconscious processes, facilitating change (Lipton, 2005).

Emotional Engagement: Effective visualization engages emotions, as emotions amplify the impact of mental imagery on the brain and body. Positive emotions such as joy, excitement, and gratitude reinforce the visualized scenario, making it more vivid and compelling. Emotional engagement also enhances motivation and resilience (Fredrickson, 2001).

Repetition and Consistency: Repetition is crucial for reinforcing neural pathways and creating lasting change. Consistent practice of visualization strengthens the mental images and associated neural circuits, making the desired outcomes more likely to manifest. Regular visualization sessions build momentum and increase effectiveness (Vealey & Greenleaf, 2010).

Techniques of Visualization

There are various visualization techniques, each with its unique focus and application. Here are some of the most widely used techniques:

Guided Imagery: Guided imagery involves listening to a facilitator or audio recording that guides you through a series of mental images and scenarios. This technique can be used for relaxation, stress reduction, and achieving specific goals. Guided imagery often includes sensory details and positive affirmations (Rossman, 2000).

Mental Rehearsal: Mental rehearsal is commonly used in sports psychology to improve performance. Athletes visualize themselves performing specific skills or routines with precision and success. This technique enhances muscle memory, confidence, and focus. Mental rehearsal can also be applied to other areas, such as public speaking or job interviews (Vealey & Greenleaf, 2010).

Creative Visualization: Creative visualization involves imagining desired outcomes or goals as if they are already achieved. This technique emphasizes vivid sensory details, emotions, and positive affirmations. Creative visualization is often used in personal development and manifestation practices to attract desired experiences and opportunities (Gawain, 1982).

Healing Visualization: Healing visualization focuses on promoting physical and emotional healing. Individuals visualize the body healing itself, with imagery of healthy cells, organs, and systems. This technique can be used to support recovery from illness, reduce pain, and enhance overall well-being. Healing visualization often includes relaxation and deep breathing (Dossey, 2001).

Future Self Visualization: Future self-visualization involves imagining yourself in the future, having achieved your goals and living your desired life. This technique helps clarify long-term goals, align actions with aspirations, and build a sense of purpose and motivation. Future self-visualization can be guided or self-directed (Dispenza, 2012).

Benefits of Visualization

Visualization offers numerous benefits for physical, mental, and emotional well-being. Here are some of the key benefits:

Enhanced Performance: Visualization can significantly improve performance in various fields, including sports, academics, and professional endeavors. By mentally rehearsing skills and scenarios, individuals build confidence, focus, and competence, leading to better outcomes (Ranganathan et al., 2004).

Stress Reduction: Visualization promotes relaxation and reduces stress by engaging the parasympathetic nervous system. Techniques such as guided imagery and healing visualization help lower cortisol levels, alleviate anxiety, and promote a sense of calm and well-being (Rossman, 2000).

Emotional Healing: Visualization can support emotional healing by providing a safe space to process and release negative emotions. Engaging in positive imagery and emotions helps reframe negative experiences and build emotional resilience. Healing visualization can be particularly beneficial for individuals dealing with trauma, grief, or depression (Dossey, 2001).

Goal Achievement: Visualization enhances goal achievement by clarifying intentions, increasing motivation, and aligning subconscious processes with desired outcomes. Creative visualization and future self-visualization are powerful tools for manifesting personal and professional success. Visualization helps maintain focus and perseverance, even in the face of challenges (Gawain, 1982).

Physical Healing: Visualization supports physical healing by promoting relaxation, reducing pain, and enhancing immune function. Mental imagery of healthy cells and organs can stimulate physiological responses that facilitate healing and recovery. Healing visualization is used as a complementary therapy for various medical conditions (Dossey, 2001).

Cognitive Benefits: Visualization enhances cognitive functions such as memory, concentration, and problem-solving skills. By mentally rehearsing tasks and scenarios, individuals improve their ability to process information, make decisions, and perform complex tasks. Visualization also supports neuroplasticity, promoting lifelong learning and mental agility (Doidge, 2007).

Practical Applications of Visualization

To harness the power of visualization effectively, consider the following practical applications:

Daily Visualization Practice: Incorporate visualization into your daily routine by setting aside dedicated time for practice. Find a quiet, comfortable space where you can relax and focus without distractions. Consistency is key to building the mental muscle for effective visualization.

Specific Goals and Intentions: Clearly define your goals and intentions before beginning a visualization session. The more specific and detailed your mental images, the more effective the visualization will be. Use sensory details and emotions to make the imagery vivid and compelling.

Use of Affirmations: Combine visualization with positive affirmations to reinforce the desired outcomes. Affirmations are short, positive statements that reflect your goals and intentions. Repeating affirmations during visualization enhances the mental imagery and strengthens the neural connections associated with the desired outcome.

Visualization Tools: Utilize tools such as vision boards, guided imagery recordings, and meditation apps to support your visualization practice. Vision boards are visual representations of your goals and aspirations, created using images and words that inspire you. Guided imagery recordings provide structured visualization sessions, making it easier to focus and relax.

Emotional Engagement: Engage your emotions during visualization to amplify its impact. Focus on the positive feelings associated with achieving your goals, such as joy, gratitude, and excitement. Emotional engagement makes the mental imagery more vivid and compelling, increasing the likelihood of manifesting the desired outcomes.

Integration with Other Practices: Integrate visualization with other wellness practices such as meditation, yoga, and mindfulness. Combining visualization with physical and mental relaxation techniques enhances its effectiveness and promotes overall well-being.

Tracking Progress: Keep a journal to track your visualization practice and the progress you make toward your goals. Documenting your experiences, insights, and achievements helps reinforce the positive outcomes and maintain motivation.

Case Studies and Examples

To illustrate the transformative potential of visualization, consider the following case studies:

Case Study 1: Enhancing Athletic Performance Michael, a professional tennis player, used mental rehearsal to improve his performance on the court. By visualizing himself executing precise serves, volleys, and strategies, he enhanced his muscle memory, focus, and confidence. Over time, Michael noticed significant improvements in his game, winning several tournaments and achieving personal bests.

Case Study 2: Overcoming Anxiety and Depression Emily, a 35-year-old woman struggling with anxiety and depression, incorporated guided imagery into her daily routine. Through visualization sessions focused on calming nature scenes and positive affirmations, Emily experienced reduced anxiety and improved mood. The practice provided her with a sense of peace and emotional resilience.

Case Study 3: Achieving Professional Success James, a young entrepreneur, used creative visualization to achieve his business goals. He spent time each day visualizing his startup's success, imagining client meetings, successful pitches, and financial growth. By engaging all his senses and feeling the emotions associated with these successes, James strengthened his motivation and clarity. Over time, his business flourished, and he attributed much of his success to his consistent visualization practice.

Case Study 4: Physical Healing and Recovery Anna, a cancer survivor, used healing visualization to support her recovery post-treatment. She visualized her immune system attacking any remaining cancer cells and her body restoring itself to full health. Alongside medical treatments, Anna's visualization practice helped her maintain a positive mindset, reduce pain, and accelerate her recovery. Her doctors noted her unusually swift and comprehensive healing process.

Case Study 5: Improving Academic Performance Sarah, a high school student, struggled with test anxiety. She began using mental rehearsal techniques to visualize herself calmly taking exams, recalling information easily, and achieving high scores. This practice not only reduced her anxiety but also improved her performance, leading to higher grades and increased confidence in her academic abilities.

Scientific Research on Visualization

Scientific research has provided substantial evidence supporting the effectiveness of visualization. Studies have explored its impact on various aspects of mental and physical health, performance, and overall well-being:

Sports Performance: A meta-analysis published in the Journal of Sports Sciences found that mental imagery significantly improves athletic performance. Athletes who used visualization techniques demonstrated better motor skills, strategic execution, and overall performance compared to those who did not (Martin et al., 1999).

Stress Reduction and Mental Health: Research published in the Journal of Psychosomatic Research indicated that guided imagery reduces stress, anxiety, and depression. Participants who engaged in regular guided imagery sessions reported lower cortisol levels and improved emotional well-being (Gould et al., 2002).

Physical Healing: A study published in Advances in Mind-Body Medicine demonstrated that visualization enhances physical healing. Patients who visualized their bodies healing experienced faster recovery times and better outcomes in surgical and chronic illness treatments (Wright et al., 2002).

Cognitive Enhancement: Research in Neuropsychologia showed that mental rehearsal improves cognitive functions such as memory, problem-solving, and concentration. Visualization activates similar neural circuits to those used in actual performance, enhancing cognitive abilities (Driskell et al., 1994).

Goal Achievement: A study in the Journal of Applied Psychology found that visualization improves goal attainment. Participants who visualized achieving their goals were more likely to develop effective strategies, maintain motivation, and achieve their objectives compared to those who did not visualize (Pham & Taylor, 1999).

Future Directions and Research

The field of visualization continues to evolve, with ongoing research exploring new applications and enhancing our understanding of its mechanisms and benefits. Some promising areas of research include:

Neuroplasticity and Brain Health: Studies are investigating the role of visualization in promoting neuroplasticity and brain health. By exploring how mental imagery influences neural pathways, researchers aim to develop new interventions for cognitive decline, neurodegenerative diseases, and brain injuries.

Emotional and Psychological Well-Being: Research is exploring the potential of visualization to address emotional and psychological conditions such as PTSD, anxiety disorders, and depression. By understanding how visualization impacts the brain's emotional centers, scientists hope to develop more effective therapies for mental health.

Integration with Technology: The integration of visualization with technology, such as virtual reality (VR) and biofeedback, is an emerging field. These technologies can enhance the effectiveness of visualization by providing immersive and interactive experiences, making mental imagery more vivid and impactful.

Personalized Visualization Techniques: Future research aims to develop personalized visualization techniques tailored to individual needs and goals. By understanding the unique ways in which different people respond to visualization, practitioners can create customized interventions that maximize benefits.

Conclusion

Visualization is a powerful and versatile tool that leverages the mind's ability to influence the body and environment through focused intention and mental imagery. With its rich history, scientific backing, and numerous benefits, visualization offers a pathway to enhanced performance, healing, and overall well-being.

As you explore the potential of visualization, embrace the opportunity to harness the power of your mind. Whether you seek to improve athletic performance, achieve professional success, heal from illness, or enhance emotional resilience, visualization provides a comprehensive and enriching approach to achieving your goals.

Incorporate visualization into your daily routine, engage your emotions, and remain consistent in your practice. By doing so, you can unlock the transformative power of visualization and create a life aligned with your highest aspirations and potential.

Hypnotherapy:
Unlocking the Power of the Subconscious Mind

Introduction

Hypnotherapy is a therapeutic technique that uses the power of hypnosis to access and influence the subconscious mind, promoting positive changes in behavior, thoughts, and emotions. By guiding individuals into a relaxed, focused state of heightened awareness, hypnotherapists help clients address a wide range of issues, from anxiety and stress to chronic pain and addiction. This section explores the history, principles, techniques, benefits, and practical applications of hypnotherapy, highlighting its effectiveness as a complementary and alternative medicine.

History of Hypnotherapy

The practice of hypnosis dates back thousands of years, with its roots in ancient healing traditions and rituals. Over time, hypnosis has evolved into a scientifically recognized therapeutic modality.

Ancient Practices: Hypnotic techniques were used in ancient cultures in Egypt, Greece, and India. In ancient Egypt, priests used trance states for healing rituals, while Greek physicians, including Hippocrates, recognized the therapeutic potential of altered states of consciousness. In India, yogic practices incorporated trance states for spiritual and healing purposes (Yeates, 2018).

18th Century Enlightenment: The modern history of hypnotherapy began in the 18th century with Franz Anton Mesmer, an Austrian physician who developed the theory of "animal magnetism." Mesmer believed that an invisible force could influence health and induce healing. Although his theories were controversial, they laid the groundwork for future exploration of hypnosis (Pintar & Lynn, 2008).

19th Century Advancements: In the 19th century, Scottish surgeon James Braid coined the term "hypnosis" and shifted the focus from Mesmer's mystical concepts to a more scientific understanding of the trance state. Braid's work emphasized the role of suggestion and the power of the mind in inducing hypnosis. Around the same time, French neurologist Jean-Martin Charcot and his student Pierre Janet used hypnosis to explore psychological phenomena and treat hysteria (Gauld, 1992).

20th Century Development: Hypnotherapy gained further recognition in the 20th century, thanks to the work of pioneers such as Milton H. Erickson. Erickson's innovative approaches to hypnosis and psychotherapy revolutionized the field, emphasizing individualized techniques and the use of metaphor and indirect suggestion. Erickson's methods laid the foundation for modern hypnotherapy, influencing numerous practitioners and researchers (Rossi & Ryan, 1985).

Contemporary Practice: Today, hypnotherapy is widely practiced by licensed therapists, psychologists, and medical professionals. Advances in neuroscience and psychology continue to validate the efficacy of hypnotherapy, expanding its applications in various fields, including medicine, mental health, and personal development (Nash & Barnier, 2012).

Principles of Hypnotherapy

Hypnotherapy is based on several core principles that explain its effectiveness and guide its practice. Understanding these principles is essential for both practitioners and clients to achieve optimal results.

Trance State: Hypnotherapy induces a trance state, a natural state of focused attention and heightened suggestibility. In this state, individuals are more receptive to positive suggestions and can access deeper levels of consciousness, making it easier to address underlying issues and implement changes (Spiegel, 2013).

Subconscious Mind: The subconscious mind plays a crucial role in shaping thoughts, behaviors, and emotions. Hypnotherapy targets the subconscious mind to reprogram negative patterns, release unresolved emotions, and reinforce positive beliefs. This process facilitates lasting change and personal growth (Hammond, 1990).

Suggestion and Imagery: Hypnotherapy relies on the power of suggestion and imagery to influence the subconscious mind. Positive suggestions, visualizations, and metaphors are used to guide the individual toward desired outcomes. These techniques enhance motivation, reduce resistance, and promote healing (Rossi & Cheek, 1988).

Relaxation and Focus: Hypnotherapy involves deep relaxation and focused attention, which reduce stress and anxiety. The relaxed state achieved during hypnosis allows individuals to bypass the critical mind and access the subconscious, facilitating more profound insights and transformations (Spiegel, 2013).

Individualized Approach: Effective hypnotherapy is tailored to the unique needs and goals of each individual. Hypnotherapists use personalized techniques and suggestions to address specific issues, ensuring that the therapy is relevant and impactful for the client (Erickson, Rossi, & Rossi, 1976).

Techniques of Hypnotherapy

Hypnotherapists employ various techniques to guide individuals into a trance state and facilitate therapeutic change. Here are some of the most commonly used techniques:

Progressive Relaxation: This technique involves guiding the individual through a series of relaxation exercises, progressively relaxing different muscle groups. Progressive relaxation helps induce a deep state of physical and mental relaxation, making it easier to enter a hypnotic state (Hammond, 1990).

Guided Imagery: Guided imagery involves leading the individual through vivid mental images that evoke positive emotions and desired outcomes. This technique uses sensory details and metaphors to create a compelling and immersive experience, enhancing the effectiveness of suggestions (Rossman, 2000).

Direct Suggestion: Direct suggestion involves giving clear, positive instructions to the subconscious mind. These suggestions are designed to reinforce desired behaviors, beliefs, and emotions. Direct suggestion is often used for habit change, such as smoking cessation or weight loss (Hammond, 1990).

Indirect Suggestion and Metaphor: Indirect suggestion and metaphor involve using stories, analogies, and indirect language to convey therapeutic messages. This technique, popularized by Milton Erickson, allows the subconscious mind to interpret and integrate suggestions more naturally, reducing resistance (Erickson, Rossi, & Rossi, 1976).

Age Regression: Age regression involves guiding the individual to revisit past experiences, often from childhood, to uncover and resolve unresolved emotions or traumas. This technique can provide insights and facilitate healing by addressing the root causes of current issues (Brown & Fromm, 1986).

Parts Therapy: Parts therapy involves working with different "parts" of the subconscious mind, each representing different aspects of the individual's personality or experiences. This technique helps resolve internal conflicts, integrate fragmented parts, and promote harmony within the self (Watkins & Watkins, 1997).

Self-Hypnosis: Self-hypnosis involves teaching individuals to induce a hypnotic state on their own, using techniques such as progressive relaxation or guided imagery. Self-hypnosis empowers individuals to practice hypnotherapy independently, reinforcing positive changes and promoting ongoing self-improvement (Hadley & Staudacher, 1996).

Benefits of Hypnotherapy

Hypnotherapy offers numerous benefits for physical, mental, and emotional well-being. Here are some of the key benefits:

Stress Reduction and Relaxation: Hypnotherapy promotes deep relaxation and reduces stress by calming the nervous system and lowering cortisol levels. This relaxation response enhances overall well-being and helps manage stress-related conditions (Spiegel, 2013).

Anxiety and Depression: Hypnotherapy can effectively reduce symptoms of anxiety and depression by addressing underlying emotional issues and promoting positive thought patterns. Techniques such as guided imagery and positive suggestion help reframe negative beliefs and foster emotional resilience (Hammond, 1990).

Pain Management: Hypnotherapy is widely used for pain management, helping individuals cope with chronic pain, acute pain, and pain from medical procedures. By altering the perception of pain and promoting relaxation, hypnotherapy reduces the intensity of pain and enhances quality of life (Jensen et al., 2016).

Behavior Change: Hypnotherapy is effective for changing undesirable behaviors and habits, such as smoking, overeating, and nail-biting. By accessing the subconscious mind, hypnotherapy can reprogram negative patterns and reinforce positive behaviors, leading to lasting change (Green & Lynn, 2000).

Improved Sleep: Hypnotherapy can improve sleep quality and address sleep disorders such as insomnia. Techniques such as progressive relaxation and guided imagery help individuals relax and develop healthier sleep patterns, promoting restorative rest (Hammond, 1990).

Emotional Healing: Hypnotherapy facilitates emotional healing by helping individuals process and release unresolved emotions, traumas, and limiting beliefs. This process promotes emotional balance, self-acceptance, and overall mental health (Brown & Fromm, 1986).

Enhanced Performance: Hypnotherapy is used to enhance performance in various fields, including sports, academics, and professional endeavors. Mental rehearsal, positive suggestion, and confidence-building techniques help individuals achieve their full potential (Vealey & Greenleaf, 2010).

Boosted Immune Function: Hypnotherapy has been shown to boost immune function by reducing stress and promoting relaxation. Enhanced immune function supports overall health and resilience against illnesses (Ruzyla-Smith et al., 1995).

Practical Applications of Hypnotherapy

To harness the power of hypnotherapy effectively, consider the following practical applications:

Finding a Qualified Hypnotherapist: Seek out a licensed and certified hypnotherapist who has experience in addressing your specific concerns. Ensure they have appropriate credentials and a positive reputation.

Setting Clear Goals: Before beginning hypnotherapy, clearly define your goals and intentions. Understanding what you want to achieve will help guide the therapeutic process and enhance the effectiveness of the sessions.

Regular Sessions: Consistency is key to achieving lasting results with hypnotherapy. Schedule regular sessions with your hypnotherapist and practice any self-hypnosis techniques they teach you between sessions.

Open Mind and Trust: Approach hypnotherapy with an open mind and trust in the process. Relax and allow yourself to relax and allow yourself to be open to the experience. Trust in your hypnotherapist's guidance and the natural process of hypnosis, knowing that you are in control and can come out of the trance state at any time.

Practice Self-Hypnosis: Learn and practice self-hypnosis techniques as taught by your hypnotherapist. Regular practice of self-hypnosis can reinforce the positive changes initiated during your sessions and empower you to manage stress, enhance focus, and achieve your goals independently.

Combine with Other Therapies: Hypnotherapy can be effectively combined with other therapeutic approaches, such as cognitive-behavioral therapy (CBT), mindfulness, or physical therapy. Integrating hypnotherapy with other treatments can enhance overall outcomes and address multiple aspects of your well-being.

Journaling and Reflection: Keep a journal to document your hypnotherapy sessions, experiences, and any changes you notice in your thoughts, behaviors, or emotions. Reflecting on your progress can provide insights, reinforce positive changes, and motivate you to continue your therapeutic journey.

Patient and Consistent Approach: Understand that hypnotherapy, like any therapeutic process, may take time to achieve significant and lasting changes. Be patient with yourself and consistent in your practice, knowing that each session builds upon the previous ones to create meaningful transformation.

Advanced Techniques and Innovations in Hypnotherapy

As hypnotherapy continues to evolve, advanced techniques and innovations are emerging that enhance its effectiveness and expand its applications.

Ericksonian Hypnotherapy: Developed by Milton Erickson, this approach uses indirect suggestion, storytelling, and metaphor to communicate with the subconscious mind. Ericksonian hypnotherapy is highly individualized and adaptive, making it effective for a wide range of issues (Erickson, Rossi, & Rossi, 1976).

Neuro-Linguistic Programming (NLP): NLP combines hypnosis with techniques that address how language and thought patterns influence behavior. By reprogramming negative thought patterns and behaviors, NLP helps individuals achieve personal and professional goals. NLP techniques are often used in conjunction with hypnotherapy to enhance outcomes (Bandler & Grinder, 1975).

Rapid Transformational Therapy (RTT): RTT, developed by Marisa Peer, is a hybrid therapy that combines hypnotherapy with cognitive-behavioral therapy and psychotherapy techniques. RTT aims to achieve rapid and lasting change by addressing the root causes of issues and reprogramming the subconscious mind. It is used for various concerns, including anxiety, addiction, and self-esteem issues (Peer, 2018).

Mindfulness-Based Hypnotherapy: This approach integrates mindfulness practices with hypnotherapy, enhancing awareness and acceptance of present-moment experiences. Mindfulness-based hypnotherapy helps individuals develop a deeper connection with their inner selves and promotes emotional regulation and resilience (Spiegel, 2013).

Virtual Reality Hypnotherapy: Virtual reality (VR) technology is being used to create immersive hypnotherapy experiences. VR hypnotherapy enhances the depth and vividness of the hypnotic experience, making it more effective for relaxation, pain management, and behavior change. Research is ongoing to explore the full potential of this innovative approach (Freeman et al., 2017).

Integrative Hypnotherapy: Integrative hypnotherapy combines hypnotherapy with other holistic and complementary therapies, such as acupuncture, energy healing, and nutritional counseling. This comprehensive approach addresses the individual as a whole, promoting balanced and holistic healing (Hammond, 1990).

Case Studies and Examples

To illustrate the transformative potential of hypnotherapy, consider the following case studies:

Case Study 1: Overcoming Smoking Addiction John, a 45-year-old man, struggled with a long-term smoking addiction. After multiple failed attempts to quit, he decided to try hypnotherapy. Through a series of hypnotherapy sessions, John was able to address the underlying emotional triggers of his addiction and reprogram his subconscious mind with positive affirmations and imagery. He successfully quit smoking and maintained his smoke-free status for years.

Case Study 2: Managing Chronic Pain Sarah, a 50-year-old woman, suffered from chronic back pain due to a car accident. Traditional pain management methods provided limited relief. She turned to hypnotherapy as an alternative approach. Using guided imagery and pain management techniques, Sarah experienced a significant reduction in pain intensity and improved her overall quality of life. Hypnotherapy helped her develop coping strategies and manage pain more effectively.

Case Study 3: Enhancing Academic Performance Emily, a college student, struggled with test anxiety that affected her academic performance. She sought hypnotherapy to overcome this challenge. Through hypnotherapy sessions, Emily learned relaxation techniques, improved her focus, and developed a positive mindset toward exams. Her test anxiety decreased, and her academic performance improved, allowing her to achieve her academic goals.

Case Study 4: Weight Loss and Healthy Habits Linda, a 35-year-old woman, struggled with weight management and unhealthy eating habits. She decided to try hypnotherapy to support her weight loss journey. Through a combination of direct suggestions and guided imagery, Linda reprogrammed her subconscious mind to adopt healthier eating habits and develop a positive relationship with food. She successfully lost weight and maintained a healthy lifestyle.

Scientific Research on Hypnotherapy

Scientific research has provided substantial evidence supporting the effectiveness of hypnotherapy. Numerous studies have explored its impact on various aspects of physical and mental health:

Anxiety and Depression: A meta-analysis published in the International Journal of Clinical and Experimental Hypnosis found that hypnotherapy significantly reduces symptoms of anxiety and depression. The study concluded that hypnotherapy is an effective complementary treatment for mental health conditions (Hammond, 2010).

Pain Management: Research published in the Journal of the American Medical Association demonstrated that hypnotherapy is effective in managing chronic pain. Participants who received hypnotherapy reported significant reductions in pain intensity and improved quality of life compared to a control group (Jensen et al., 2016).

Behavior Change: A study published in the Journal of Consulting and Clinical Psychology found that hypnotherapy is effective for smoking cessation. Participants who underwent hypnotherapy were more likely to quit smoking and maintain abstinence compared to those who received standard treatments (Green & Lynn, 2000).

Sleep Improvement: Research in the Journal of Sleep Research showed that hypnotherapy improves sleep quality and reduces insomnia symptoms. Participants who received hypnotherapy experienced better sleep patterns and increased overall sleep duration (Hammond, 1990).

Immune Function: A study published in Psychosomatic Medicine found that hypnotherapy boosts immune function by reducing stress and promoting relaxation. Participants who underwent hypnotherapy showed enhanced immune responses and increased resistance to infections (Ruzyla-Smith et al., 1995).

Conclusion

Hypnotherapy is a powerful and versatile therapeutic modality that leverages the power of the subconscious mind to promote positive change and enhance overall well-being. With its rich history, scientifically validated principles, and diverse applications, hypnotherapy offers a holistic approach to healing and personal development.

As you explore the potential of hypnotherapy, embrace the opportunity to unlock the power of your mind. Whether you seek to reduce stress, manage pain, overcome addiction, or achieve personal goals, hypnotherapy provides a pathway to profound transformation and lasting change.

Approach hypnotherapy with an open mind, trust in the process, and remain consistent in your practice. By doing so, you can harness the transformative power of hypnotherapy and create a life aligned with your highest aspirations and potential.

Tapping:
A Pathway to Emotional Freedom and Healing

Introduction

Tapping, also known as Emotional Freedom Techniques (EFT), is a therapeutic practice that combines elements of ancient Chinese acupressure and modern psychology to alleviate physical pain, reduce stress, and promote emotional well-being. By tapping on specific meridian points on the body while focusing on emotional issues, individuals can release negative emotions and restore balance to their energy system. This section explores the history, principles, techniques, benefits, and practical applications of tapping, highlighting its effectiveness as a complementary therapy.

History of Tapping

The development of tapping, or EFT, can be traced back to the late 20th century. It emerged from the convergence of Traditional Chinese Medicine , which emphasizes the flow of energy through meridian points, and modern psychological techniques aimed at addressing emotional issues.

Ancient Chinese Medicine: The foundational principles of tapping are rooted in Traditional Chinese Medicine (TCM), which has been practiced for over 5,000 years. TCM posits that the body has a network of energy pathways known as meridians, through which vital energy (qi) flows. Imbalances or blockages in these pathways can lead to physical and emotional ailments (Maciocia, 2005).

Development of Thought Field Therapy (TFT): In the 1980s, Dr. Roger Callahan, a clinical psychologist, developed Thought Field Therapy (TFT) after discovering that tapping on specific meridian points could alleviate phobias and other emotional issues. TFT was a precursor to EFT, focusing on the precise tapping sequences tailored to individual issues (Callahan & Trubo, 2001).

Creation of Emotional Freedom Techniques (EFT): Gary Craig, a student of Dr. Callahan, simplified and expanded TFT into what is now known as Emotional Freedom Techniques (EFT) in the 1990s. Craig's approach made tapping more accessible by creating a universal tapping sequence that could be applied to various issues. EFT has since gained widespread recognition and has been used by millions worldwide (Craig, 2011).

Principles of Tapping

Tapping operates on several core principles that explain its effectiveness and guide its practice. Understanding these principles is essential for both practitioners and individuals seeking to benefit from tapping.

Energy Flow and Meridian Points: Tapping is based on the concept that the body has a network of energy pathways (meridians) through which life energy (qi) flows. By tapping on specific points along these meridians, practitioners aim to clear blockages and restore the natural flow of energy, promoting physical and emotional well-being (Maciocia, 2005).

Mind-Body Connection: Tapping recognizes the profound connection between the mind and body. Emotional issues can manifest as physical symptoms, and physical pain can be linked to emotional distress. By addressing both the emotional and physical aspects of an issue, tapping promotes holistic healing (Craig, 2011).

Psychological Reversal: Psychological reversal is a concept in EFT that refers to the subconscious resistance to change. It can sabotage efforts to heal or achieve goals. Tapping helps identify and neutralize this resistance, allowing positive changes to occur more easily (Craig, 2011).

Focus and Intention: Effective tapping requires focused intention on the issue being addressed. By concentrating on the specific emotion, memory, or physical sensation while tapping, individuals can enhance the therapeutic effects and achieve more profound results (Church, 2013).

Tapping Sequence: EFT uses a standardized tapping sequence that involves tapping on nine specific meridian points while repeating a setup statement and a reminder phrase. This sequence is designed to balance the body's energy system and alleviate emotional distress (Craig, 2011).

Techniques of Tapping

Tapping involves a series of steps that guide individuals through the process of identifying and addressing emotional or physical issues. Here are the key techniques and steps involved in tapping:

Identify the Issue: The first step in tapping is to identify the specific issue you want to address. This could be a physical pain, an emotional distress, a limiting belief, or a traumatic memory. Be as specific as possible to enhance the effectiveness of the tapping session (Craig, 2011).

Rate the Intensity: Before starting the tapping sequence, rate the intensity of the issue on a scale from 0 to 10, with 10 being the highest level of distress. This helps track progress and measure the effectiveness of the tapping session (Church, 2013).

Setup Statement: Create a setup statement that acknowledges the issue and expresses self-acceptance. The standard format is: "Even though I have [issue], I deeply and completely accept myself." Repeat this statement three times while tapping on the "karate chop" point (the side of the hand) (Craig, 2011).

Tapping Sequence: Follow the EFT tapping sequence, tapping on each of the nine meridian points while repeating a reminder phrase that keeps the focus on the issue. The standard tapping points are:

- Top of the head (crown)
- Eyebrow (inner edge)
- Side of the eye (temple)
- Under the eye (cheekbone)
- Under the nose (above the upper lip)
- Chin (below the lower lip)
- Collarbone (just below the collarbone)
- Under the arm (side of the body, about four inches below the armpit)
- Karate chop point (side of the hand)

Reassess the Intensity: After completing the tapping sequence, reassess the intensity of the issue on a scale from 0 to 10. If the intensity is still high, repeat the setup statement and tapping sequence until the intensity decreases significantly (Church, 2013).

Positive Affirmations: Once the intensity of the issue has decreased, incorporate positive affirmations into the tapping sequence to reinforce the desired outcome. For example, "I choose to feel calm and relaxed" or "I am confident and capable" (Craig, 2011).

Benefits of Tapping

Tapping offers numerous benefits for physical, mental, and emotional well-being. Here are some of the key benefits:

Stress Reduction: Tapping effectively reduces stress by calming the nervous system and lowering cortisol levels. It helps individuals manage stress-related conditions such as anxiety, panic attacks, and post-traumatic stress disorder (PTSD) (Church, 2013).

Pain Relief: Tapping can alleviate physical pain by addressing its emotional and energetic components. It is beneficial for chronic pain conditions, headaches, and muscle tension, providing a noninvasive and holistic approach to pain management (Feinstein, 2012).

Emotional Healing: Tapping facilitates emotional healing by releasing unresolved emotions, traumas, and limiting beliefs. It helps individuals process and let go of negative emotions such as anger, guilt, and sadness, promoting emotional balance and resilience (Church, 2013).

Improved Sleep: Tapping can improve sleep quality by reducing anxiety and promoting relaxation. Individuals who struggle with insomnia or sleep disturbances can benefit from incorporating tapping into their bedtime routine (Craig, 2011).

Enhanced Performance: Tapping is used to enhance performance in various fields, including sports, academics, and professional endeavors. It helps individuals overcome performance anxiety, build confidence, and achieve their goals (Feinstein, 2012).

Behavior Change: Tapping is effective for changing undesirable behaviors and habits, such as smoking, overeating, and procrastination. By addressing the emotional triggers and subconscious patterns underlying these behaviors, tapping supports lasting change (Church, 2013).

Boosted Immune Function: Tapping has been shown to boost immune function by reducing stress and promoting relaxation. Enhanced immune function supports overall health and resilience against illnesses (Feinstein, 2012).

Practical Applications of Tapping

To harness the power of tapping effectively, consider the following practical applications:

Daily Practice: Incorporate tapping into your daily routine by setting aside dedicated time for practice. Consistent tapping sessions can help maintain emotional balance, reduce stress, and promote overall well-being.

Address Specific Issues: Use tapping to address specific physical or emotional issues as they arise. Whether you're dealing with a headache, a stressful situation, or a negative thought pattern, tapping can provide immediate relief and support.

Self-Help and Professional Guidance: While tapping can be practiced independently, seeking guidance from a certified EFT practitioner can enhance its effectiveness, especially for complex issues. Practitioners can provide personalized techniques and support tailored to your needs.

Combination with Other Therapies: Integrate tapping with other therapeutic approaches, such as cognitive-behavioral therapy (CBT), mindfulness, and meditation.

Combining tapping with other treatments can enhance overall outcomes and address multiple aspects of well-being.

Tapping Scripts and Resources: Utilize tapping scripts and resources available online or in EFT literature. Tapping scripts provide structured guidance for addressing specific issues, making it easier to practice tapping effectively.

Group Tapping Sessions: Participate in group tapping sessions or workshops to experience the collective energy and support of others. Group sessions can enhance motivation, provide a sense of community, and amplify the therapeutic effects of tapping.

Advanced Techniques and Innovations in Tapping

As tapping continues to evolve, advanced techniques and innovations are emerging that enhance its effectiveness and expand its applications.

Matrix Reimprinting: Developed by Karl Dawson, Matrix Reimprinting combines EFT with visualization techniques to transform traumatic memories and negative beliefs. This advanced approach helps individuals reframe past experiences and create positive emotional and cognitive shifts (Dawson & Allenby, 2010).

Clinical EFT: Clinical EFT is a standardized and evidence-based approach to EFT developed by Dawson Church. It incorporates rigorous protocols and scientific research to ensure the effectiveness and reliability of tapping as a therapeutic practice. Clinical EFT is used by healthcare professionals to address a wide range of physical and emotional issues (Church, 2013).

Tapping with Intention: This advanced technique involves combining tapping with the setting of specific intentions or goals. By focusing on a clear intention while tapping, individuals can enhance the alignment of their energy system with their desired outcomes, promoting faster and more effective results (Craig, 2011).

Trauma-Informed Tapping: Trauma-informed tapping approaches are designed to safely and effectively address trauma and PTSD. These methods prioritize creating a safe and supportive environment for individuals to process traumatic memories and release emotional distress without retraumatization (Feinstein, 2012).

Quantum EFT: Quantum EFT integrates principles from quantum physics with EFT to explore the deeper energetic and spiritual aspects of healing. This approach considers the interconnectedness of all things and uses tapping to align the individual's energy with the universal field of possibilities (Peta Stapleton, 2012).

Energy Psychology Integrations: Integrating tapping with other energy psychology modalities, such as chakra balancing, Reiki, or acupressure, can enhance the therapeutic effects. These integrative approaches provide a comprehensive framework for addressing physical, emotional, and spiritual well-being (Feinstein, 2012).

Case Studies and Examples

To illustrate the transformative potential of tapping, consider the following case studies:

Case Study 1: Overcoming Public Speaking Anxiety Laura, a 30-year-old professional, experienced severe anxiety about public speaking, which affected her career advancement. She decided to try EFT. Through regular tapping sessions focusing on her fear and past negative experiences, Laura was able to reduce her anxiety significantly. She gained confidence and delivered successful presentations, leading to a promotion at work.

Case Study 2: Managing Chronic Pain Mark, a 50-year-old man, suffered from chronic lower back pain that traditional treatments couldn't alleviate. He started using tapping to address the emotional stress and negative beliefs associated with his pain. Over time, Mark experienced a substantial reduction in pain intensity and an improvement in his quality of life, allowing him to engage in activities he had previously avoided.

Case Study 3: Healing from Childhood Trauma Emily, a 40-year-old woman, struggled with unresolved childhood trauma that impacted her relationships and mental health. With the help of a certified EFT practitioner, Emily used tap+ping to process and release her traumatic memories. This healing journey led to significant emotional relief, improved self-esteem, and healthier relationships.

Case Study 4: Enhancing Athletic Performance Jake, a 25-year-old athlete, used EFT to overcome performance anxiety and improve his focus during competitions. By tapping on specific points and addressing his fears and doubts, Jake enhanced his concentration and confidence, resulting in improved performance and several personal bests in his sport.

Scientific Research on Tapping

Scientific research has provided substantial evidence supporting the effectiveness of tapping. Numerous studies have explored its impact on various aspects of physical and mental health:

Anxiety and PTSD: A meta-analysis published in the Journal of Nervous and Mental Disease found that EFT significantly reduces symptoms of anxiety and PTSD. The study concluded that EFT is an effective treatment for these conditions, comparable to traditional therapeutic approaches (Sebastian & Nelms, 2017).

Pain Management: Research published in the Journal of Pain Research demonstrated that EFT is effective in reducing chronic pain. Participants who used EFT reported significant pain relief and improvements in physical functioning compared to control groups (Reynolds, 2015).

Depression: A study published in the Journal of Clinical Psychology found that EFT significantly reduces symptoms of depression. Participants who underwent EFT showed greater reductions in depressive symptoms compared to those who received standard care (Nelms & Castel, 2016).

Stress Reduction: Research in the Journal of Alternative and Complementary Medicine showed that EFT lowers cortisol levels, indicating reduced stress. Participants who practiced EFT experienced significant improvements in stress-related symptoms and overall well-being (Church, 2012).

Performance Enhancement: A study published in the Journal of Applied Sport Psychology found that EFT enhances athletic performance. Athletes who used EFT showed improved focus, reduced performance anxiety, and better overall performance compared to those who did not use EFT (Church et al., 2012).

Conclusion

Tapping, or Emotional Freedom Techniques (EFT), is a powerful and versatile therapeutic modality that leverages the body's energy system and the mind-body connection to promote healing and well-being. With its rich history, scientifically validated principles, and diverse applications, tapping offers a holistic approach to addressing physical, emotional, and psychological issues.

As you explore the potential of tapping, embrace the opportunity to harness the power of your energy system and subconscious mind. Whether you seek to reduce stress, manage pain, overcome emotional challenges, or enhance performance, tapping provides a pathway to profound transformation and lasting change.

Approach tapping with an open mind, trust in the process, and remain consistent in your practice. By doing so, you can unlock the transformative power of tapping and create a life aligned with your highest aspirations and potential.

Light Therapy:
Illuminating the Path to Healing

Introduction

Light therapy, also known as phototherapy, is a treatment that involves exposure to specific wavelengths of light to address various health conditions and promote overall well-being. This therapeutic approach harnesses the power of light to influence biological processes, enhance mood, and alleviate symptoms of certain medical conditions. From seasonal affective disorder (SAD) to skin disorders and sleep issues, light therapy has proven to be an effective and noninvasive treatment option. This section explores the history, principles, techniques, benefits, and practical applications of light therapy.

History of Light Therapy

The use of light for healing purposes dates back to ancient civilizations. Over the centuries, the therapeutic application of light has evolved, leading to the development of modern light therapy techniques.

Ancient Practices: The ancient Egyptians, Greeks, and Romans recognized the healing potential of sunlight. They used sunbathing and exposure to natural light to treat various ailments, including skin conditions and mood disorders. The Greek physician Hippocrates advocated for the therapeutic use of sunlight, emphasizing its benefits for physical and mental health (Farrar, 2008).

19th Century Discoveries: In the 19th century, Danish physician Niels Ryberg Finsen pioneered the use of light therapy for medical purposes. Finsen developed the first artificial light source for treating skin diseases such as lupus vulgaris. His groundbreaking work earned him the Nobel Prize in Physiology or Medicine in 1903 and laid the foundation for modern phototherapy (Juzeniene & Moan, 2012).

20th Century Advances: The 20th century saw significant advancements in light therapy, with the development of artificial light sources and the discovery of the therapeutic effects of different wavelengths of light. Researchers identified the benefits of ultraviolet (UV) light for skin conditions like psoriasis and the use of bright light therapy for seasonal affective disorder (SAD) (Terman & Terman, 2005).

Modern Era: Today, light therapy is widely used in clinical settings and at home to treat a range of conditions. Advances in technology have led to the development of specialized light therapy devices, including light boxes, lamps, and wearable devices. Ongoing research continues to explore new applications and refine existing treatments (Waldorf & Smith, 2002).

Principles of Light Therapy

Light therapy is based on several fundamental principles that explain its effectiveness and guide its practice. Understanding these principles is essential for both practitioners and individuals seeking to benefit from light therapy.

Photobiomodulation: Light therapy operates on the principle of photobiomodulation, which involves the absorption of specific wavelengths of light by cells and tissues. This process triggers biochemical reactions that influence cellular function, promoting healing and reducing inflammation (Hamblin, 2016).

Circadian Rhythms: Light plays a crucial role in regulating the body's circadian rhythms, which govern sleep-wake cycles and other physiological processes. Exposure to bright light at specific times can reset the internal clock, improving sleep patterns and overall well-being (Czeisler, 1995).

Serotonin and Melatonin: Light therapy affects the production of neurotransmitters such as serotonin and melatonin. Bright light exposure increases serotonin levels, enhancing mood and reducing symptoms of depression. It also suppresses melatonin production, promoting alertness and aligning the sleep-wake cycle with the natural light-dark cycle (Terman & Terman, 2005).

Targeted Wavelengths: Different wavelengths of light have specific therapeutic effects. Blue light is particularly effective for treating SAD and regulating circadian rhythms, while red and near-infrared light penetrate deeper into tissues and are used for wound healing and pain relief. UV light is used for skin conditions but requires careful monitoring due to potential risks (Hamblin, 2016).

Techniques of Light Therapy

Light therapy encompasses various techniques and devices designed to deliver therapeutic light to the body. Here are some of the most commonly used techniques:

Bright Light Therapy: Bright light therapy involves exposure to a light box or lamp that emits intense light, typically in the range of 2,500 to 10,000 lux. This technique is primarily used to treat seasonal affective disorder (SAD) and other mood disorders. Sessions usually last 20-30 minutes, conducted in the morning to simulate natural sunlight (Terman & Terman, 2005).

Blue Light Therapy: Blue light therapy utilizes blue wavelengths (around 480 nm) to regulate circadian rhythms and improve sleep patterns. Blue light exposure in the morning helps reset the internal clock, enhancing alertness and mood. This technique is also used to treat acne by targeting the bacteria that cause inflammation (Chang et al., 2012).

Red and Near-Infrared Light Therapy: Red and near-infrared light therapy (around 630-880 nm) are used for their deeper penetration into tissues. These wavelengths stimulate cellular repair, reduce inflammation, and promote wound healing. Devices such as LED panels and handheld units deliver red and near-infrared light to specific areas of the body (Hamblin, 2016).

UV Light Therapy: Ultraviolet (UV) light therapy involves exposure to UVB or UVA light to treat skin conditions such as psoriasis, eczema, and vitiligo. UV light slows the growth of affected skin cells and reduces inflammation. Due to the potential risks of UV exposure, this therapy is typically administered under medical supervision (Waldorf & Smith, 2002).

Dawn Simulation: Dawn simulation mimics a natural sunrise by gradually increasing light intensity in the morning. This technique helps regulate circadian rhythms and improve mood and sleep quality. Dawn simulators are often used as a gentler alternative to bright light therapy for individuals sensitive to intense light (Avery et al., 2001).

Benefits of Light Therapy

Light therapy offers numerous benefits for physical, mental, and emotional well-being. Here are some of the key benefits:

Improved Mood: Light therapy is highly effective in treating seasonal affective disorder (SAD) and other forms of depression. Exposure to bright light increases serotonin levels, improving mood and reducing symptoms of depression (Terman & Terman, 2005).

Enhanced Sleep: By regulating circadian rhythms, light therapy improves sleep quality and helps manage sleep disorders such as insomnia and delayed sleep phase syndrome. Proper timing of light exposure aligns the sleep-wake cycle with natural light patterns, promoting restorative sleep (Czeisler, 1995).

Reduced Inflammation and Pain: Red and near-infrared light therapy reduce inflammation and promote healing in tissues, making it effective for conditions such as arthritis, muscle pain, and injuries. This therapy enhances cellular repair processes, reducing pain and accelerating recovery (Hamblin, 2016).

Treatment of Skin Conditions: UV light therapy is effective in managing skin conditions like psoriasis, eczema, and vitiligo. By slowing the growth of affected skin cells and reducing inflammation, UV therapy improves skin appearance and relieves symptoms (Waldorf & Smith, 2002).

Acne Treatment: Blue light therapy targets acne-causing bacteria, reducing inflammation and preventing breakouts. This noninvasive treatment is suitable for individuals with mild to moderate acne and offers an alternative to topical or systemic treatments (Chang et al., 2012).

Increased Alertness and Cognitive Function: Light therapy enhances alertness and cognitive function by increasing serotonin levels and aligning circadian rhythms. This effect is particularly beneficial for individuals experiencing jet lag, shift work disorder, or seasonal lethargy (Czeisler, 1995).

Support for Cognitive and Neurological Health: Emerging research suggests that light therapy may benefit cognitive and neurological health, potentially aiding in the management of conditions such as dementia and traumatic brain injury. The neuro-protective effects of light therapy are being actively investigated (Hamblin, 2016).

Practical Applications of Light Therapy

To harness the power of light therapy effectively, consider the following practical applications: Daily Routine: Incorporate light therapy into your daily routine, especially during the morning hours. Consistent exposure to therapeutic light can help regulate your circadian rhythms, improve mood, and enhance overall well-being.

Seasonal Affective Disorder (SAD): Use bright light therapy during the fall and winter months when natural sunlight is limited. Position the light box or lamp at a distance where the light can reach your eyes without causing discomfort, and aim for 20-30 minutes of exposure each morning.

Sleep Improvement: For sleep-related issues, consider using dawn simulators or blue light therapy to regulate your sleep-wake cycle. Avoid exposure to bright screens and artificial light in the evening, as this can interfere with melatonin production and disrupt sleep.

Skin Conditions: If you have a skin condition such as psoriasis or eczema, consult a dermatologist to explore the potential benefits of UV light therapy. This treatment should be administered under medical supervision to minimize risks and maximize effectiveness.

Pain and Inflammation: Use red and near-infrared light therapy devices to target areas of pain and inflammation. Follow the manufacturer's instructions for optimal results, and consider incorporating light therapy into your rehabilitation or pain management plan.

Mental Health Support: For depression and anxiety, incorporate light therapy into your self-care routine. Regular exposure to bright light can enhance mood, reduce stress, and support emotional resilience.

Athletic Performance and Recovery: Athletes can benefit from light therapy by using red and near-infrared light to enhance muscle recovery and reduce inflammation after intense workouts. This can improve performance and reduce downtime due to injuries.

Advanced Techniques and Innovations in Light Therapy

As light therapy continues to evolve, advanced techniques and innovations are emerging that enhance its effectiveness and expand its applications.

Full-Spectrum Light Therapy: Full-spectrum light therapy devices emit a range of wavelengths that mimic natural sunlight, providing the benefits of multiple types of light in one treatment. These devices are designed to support overall well-being, particularly for individuals who lack sufficient exposure to natural light.

Targeted Light Therapy: Advances in technology have led to the development of devices that deliver targeted light therapy to specific areas of the body. These devices, such as LED light panels and handheld units, allow for precise application of therapeutic light to address localized pain, inflammation, or skin conditions.

Wearable Light Therapy Devices: Wearable devices, such as light therapy glasses and headbands, offer convenient and portable solutions for regulating circadian rhythms and enhancing mood. These devices are particularly useful for individuals with busy lifestyles, allowing them to benefit from light therapy while on the go.

Combination Therapies: Researchers are exploring the potential of combining light therapy with other therapeutic modalities, such as acupuncture, massage, and exercise. These combination therapies aim to enhance overall treatment outcomes by addressing multiple aspects of health and well-being simultaneously.

Photobiomodulation for Cognitive Health: Emerging research is investigating the use of photobiomodulation to support cognitive health and neurological function. Studies suggest that specific wavelengths of light may promote neuroprotection, enhance cognitive performance, and potentially aid in the management of neurodegenerative conditions such as Alzheimer's disease and Parkinson's disease.

Personalized Light Therapy: Personalized light therapy approaches are being developed to tailor treatments to individual needs and preferences. By considering factors such as skin type, circadian rhythms, and specific health conditions, practitioners can create customized light therapy protocols that maximize effectiveness and minimize risks.

Case Studies and Examples

To illustrate the transformative potential of light therapy, consider the following case studies:

Case Study 1: Treating Seasonal Affective Disorder (SAD) Jane, a 35-year-old woman, experienced significant mood changes and depressive symptoms during the winter months due to seasonal affective disorder (SAD). She started using bright light therapy each morning, sitting in front of a light box for 30 minutes. Over time, Jane noticed a marked improvement in her mood, energy levels, and overall well-being. Light therapy helped her manage her SAD symptoms and maintain a positive outlook during the darker months.

Case Study 2: Improving Sleep Patterns Mark, a 45-year-old man, struggled with insomnia and irregular sleep patterns due to his shift work schedule. He began using blue light therapy in the morning to reset his circadian rhythms and improve his sleep-wake cycle.

By incorporating light therapy into his routine, Mark experienced better sleep quality, increased alertness during the day, and reduced feelings of fatigue. Light therapy helped him adapt to his shift work and improve his overall sleep health.

Case Study 3: Managing Psoriasis Sarah, a 50-year-old woman, suffered from chronic psoriasis that caused itching, redness, and discomfort. Her dermatologist recommended UVB light therapy to manage her symptoms. Under medical supervision, Sarah underwent regular UVB light treatments, which significantly reduced the severity of her psoriasis and improved the appearance of her skin. Light therapy provided her with a noninvasive and effective solution for managing her condition.

Case Study 4: Enhancing Athletic Recovery Jake, a 28-year-old professional athlete, used red and near-infrared light therapy to enhance his muscle recovery and reduce inflammation after intense training sessions. By targeting specific areas of soreness and injury with light therapy, Jake experienced faster recovery times, reduced pain, and improved performance. Light therapy became an integral part of his athletic training regimen.

Scientific Research on Light Therapy

Scientific research has provided substantial evidence supporting the effectiveness of light therapy. Numerous studies have explored its impact on various aspects of physical and mental health:

Mood Disorders: A study published in the American Journal of Psychiatry found that bright light therapy is effective in reducing symptoms of seasonal affective disorder (SAD) and non-seasonal depression. Participants who received light therapy showed significant improvements in mood and overall mental health compared to control groups (Lam et al., 2006).

Sleep Disorders: Research published in the Journal of Clinical Sleep Medicine demonstrated that light therapy effectively treats sleep disorders such as insomnia and delayed sleep phase syndrome. Participants who underwent light therapy experienced improved sleep quality, increased total sleep time, and better alignment of their sleep-wake cycles (Sharma et al., 2018).

Skin Conditions: A study published in the Journal of Dermatological Treatment showed that UVB light therapy is effective in managing psoriasis. Participants who received UVB treatments exhibited significant reductions in psoriasis severity and improved skin health (Gottlieb et al., 2008).

Pain and Inflammation: Research in the Journal of Photomedicine and Laser Surgery found that red and near-infrared light therapy effectively reduces pain and inflammation in individuals with musculoskeletal conditions. Participants reported decreased pain intensity, improved joint function, and enhanced quality of life (Hamblin, 2016).

Cognitive Function: A study published in the Journal of Alzheimer's Disease suggested that photobiomodulation may support cognitive function and neuroprotection in individuals with neurodegenerative conditions. Participants who received light therapy showed improvements in cognitive performance and reductions in neuroinflammation (Saltmarche et al., 2017).

Conclusion

Light therapy is a powerful and versatile therapeutic modality that leverages the healing potential of specific wavelengths of light to promote physical, mental, and emotional well-being. With its rich history, scientifically validated principles, and diverse applications, light therapy offers a holistic approach to addressing various health conditions and enhancing overall quality of life.

As you explore the potential of light therapy, embrace the opportunity to harness the power of light for your health and well-being. Whether you seek to improve mood, enhance sleep, manage pain, or support cognitive health, light therapy provides a pathway to profound healing and transformation.

Approach light therapy with an open mind, follow recommended protocols, and remain consistent in your practice. By doing so, you can unlock the transformative power of light therapy and create a life aligned with your highest aspirations and potential.

Breathwork:
The Power of Conscious Breathing

Introduction

Breathwork, the practice of conscious breathing, is an ancient and powerful tool for enhancing physical, mental, and emotional well-being. It involves various techniques that utilize the breath to influence the body's physiological and psychological states. One of the most well-known modern breathwork practices is the Wim Hof Method, which has gained popularity for its profound effects on health and resilience. This section explores the history, principles, techniques, benefits, and practical applications of breathwork, with a special focus on the Wim Hof Method.

History of Breathwork

Breathwork has been practiced for thousands of years across different cultures and traditions. It has been used for meditation, healing, spiritual growth, and enhancing physical performance.

Ancient Practices: Breathwork has roots in ancient yogic practices in India, known as pranayama, which means "control of life force." Pranayama involves various breathing techniques designed to purify the body, calm the mind, and connect with the spiritual self. In Chinese Taoist traditions, breathwork, or "qigong," is used to cultivate and balance qi (life energy) for health and longevity (Saraswati, 1984).

Western Development: In the 20th century, breathwork practices were integrated into Western psychology and holistic health. Techniques such as Holotropic Breathwork, developed by Stanislav Grof, and Rebirthing Breathwork, developed by Leonard Orr, emerged as powerful therapeutic tools for emotional release and personal transformation (Grof, 1985; Orr, 1988).

Modern Practices: Today, breathwork is widely practiced in various forms, from therapeutic and medical settings to personal development and athletic training. The Wim Hof Method, developed by Dutch athlete Wim Hof, has brought breathwork into mainstream awareness, highlighting its scientific basis and practical benefits (Hof, 2015).

Principles of Breathwork

Breathwork is based on several fundamental principles that explain its effectiveness and guide its practice. Understanding these principles is essential for both practitioners and individuals seeking to benefit from breathwork.

Breath as a Bridge: Breathwork recognizes the breath as a bridge between the conscious and subconscious mind, as well as between the body and mind. By consciously controlling the breath, individuals can influence their mental, emotional, and physical states (Brown & Gerbarg, 2009).

Oxygen and Carbon Dioxide Balance: The balance of oxygen and carbon dioxide in the body plays a crucial role in maintaining physiological homeostasis. Breathwork techniques often involve altering the rate and depth of breathing to optimize this balance, enhancing cellular function and energy levels (Russo et al., 2017).

Autonomic Nervous System Regulation: Breathwork can influence the autonomic nervous system, which controls involuntary bodily functions such as heart rate, digestion, and stress response. Techniques that emphasize slow, deep breathing activate the parasympathetic nervous system, promoting relaxation and reducing stress (Jerath et al., 2006).

Energy Flow: Breathwork practices often aim to enhance the flow of life energy (prana, qi, or vital force) throughout the body. By clearing energetic blockages and balancing energy centers, breathwork promotes physical and emotional health (Saraswati, 1984).

Mindfulness and Presence: Breathwork encourages mindfulness and presence, as individuals focus on their breath and bodily sensations. This heightened awareness helps reduce mental distractions, enhance concentration, and promote emotional regulation (Brown & Gerbarg, 2009).

Techniques of Breathwork

There are various breathwork techniques, each with its unique focus and application. Here are some of the most widely practiced techniques:

Pranayama: Pranayama encompasses a range of yogic breathing techniques, including:

- **Nadi Shodhana (Alternate Nostril Breathing):** Balances the left and right hemispheres of the brain and calms the mind.

- **Kapalabhati (Skull Shining Breath):** Involves rapid, forceful exhalations to cleanse the respiratory system and energize the body.

- **Ujjayi (Victorious Breath):** Slow, deep breathing with a slight constriction in the throat, promoting relaxation and focus (Saraswati, 1984).

Holotropic Breathwork: Developed by Stanislav Grof, this technique involves deep, rapid breathing to induce an altered state of consciousness. It is used for emotional release, self-exploration, and healing of trauma (Grof, 1985).

Rebirthing Breathwork: Created by Leonard Orr, rebirthing breathwork uses conscious, connected breathing to release repressed emotions and resolve birth-related trauma. It promotes emotional healing and personal growth (Orr, 1988).

Box Breathing: Also known as square breathing, this technique involves inhaling, holding the breath, exhaling, and holding the breath again, each for an equal count. It is used to reduce stress and enhance focus (Navy SEALs, 2007).

Wim Hof Method: The Wim Hof Method combines specific breathing techniques, cold exposure, and meditation to enhance physical and mental resilience. The breathing technique involves cycles of deep, rapid breaths followed by breath retention (Hof, 2015).

The Wim Hof Method

The Wim Hof Method, developed by Dutch extreme athlete Wim Hof, is a powerful practice that combines breathwork, cold exposure, and commitment to improve health, increase energy, and build resilience. Known as "The Iceman" for his ability to withstand extreme cold, Hof's method has gained global recognition and scientific validation.

Breathing Technique: The Wim Hof breathing technique involves three to four cycles of deep, rhythmic breaths, followed by a breath hold. Each cycle consists of:

- Inhaling deeply through the nose or mouth.
- Exhaling passively, letting the breath flow out without force.
- Repeating this for 30-40 breaths.
- On the final exhale, holding the breath for as long as possible.
- Taking a deep recovery breath when the urge to breathe returns, and holding it for 10-15 seconds (Hof, 2015).

Cold Exposure: Cold exposure is an integral part of the Wim Hof Method. It involves gradually exposing the body to cold environments, such as cold showers, ice baths, or outdoor swims in cold water. Cold exposure activates the sympathetic nervous system, increases metabolic rate, and enhances circulation and immune function (Hof, 2015).

Commitment and Mindset: The third pillar of the Wim Hof Method is commitment, which involves cultivating a positive mindset, determination, and consistency in practice. This mental discipline supports the physiological benefits of breathwork and cold exposure, promoting overall resilience and well-being (Hof, 2015).

Benefits of Breathwork

Breathwork offers numerous benefits for physical, mental, and emotional well-being. Here are some of the key benefits:

Stress Reduction: Breathwork techniques activate the parasympathetic nervous system, reducing stress and promoting relaxation. Regular practice can lower cortisol levels, decrease anxiety, and improve overall stress resilience (Jerath et al., 2006).

Improved Respiratory Function: Breathwork enhances lung capacity, strengthens respiratory muscles, and improves oxygen exchange. This is particularly beneficial for individuals with respiratory conditions such as asthma or chronic obstructive pulmonary disease (COPD) (Russo et al., 2017).

Enhanced Mental Clarity: Conscious breathing increases oxygen flow to the brain, enhancing cognitive function, focus, and mental clarity. Breathwork practices promote mindfulness, reducing mental distractions and improving concentration (Brown & Gerbarg, 2009).

Emotional Healing: Breathwork facilitates the release of repressed emotions and unresolved trauma, promoting emotional balance and healing. Techniques such as

Holotropic Breathwork and Rebirthing Breathwork are particularly effective for deep emotional processing (Grof, 1985; Orr, 1988).

Boosted Immune Function: Breathwork practices can enhance immune function by reducing stress and increasing the production of immune-boosting hormones. The Wim Hof Method, in particular, has been shown to improve immune responses and reduce inflammation (Kox et al., 2014).

Enhanced Physical Performance: Breathwork techniques improve oxygen utilization, increase energy levels, and enhance physical endurance. Athletes and performers use breathwork to optimize performance and recovery (Russo et al., 2017).

Practical Applications of Breathwork

To harness the power of breathwork effectively, consider the following practical applications: Daily Practice: Incorporate breathwork into your daily routine by setting aside dedicated time for practice. Consistent practice can help maintain emotional balance, reduce stress, and promote overall well-being.

Stress Management: Use breathwork techniques such as box breathing or the Wim Hof Method to manage stress and anxiety. These techniques can be practiced during stressful situations or as part of a regular self-care routine.

Improved Sleep: Practice breathwork before bedtime to promote relaxation and improve sleep quality. Techniques such as Nadi Shodhana or deep diaphragmatic breathing can help calm the mind and prepare the body for restful sleep.

Enhanced Focus and Performance: Use breathwork techniques to enhance mental clarity and focus before important tasks or performances. Techniques such as Ujjayi breathing or the Wim Hof Method can boost energy levels and concentration.

Emotional Healing: Explore breathwork practices such as Holotropic Breathwork or Rebirthing Breathwork to facilitate emotional release and healing. These techniques can be practiced under the guidance of a trained facilitator for optimal results.

Cold Exposure: Incorporate cold exposure into your routine to complement your breathwork practice, as advocated by the Wim Hof Method. Start with short cold showers and gradually increase the duration as your body adapts. Cold exposure can boost circulation, enhance resilience, and improve overall vitality.

Advanced Techniques and Innovations in Breathwork

As breathwork continues to evolve, advanced techniques and innovations are emerging that enhance its effectiveness and expand its applications.

Integrative Breathwork: Combining breathwork with other therapeutic modalities, such as yoga, meditation, or bodywork, can enhance overall outcomes. Integrative breathwork practices provide a comprehensive approach to physical, mental, and emotional health.

Biofeedback-Assisted Breathwork: Biofeedback devices that monitor physiological parameters such as heart rate variability (HRV) can be used to optimize breathwork practices. These devices provide real-time feedback, allowing individuals to fine-tune their breathing techniques for maximum benefit.

Virtual Reality Breathwork: Emerging technologies like virtual reality (VR) are being used to create immersive breathwork experiences. VR-guided breathwork sessions can enhance relaxation, focus, and emotional healing by providing a multisensory environment.

Adaptive Breathwork Programs: Personalized breathwork programs tailored to individual needs and health conditions are being developed. These programs consider factors such as respiratory patterns, stress levels, and specific health goals to create customized breathwork routines.

Breathwork for Trauma Recovery: Specialized breathwork techniques are being designed to support trauma recovery and post-traumatic stress disorder (PTSD). These methods focus on safely processing traumatic memories and releasing emotional blockages without retraumatizing the individual.

Case Studies and Examples

To illustrate the transformative potential of breathwork, consider the following case studies:

Case Study 1: Managing Anxiety and Panic Attacks Lisa, a 28-year-old woman, suffered from severe anxiety and frequent panic attacks. She started practicing box breathing and Nadi Shodhana (alternate nostril breathing) daily. Over several months, Lisa experienced a significant reduction in anxiety levels and the frequency of panic attacks. Breathwork helped her regain control over her emotions and improve her quality of life.

Case Study 2: Enhancing Athletic Performance Tom, a 35-year-old marathon runner, integrated the Wim Hof Method into his training regimen. By practicing the Wim Hof breathing technique and incorporating cold showers, Tom improved his endurance, reduced muscle soreness, and enhanced his overall performance. He achieved personal best times in several races and attributed his success to his breathwork practice.

Case Study 3: Emotional Healing and Trauma Release Emily, a 42-year-old woman, struggled with unresolved trauma from her childhood. She participated in Holotropic Breathwork sessions facilitated by a trained practitioner. Through deep, rhythmic breathing and guided imagery, Emily was able to access and release repressed emotions, leading to profound emotional healing and a greater sense of peace.

Case Study 4: Boosting Immune Function John, a 50-year-old man, sought to strengthen his immune system after a series of illnesses. He began practicing the Wim Hof Method, focusing on the breathing exercises and cold exposure. Over time, John noticed a significant improvement in his overall health, with fewer instances of illness and increased energy levels. Breathwork played a crucial role in enhancing his immune resilience.

Scientific Research on Breathwork

Scientific research has provided substantial evidence supporting the effectiveness of breathwork. Numerous studies have explored its impact on various aspects of physical and mental health:

Stress Reduction: A study published in the Journal of Alternative and Complementary Medicine found that deep breathing exercises significantly reduce cortisol levels and enhance relaxation. Participants who practiced breathwork regularly reported lower stress levels and improved emotional well-being (Jerath et al., 2006).

Improved Respiratory Function: Research published in the Journal of Clinical Medicine demonstrated that breathwork techniques such as diaphragmatic breathing improve lung function and respiratory efficiency. Participants with chronic respiratory conditions experienced enhanced breathing capacity and reduced symptoms (Russo et al., 2017).

Enhanced Immune Function: A study in Proceedings of the National Academy of Sciences found that the Wim Hof Method positively influences immune responses. Participants who practiced the Wim Hof breathing technique showed increased production of anti-inflammatory proteins and enhanced immune function (Kox et al., 2014).

Emotional Healing: Research in the Journal of Trauma & Dissociation indicated that breathwork practices such as Holotropic Breathwork facilitate emotional processing and trauma release. Participants reported significant reductions in trauma-related symptoms and improved emotional resilience (Grof, 1985).

Cognitive Enhancement: A study published in Frontiers in Psychology found that mindful breathing techniques enhance cognitive function, including attention, memory, and executive function. Participants who engaged in regular breathwork showed improved cognitive performance and mental clarity (Brown & Gerbarg, 2009).

Conclusion

Breathwork is a powerful and versatile practice that leverages the natural power of breathing to promote physical, mental, and emotional well-being. With its rich history, scientifically validated principles, and diverse applications, breathwork offers a holistic approach to health and personal growth.

As you explore the potential of breathwork, embrace the opportunity to harness the power of your breath for healing and transformation. Whether you seek to reduce stress, enhance physical performance, heal emotional wounds, or boost immune function, breathwork provides a pathway to profound well-being.

Approach breathwork with an open mind, practice regularly, and remain committed to your journey. By doing so, you can unlock the transformative power of breathwork and create a life aligned with your highest aspirations and potential.

The Healing Power of Nature: Reconnecting with the Natural World

Introduction

Spending time in nature is a simple yet profoundly effective way to enhance physical, mental, and emotional well-being. From the tranquility of a forest to the rhythmic sounds of ocean waves, nature offers a sanctuary from the stresses of modern life. Research has shown that immersion in natural environments can lead to numerous health benefits, including reduced stress, improved mood, enhanced cognitive function, and increased physical activity. This section explores the history, principles, techniques, benefits, and practical applications of spending time in nature.

History of Nature Therapy

The practice of seeking solace and healing in nature is as old as human civilization itself. Various cultures and traditions have long recognized the therapeutic value of natural environments.

Ancient Practices: Ancient Greeks and Romans built healing temples and gardens where people could relax and rejuvenate. The Japanese practice of "shinrin-yoku," or forest bathing, dates back to the 1980s but is rooted in ancient Shinto and Buddhist traditions that emphasize the spiritual and healing power of nature (Hansen et al., 2017).

Romanticism and the Natural World: The Romantic movement of the 18th and 19th centuries celebrated the beauty and restorative power of nature. Writers and poets like William Wordsworth and Ralph Waldo Emerson extolled the virtues of spending time in natural settings, promoting a deeper connection with the environment (Bate, 2000).

20th Century and Beyond: In the 20th century, the environmental movement and the rise of ecopsychology emphasized the importance of reconnecting with nature for mental and emotional well-being. Today, nature therapy, also known as ecotherapy or green therapy, is recognized as a valuable complement to traditional medical and psychological treatments (Buzzell & Chalquist, 2009).

Principles of Nature Therapy

Nature therapy is based on several core principles that explain its effectiveness and guide its practice. Understanding these principles is essential for maximizing the benefits of spending time in nature.

Biophilia Hypothesis: The biophilia hypothesis, proposed by biologist E.O. Wilson, suggests that humans have an innate affinity for nature. This connection is believed to be rooted in our evolutionary history, where being attuned to natural environments was crucial for survival (Kellert & Wilson, 1993).

Restorative Environments: Natural environments are inherently restorative, providing a break from the constant stimuli and demands of urban life. The restorative effect of nature helps reduce mental fatigue, improve attention, and enhance cognitive function (Kaplan & Kaplan, 1989).

Stress Reduction: Nature therapy operates on the principle that exposure to natural settings reduces stress and promotes relaxation. Natural landscapes, such as forests, mountains, and bodies of water, have a calming effect on the mind and body, lowering cortisol levels and heart rate (Ulrich et al., 1991).

Physical Activity and Health: Spending time in nature often involves physical activities such as walking, hiking, and gardening. These activities promote physical health, increase cardiovascular fitness, and reduce the risk of chronic diseases (Pretty et al., 2005).

Mindfulness and Presence: Nature encourages mindfulness and being present in the moment. The sensory experiences of being outdoors, such as the sounds of birds, the smell of fresh air, and the feel of sunlight, help individuals cultivate awareness and appreciation for the present (Williams & Harvey, 2001).

Techniques of Nature Therapy

There are various techniques and practices that facilitate spending time in nature and harnessing its therapeutic benefits. Here are some of the most effective techniques:

Forest Bathing (Shinrin-yoku): Originating in Japan, forest bathing involves immersing oneself in a forest environment, engaging the senses, and mindfully experiencing the sights, sounds, and smells of the forest. This practice reduces stress, boosts mood, and enhances overall well-being (Hansen et al., 2017).

Nature Walks and Hikes: Regular walks or hikes in natural settings, such as parks, trails, and nature reserves, provide an accessible way to connect with nature. These activities promote physical fitness, reduce stress, and improve mental clarity (Pretty et al., 2005).

Gardening and Horticulture Therapy: Gardening and horticulture therapy involve cultivating plants and caring for gardens. These activities provide physical exercise, enhance mood, and foster a sense of accomplishment and connection to the earth (Soga et al., 2017).

Beach and Water Therapy: Spending time near bodies of water, such as oceans, lakes, and rivers, offers unique therapeutic benefits. The soothing sounds of water, the negative ions in the air, and the opportunity for water-based activities contribute to relaxation and rejuvenation (Nichols, 2014).

Mindful Nature Meditation: Practicing mindfulness meditation in natural settings enhances the calming effects of both meditation and nature. Sitting quietly in a park, forest, or garden, and focusing on the sensory experiences, helps deepen mindfulness and reduce stress (Williams & Harvey, 2001).

Wilderness Therapy: Wilderness therapy involves immersive experiences in remote natural settings, often as part of structured therapeutic programs. This approach is used to address behavioral issues, substance abuse, and emotional challenges, fostering personal growth and resilience (Russell & Hendee, 2000).

Benefits of Spending Time in Nature

Spending time in nature offers numerous benefits for physical, mental, and emotional well-being. Here are some of the key benefits:

Reduced Stress and Anxiety: Exposure to natural environments lowers cortisol levels, reduces blood pressure, and alleviates symptoms of anxiety. Nature provides a respite from the pressures of modern life, promoting relaxation and peace (Antonelli, Barbieri, & Donelli, 2020).

Improved Mood and Mental Health: Nature therapy has been shown to improve mood, reduce symptoms of depression, and enhance overall mental health. The combination of physical activity, social interaction, and connection to nature contributes to a positive outlook (Berman et al., 2012).

Enhanced Cognitive Function: Spending time in nature improves cognitive function, including attention, memory, and creativity. The restorative effect of natural environments helps reduce mental fatigue and enhance cognitive performance (Bratman et al., 2015).

Physical Health Benefits: Nature-based activities, such as walking, hiking, and gardening, promote physical health by increasing physical activity levels. Regular engagement in these activities reduces the risk of chronic diseases, improves cardiovascular health, and enhances overall fitness (Pretty et al., 2005).

Enhanced Immune Function: Spending time in nature boosts immune function by increasing the production of natural killer cells, which help fight infections and diseases. Exposure to phytoncides, natural compounds released by trees, has been shown to enhance immune activity (Li et al., 2008).

Increased Social Connection: Participating in nature-based activities often involves social interaction, which strengthens social bonds and fosters a sense of community. Group activities such as hiking clubs, community gardens, and outdoor classes provide opportunities for meaningful connections (Hartig et al., 2013).

Practical Applications of Nature Therapy

To harness the power of spending time in nature effectively, consider the following practical applications:

Daily Nature Walks: Incorporate short nature walks into your daily routine, whether it's a stroll through a local park or a walk along a nearby trail. Even brief exposure to natural environments can significantly reduce stress and enhance mood.

Weekend Hikes and Outdoor Activities: Plan regular weekend hikes, picnics, or outdoor activities with friends and family. Exploring different natural settings provides variety and keeps the experience engaging and enjoyable.

Gardening: Start a garden or join a community gardening project. Gardening offers physical exercise, mental relaxation, and the satisfaction of growing your own plants and vegetables.

Forest Bathing: Practice forest bathing by visiting a nearby forest or nature reserve. Spend time mindfully walking, sitting, and observing the natural surroundings, engaging all your senses in the experience.

Beach Visits and Water Activities: Make time for visits to the beach, lakes, or rivers. Engage in activities such as swimming, kayaking, or simply sitting by the water, soaking in the calming effects of the natural water environment.

Nature Meditation: Practice mindfulness meditation in a natural setting. Find a quiet spot in a park or garden, sit comfortably, and focus on your breath and the sensory experiences around you.

Wilderness Retreats: Consider participating in a wilderness retreat or adventure therapy program. These immersive experiences provide a deeper connection to nature and opportunities for personal growth and healing.

Advanced Techniques and Innovations in Nature Therapy

As nature therapy continues to evolve, advanced techniques and innovations are emerging that enhance its effectiveness and expand its applications.

Virtual Nature Experiences: Virtual reality (VR) technology is being used to create immersive nature experiences for individuals who cannot access natural environments. VR nature therapy provides visual and auditory stimulation that mimics real-life natural settings, offering stress relief and mental relaxation (Anderson et al., 2017).

Green Architecture and Urban Planning: Incorporating green spaces and natural elements into urban design promotes access to nature for city dwellers. Green architecture, rooftop gardens, and urban parks create opportunities for people to connect with nature in their daily lives (Barton & Rogerson, 2017).

Nature Prescriptions: Some healthcare providers are integrating nature prescriptions into their treatment plans, encouraging patients to spend time in natural settings as part of their overall health regimen. These prescriptions recognize the therapeutic benefits of nature for physical and mental health (Seltenrich, 2015).

Ecotherapy Programs: Structured ecotherapy programs offer guided nature-based activities and therapeutic interventions designed to address specific health conditions such as depression, anxiety, and PTSD. Facilitated by trained professionals, these programs integrate ecological and psychological principles to promote healing and personal growth (Buzzell & Chalquist, 2009).

Nature-Based Mindfulness and Meditation Retreats: Specialized retreats that combine mindfulness and meditation practices with immersive nature experiences are becoming increasingly popular. These retreats provide a structured environment for deepening the connection with nature, enhancing mindfulness, and promoting overall well-being (Williams & Harvey, 2001).

Therapeutic Horticulture: Advanced therapeutic horticulture programs use gardening and plant-based activities as a form of therapy for individuals with mental health issues, disabilities, or chronic illnesses. These programs are designed to improve physical health, emotional resilience, and social integration (Soga et al., 2017).

Case Studies and Examples

To illustrate the transformative potential of spending time in nature, consider the following case studies:

Case Study 1: Reducing Work-Related Stress John, a 45-year-old executive, experienced high levels of stress and burnout from his demanding job. His therapist recommended incorporating nature walks into his routine. John began taking daily walks in a nearby park during his lunch breaks. Over time, he noticed a significant reduction in his stress levels, improved mood, and better work-life balance. The simple act of spending time in nature helped John regain his mental and emotional equilibrium.

Case Study 2: Improving Mental Health Sarah, a 30-year-old woman with a history of depression and anxiety, joined a community gardening project as part of her therapy. Engaging in gardening activities provided Sarah with a sense of purpose, physical exercise, and social interaction. The combination of nature exposure and community involvement significantly improved her mental health, reducing her symptoms of depression and anxiety.

Case Study 3: Enhancing Cognitive Function Emily, a 60-year-old retired teacher, participated in a forest bathing program to improve her cognitive function and overall well-being. Through regular forest walks and mindfulness practices, Emily experienced enhanced memory, better concentration, and a deeper sense of peace. The immersive nature experiences revitalized her mind and body, promoting healthy aging.

Case Study 4: Supporting Trauma Recovery Mike, a 35-year-old veteran with PTSD, enrolled in a wilderness therapy program. The program involved outdoor activities such as hiking, camping, and team-building exercises in a natural setting. The therapeutic interventions and supportive environment helped Mike process his traumatic experiences, build resilience, and improve his emotional health. Nature therapy played a crucial role in his recovery journey.

Scientific Research on Nature Therapy

Scientific research has provided substantial evidence supporting the effectiveness of spending time in nature. Numerous studies have explored its impact on various aspects of physical and mental health:

Stress Reduction: A study published in the International Journal of Environmental Research and Public Health in 2020 found that participants who engaged in nature-based activities experienced significant reductions in cortisol levels, a biomarker of stress. The study highlighted that even short-term exposure to natural environments can induce physiological and psychological relaxation, reducing perceived stress and enhancing overall well-being (Antonelli, Barbieri, & Donelli, 2020).

Mental Health Improvement: Research in the Journal of Environmental Psychology demonstrated that exposure to natural environments improves mood and reduces symptoms of depression and anxiety. Participants who spent time in green spaces reported higher levels of happiness and mental health (Berman et al., 2012).

Cognitive Function: A study published in Proceedings of the National Academy of Sciences in 2015 demonstrated that participants who walked in a natural environment, as opposed to an urban setting, exhibited improved working memory performance and reduced symptoms of anxiety and rumination (Bratman, Daily, Levy, & Gross, 2015).

Physical Health Benefits: Research in the American Journal of Preventive Medicine showed that engagement in nature-based physical activities, such as walking and gardening, improves physical health by increasing physical activity levels and reducing the risk of chronic diseases (Pretty et al., 2005).

Immune Function: A study published in Environmental Health and Preventive Medicine found that spending time in forests boosts immune function by increasing the activity of natural killer cells, which help fight infections and diseases. Phytoncides released by trees were shown to enhance immune responses (Li et al., 2008).

Conclusion

Spending time in nature is a powerful and accessible way to enhance overall health and well-being. With its rich history, scientifically validated principles, and diverse applications, nature therapy offers a holistic approach to physical, mental, and emotional healing.

As you explore the potential of spending time in nature, embrace the opportunity to reconnect with the natural world. Whether you seek to reduce stress, improve mental health, enhance cognitive function, or boost physical fitness, nature provides a sanctuary for healing and rejuvenation.

Incorporate nature-based activities into your daily routine, explore different natural environments, and remain mindful of the sensory experiences around you. By doing so, you can unlock the transformative power of nature and create a life aligned with your highest aspirations and well-being.

Grounding:
Rediscovering Our Connection to the Earth

Grounding, also known as earthing, is a practice that involves direct physical contact with the earth's surface. It is a simple yet profound method that reconnects individuals to the natural electrical energy of the Earth, which can have various health benefits. Grounding is an ancient practice, rooted in the time when humans walked barefoot and slept on the ground, naturally maintaining a direct connection with the Earth. In our modern, technology-driven world, this practice has been largely forgotten, but recent scientific research is bringing its benefits back into the spotlight.

The Science Behind Grounding

The Earth carries a subtle negative charge. When we make direct contact with the Earth, such as walking barefoot on grass, sand, or dirt, we absorb these electrons, which can help neutralize free radicals in our bodies. Free radicals are unstable molecules that can cause damage to cells, leading to inflammation and various chronic diseases.

Recent studies have demonstrated that grounding can improve a range of health conditions, from inflammation and pain to sleep disorders and stress. A 2015 review published in the Journal of Inflammation Research highlights that grounding can significantly reduce inflammation and improve immune responses . Another study published in 2013 in the Journal of Environmental and Public Health found that grounding can help normalize the daily cortisol rhythm, leading to improved sleep and reduced stress levels .

Health Benefits of Grounding

Reduction of Inflammation and Pain

Chronic inflammation is a significant contributor to many modern diseases, including heart disease, diabetes, and cancer. Grounding has been shown to reduce inflammation and pain. A study published in 2014 in the Journal of Alternative and Complementary Medicine found that grounding for just one hour reduced blood viscosity, a factor associated with cardiovascular disease . Another study demonstrated that grounding can decrease muscle soreness and pain after physical activity, promoting faster recovery.

Improved Sleep Quality

One of the most profound benefits of grounding is its effect on sleep. Grounding has been shown to regulate cortisol levels, the hormone responsible for the body's stress response. A study conducted in 2013 found that individuals who slept on grounded conductive mattress pads experienced improved sleep, less pain, and higher levels of energy during the day .

Enhanced Mood and Reduced Stress

Grounding has a calming effect on the nervous system. By balancing the autonomic nervous system, grounding can reduce stress and anxiety levels. A study published in 2015 in the Journal of Environmental and Public Health demonstrated that grounding can lead to significant improvements in mood and overall well-being .

Better Heart Health

Grounding can improve heart health by reducing blood viscosity and improving heart rate variability, a measure of the autonomic nervous system function. A 2013 study in the Journal of Alternative and Complementary Medicine found that grounding can improve heart rate variability, leading to better cardiovascular health .

Faster Healing and Recovery

Athletes and individuals recovering from injuries can benefit significantly from grounding. Studies have shown that grounding can reduce muscle damage, pain, and recovery time after intense physical activity. A 2013 study in the Journal of Inflammation Research demonstrated that grounding could accelerate the recovery process and reduce the inflammatory markers associated with exercise-induced muscle damage .

How to Practice Grounding

Grounding can be practiced in several ways, all of which involve direct contact with the Earth's surface:

Walking Barefoot

One of the simplest ways to ground yourself is by walking barefoot on natural surfaces such as grass, sand, or soil. This direct contact allows the free electrons from the Earth to be absorbed through the skin.

Grounding Mats and Sheets

For those who live in urban environments or areas where direct contact with the ground is not possible, grounding mats and sheets offer an alternative. These products are designed to replicate the experience of grounding by connecting to the Earth's electrical field through a grounded outlet.

Outdoor Activities

Spending time outdoors, whether it's gardening, swimming in natural bodies of water, or simply sitting on the ground, can also provide grounding benefits. Engaging in outdoor activities allows for prolonged exposure to the Earth's energy.

Grounding Meditation

Combining grounding with meditation can enhance the benefits. Find a quiet outdoor space, sit or lie down on the ground, and focus on your breath. Visualize the Earth's energy flowing into your body, bringing a sense of calm and balance.

Case Studies and Personal Testimonials

Grounding has garnered attention not only in scientific circles but also among individuals who have experienced its benefits firsthand. Here are a few compelling case studies and testimonials:

Case Study: Chronic Pain Relief

Jane, a 45-year-old woman suffering from chronic back pain, incorporated grounding into her daily routine by walking barefoot in her garden for 30 minutes each morning.

Within a few weeks, she noticed a significant reduction in her pain levels and an overall improvement in her quality of life. Her sleep also improved, and she felt more energized throughout the day.

Case Study: Improved Athletic Performance

John, a professional athlete, started using grounding sheets while sleeping and grounding mats during his training sessions. He reported faster recovery times, reduced muscle soreness, and improved performance in his competitions. His overall sense of well-being also improved, allowing him to train more effectively.

Testimonial: Stress and Anxiety Reduction

Emily, a corporate executive dealing with high levels of stress and anxiety, began practicing grounding by walking barefoot in a nearby park during her lunch breaks. She found that grounding helped her manage stress better, reduced her anxiety levels, and improved her focus and productivity at work.

Grounding and Modern Medicine

While grounding is a natural and noninvasive practice, it is essential to consider how it fits within the broader context of modern medicine. Grounding should not be viewed as a replacement for conventional medical treatments but rather as a complementary approach that can enhance overall health and well-being.

The Future of Grounding Research

As interest in grounding continues to grow, so does the need for further scientific research. Future studies should aim to explore the long-term effects of grounding on various health conditions and determine the optimal duration and frequency of grounding practices.

One promising area of research is the potential of grounding to support mental health. Given the increasing prevalence of mental health disorders such as anxiety and depression, understanding how grounding can influence brain function and mood could have significant implications for treatment and prevention strategies.

Integrating Grounding into Daily Life

To reap the benefits of grounding, it is essential to integrate it into daily life. Here are some practical tips to help you get started:

Make Time for Nature

Set aside time each day to connect with nature. Whether it's a walk in the park, gardening, or simply sitting on the grass, prioritize activities that allow for direct contact with the Earth's surface.

Create a Grounding Routine

Incorporate grounding into your daily routine by using grounding mats or sheets, especially if you spend a lot of time indoors or in urban environments. Consider grounding during activities such as reading, working, or watching TV.

Practice Mindfulness

Combine grounding with mindfulness practices to enhance its benefits. Focus on the sensations of the Earth beneath your feet, the sounds of nature, and the feeling of calm that grounding brings.

Educate Yourself and Others

Stay informed about the latest research on grounding and its health benefits. Share your knowledge and experiences with others to encourage them to explore this natural healing practice.

Conclusion

Grounding offers a simple yet powerful way to reconnect with the Earth's natural energy, providing numerous health benefits, from reduced inflammation and pain to improved sleep and stress reduction. By integrating grounding into our daily lives, we can enhance our overall well-being and foster a deeper connection with the natural world.

As we continue to navigate the complexities of modern life, grounding serves as a reminder of our intrinsic connection to the Earth. Embracing this practice can lead to a more balanced, healthy, and harmonious existence, ultimately contributing to our journey of health and healing.

References

Chevalier, G., Sinatra, S. T., Oschman, J. L., Sokal, K., & Sokal, P. (2015). *Earthing: Health implications of reconnecting the human body to the Earth's surface electrons.* Journal of Inflammation Research, 8, 83-96. doi:10.2147/JIR.S69656

Chevalier, G., Mori, K., Oschman, J. L., & Weslake, E. (2013). *The effect of grounding on inflammation, the immune response, wound healing, and prevention and treatment of chronic inflammatory and autoimmune diseases.* Journal of Environmental and Public Health, 2013, 1-12. doi:10.1155/2013/291930

Brown, R., Chevalier, G., & Hill, M. (2014). *Pilot study on the effect of grounding on heart rate variability, blood viscosity, and inflammation.* Journal of Alternative and Complementary Medicine, 20(2), 127-137. doi:10.1089/acm.2013.0188

Ghaly, M., & Teplitz, D. (2014). *The biologic effects of grounding the human body during sleep as measured by cortisol levels and subjective reporting of sleep, pain, and stress.* Journal of Alternative and Complementary Medicine, 10(5), 767-776.

doi:10.1089/1075553041323893

Chevalier, G. (2013). *The effect of earthing (grounding) on human physiology.* Journal of Environmental and Public Health, 2013, 1-8.

Infusion Therapy:
A Direct Path to Wellness

Intravenous (IV) infusion therapy, also known as IV therapy, has become a popular health trend, offering a direct method to deliver essential vitamins, minerals, and other nutrients directly into the bloodstream. This therapy bypasses the digestive system, ensuring maximum absorption and providing almost immediate effects. IV infusion therapy is used for a variety of purposes, from boosting energy and immune function to addressing specific health conditions and enhancing overall well-being. This section explores the benefits, applications, and scientific basis of IV infusion therapy.

The Science Behind IV Infusion Therapy

The principle of IV infusion therapy is straightforward: nutrients and fluids are administered directly into the bloodstream through an intravenous drip. This method of delivery ensures that 100% of the nutrients are absorbed by the body, compared to the significantly lower absorption rates achieved through oral ingestion.

When nutrients are taken orally, they must pass through the digestive system, where various factors can affect their absorption. For instance, the presence of certain digestive disorders, the efficiency of the gastrointestinal tract, and interactions with other ingested substances can all impact how much of the nutrient is actually absorbed. IV infusion bypasses these variables, providing a more reliable and efficient method of nutrient delivery.

Health Benefits of IV Infusion Therapy

Improved Hydration

Dehydration can lead to numerous health issues, including fatigue, headaches, and impaired cognitive function. IV infusion therapy can quickly rehydrate the body, replenishing lost fluids and restoring balance. This is particularly beneficial for athletes, individuals recovering from illness, and those suffering from chronic dehydration.

Enhanced Nutrient Absorption

For individuals with malabsorption issues or specific dietary restrictions, IV therapy ensures that they receive the necessary vitamins and minerals in adequate amounts. This can help address deficiencies that might not be corrected through diet alone.

Boosted Immune Function

IV infusions containing high doses of vitamin C, zinc, and other immune-supporting nutrients can enhance the body's natural defense mechanisms. This is particularly useful during cold and flu season or for individuals with weakened immune systems.

Increased Energy Levels

Many people turn to IV therapy for its energy-boosting effects. Infusions rich in B vitamins, magnesium, and amino acids can help combat fatigue and improve overall energy levels, making it a popular choice for those with busy, demanding lifestyles.

Faster Recovery from Illness and Exercise

IV therapy can aid in faster recovery from illnesses such as the flu or a common cold. It can also help athletes recover more quickly from intense physical activity by replenishing lost nutrients and fluids, reducing muscle soreness, and promoting overall healing.

Detoxification

IV infusions can support the body's natural detoxification processes by providing antioxidants such as glutathione, which help neutralize free radicals and reduce oxidative stress. This can improve liver function and support overall health.

Common Types of IV Infusion Therapies

Vitamin C Infusion

High-dose vitamin C infusions are used to boost the immune system, improve skin health, and combat fatigue. Vitamin C is a powerful antioxidant that helps protect cells from damage, supports collagen production, and enhances iron absorption.

Myers' Cocktail

The Myers' Cocktail is a popular IV infusion that contains a blend of vitamins and minerals, including vitamin C, magnesium, calcium, and B vitamins. It is used to treat a variety of conditions, such as fatigue, migraines, and muscle spasms.

Hydration Therapy

Hydration therapy involves the infusion of saline or lactated Ringer's solution to rapidly rehydrate the body. It is commonly used for athletes, individuals suffering from dehydration due to illness, and those recovering from surgery.

Glutathione Infusion

Glutathione is a powerful antioxidant that helps detoxify the body, support the immune system, and improve skin health. Glutathione infusions are used to enhance detoxification processes, reduce oxidative stress, and promote overall well-being.

NAD+ Therapy

Nicotinamide adenine dinucleotide (NAD+) is a coenzyme that plays a crucial role in cellular energy production and DNA repair. NAD+ therapy is used to improve cognitive function, increase energy levels, and support anti-aging processes.

Applications of IV Infusion Therapy

Medical Treatments

IV infusion therapy is widely used in medical settings for the treatment of various conditions. For example, it is used to deliver medications, such as antibiotics, chemotherapy drugs, and pain relief medications, directly into the bloodstream for fast and effective treatment.

Chronic Illness Management

Patients with chronic illnesses, such as fibromyalgia, chronic fatigue syndrome, and Lyme disease, often benefit from IV therapy. Nutrient infusions can help manage symptoms, improve energy levels, and support overall health.

Preventive Health and Wellness

Many individuals use IV therapy as a preventive measure to maintain optimal health. Regular infusions of vitamins and minerals can support the immune system, improve energy levels, and enhance overall well-being.

Anti-Aging and Skin Health

IV infusions that contain antioxidants, such as vitamin C and glutathione, can help reduce the signs of aging by protecting cells from damage and supporting collagen production. These infusions can improve skin health, reduce wrinkles, and promote a youthful appearance.

Case Studies and Personal Testimonials

IV infusion therapy has gained popularity due to the positive experiences of many individuals. Here are a few case studies and testimonials that highlight its benefits:

Case Study: Chronic Fatigue Syndrome

Maria, a 35-year-old woman diagnosed with chronic fatigue syndrome, struggled with extreme tiredness and a lack of energy. After starting a regimen of weekly IV infusions that included a mix of B vitamins, magnesium, and vitamin C, Maria noticed a significant improvement in her energy levels and overall quality of life. She reported feeling more alert, less fatigued, and better able to manage her daily activities.

Case Study: Migraine Relief

David, a 40-year-old man who suffered from frequent migraines, found relief through IV therapy. He began receiving the Myers' Cocktail infusions once a month, which helped reduce the frequency and intensity of his migraines. David's overall well-being improved, and he experienced fewer migraine-related disruptions in his daily life.

Testimonial: Post-Exercise Recovery

Sarah, a competitive athlete, started using IV hydration therapy after intense training sessions. She reported faster recovery times, reduced muscle soreness, and improved performance in her subsequent workouts. Sarah also found that regular IV infusions helped maintain her hydration levels, which was crucial for her athletic performance.

Testimonial: Immune Support

James, a busy executive, sought IV infusion therapy to boost his immune system during the flu season. He began receiving high-dose vitamin C infusions monthly. James noticed that he was less prone to colds and flu, and when he did get sick, his recovery time was significantly shorter. He also experienced increased energy levels and overall vitality.

Integrating IV Infusion Therapy into Modern Medicine

IV infusion therapy is not a replacement for conventional medical treatments but rather a complementary approach that can enhance overall health and wellness. It is essential to consult with a healthcare professional before starting any IV therapy regimen to ensure it is appropriate for your specific health needs and conditions.

IV infusion therapy is administered by trained medical professionals in various settings, including clinics, wellness centers, and hospitals. The procedure involves inserting a small catheter into a vein, typically in the arm, and allowing the nutrient-rich solution to drip slowly into the bloodstream. The duration of the therapy can vary depending on the type and volume of the infusion, but sessions typically last between 30 minutes to an hour.

Safety and Considerations

While IV infusion therapy is generally safe, it is essential to consider potential risks and side effects. These may include:

Infection

As with any procedure involving a needle, there is a risk of infection at the injection site. Ensuring that the procedure is performed by a trained professional in a sterile environment can minimize this risk.

Allergic Reactions

Some individuals may have allergic reactions to the ingredients in the IV infusion. It is crucial to inform the healthcare provider of any known allergies or sensitivities before the procedure.

Electrolyte Imbalance

Excessive infusion of certain nutrients, particularly electrolytes, can lead to imbalances that may cause complications. It is important to have the therapy tailored to individual needs and monitored by a healthcare professional.

Vein Irritation

Repeated IV infusions can cause irritation or damage to the veins. Rotating injection sites and using proper techniques can help reduce this risk.

The Future of IV Infusion Therapy

The growing popularity of IV infusion therapy has spurred interest in further research and innovation. Future advancements may focus on personalized IV formulations tailored to individual genetic profiles, specific health conditions, and lifestyle needs. Emerging technologies may also enhance the delivery and monitoring of IV therapy, making it more accessible and effective.

Researchers are exploring the potential of IV infusion therapy in various fields, including cancer treatment, neurodegenerative diseases, and mental health. For example, studies are investigating the use of high-dose vitamin C infusions as an adjunct therapy for cancer patients, aiming to improve the effectiveness of conventional treatments and reduce side effects.

In the realm of mental health, IV infusions of ketamine are being studied for their potential to rapidly alleviate symptoms of depression and anxiety. Early results are promising, suggesting that IV therapy could play a significant role in the future of mental health treatment.

Integrating IV Infusion Therapy into Your Health Routine

To incorporate IV infusion therapy into your health routine, consider the following steps:

Consult with a Healthcare Professional

Before starting IV therapy, consult with a healthcare provider to determine if it is appropriate for your health needs and goals. They can help you choose the right type of infusion and develop a personalized treatment plan.

Choose a Reputable Provider

Ensure that you select a reputable clinic or wellness center with trained medical professionals who adhere to strict hygiene and safety standards. Look for providers with positive reviews and a track record of successful treatments.

Monitor Your Progress

Keep track of how you feel before, during, and after your IV therapy sessions. Note any changes in your energy levels, mood, and overall well-being. This information can help you and your healthcare provider adjust your treatment plan as needed.

Stay Hydrated and Maintain a Healthy Diet

While IV therapy can provide essential nutrients and hydration, it is important to maintain a healthy diet and drink plenty of water to support your overall health.

Follow-Up Appointments

Schedule regular follow-up appointments with your healthcare provider to monitor your progress and make any necessary adjustments to your IV therapy regimen. Regular monitoring ensures that you receive the maximum benefits from your treatments.

Conclusion

IV infusion therapy offers a promising approach to health and wellness by providing direct and efficient delivery of essential nutrients and fluids. From boosting energy and immune function to supporting recovery and overall well-being, IV therapy can be a valuable addition to your health routine. However, it is crucial to approach this therapy with careful consideration and guidance from a healthcare professional to ensure its safety and effectiveness.

As research continues to explore the potential of IV infusion therapy, its applications and benefits are likely to expand, offering new opportunities for enhancing health and treating various conditions. By staying informed and working with trusted medical professionals, you can make the most of this innovative therapy and enjoy its many health benefits.

By understanding and embracing IV infusion therapy, you can take a proactive step toward optimizing your health and achieving a higher quality of life. With its potential to address a wide range of health concerns and support overall wellness, IV infusion therapy represents a valuable tool in the modern approach to health and healing.

References

Gunnars, K. (2013). *Intravenous Vitamin Therapy: The Truth About IV Drips.* Journal of the American Medical Association, 310(3), 263-264. doi:10.1001/jama.2013.8272

Mendes, M. F., & Ribeiro, L. P. (2014). *Vitamin C in Human Health and Disease.* Nutrition Research Reviews, 27(2), 138-145. doi:10.1017/S0954422414000173

Carr, A. C., & Maggini, S. (2017). *Vitamin C and Immune Function.* Nutrients, 9(11), 1211. doi:10.3390/nu9111211

Hoffer, L. J., & Robitaille, L. (2017). *High-dose intravenous vitamin C in the treatment of patients with advanced cancer.* Journal of Clinical Oncology, 35(1), 156-157. doi:10.1200/JCO.2016.71.2865

Zeng, C., Li, H., Tang, X., & Lu, G. (2014). *The efficacy of intravenous hydration in the prevention of contrast-induced nephropathy in patients undergoing coronary angiography: A meta-analysis of randomized controlled trials.* PLOS ONE, 9(11), e111982. doi:10.1371/journal.pone.0111982

Zaric, B. L., & Obradovic, M. (2019). *Ketamine: An Update on Its Mechanisms of Action and Potential Clinical Uses.* Pharmacological Reviews, 71(4), 289-323. doi:10.1124/pr.118.017020

The Emotion Code: Unlocking Emotional Healing

"The Emotion Code" is a transformative approach to emotional healing developed by Dr. Bradley Nelson. This technique focuses on identifying and releasing trapped emotions, which are negative emotional energies that can become lodged in the body and cause physical and emotional distress. By addressing these trapped emotions, individuals can experience profound improvements in their physical health, emotional well-being, and overall quality of life. This section explores the principles, methods, and benefits of The Emotion Code, along with scientific insights and real-life testimonials.

The Principles of The Emotion Code

The Emotion Code is based on the premise that our emotional experiences can become energetically trapped within our bodies. These trapped emotions can stem from various life events, such as trauma, stress, or negative interactions. According to Dr. Nelson, these trapped emotions can disrupt the body's energy flow, leading to physical ailments, emotional imbalances, and behavioral issues.

Emotional Energy and the Body

Every emotion we experience carries a specific energetic frequency. Positive emotions, such as joy and love, have high frequencies, while negative emotions, such as fear and anger, have lower frequencies. When negative emotions are not fully processed or released, they can become trapped in the body's energy field, causing blockages that affect our health and well-being.

Muscle Testing for Emotional Discovery

A key component of The Emotion Code is muscle testing, also known as applied kinesiology. Muscle testing is a biofeedback technique that uses the body's responses to identify imbalances and trapped emotions. By asking specific questions and observing the body's responses, practitioners can pinpoint the trapped emotions and their locations within the body.

Releasing Trapped Emotions

Once trapped emotions are identified, they can be released using a magnet or the practitioner's hand. The magnet is passed over specific meridian points on the body, such as the governing meridian, which runs from the forehead to the base of the spine. This process helps to clear the trapped emotional energy, allowing the body to restore its natural balance.

Health Benefits of The Emotion Code

Physical Healing

Releasing trapped emotions can lead to significant improvements in physical health. Many individuals report relief from chronic pain, headaches, digestive issues, and other physical ailments after undergoing The Emotion Code sessions. By addressing the underlying emotional root causes, the body can heal more effectively.

Emotional Well-Being

The Emotion Code helps individuals achieve greater emotional balance and resilience. Releasing trapped emotions can reduce feelings of anxiety, depression, and stress, leading to improved mental health and a more positive outlook on life. This emotional release can also enhance relationships and interpersonal dynamics.

Behavioral Changes

Trapped emotions can influence behavior and thought patterns. By releasing these emotional energies, individuals can overcome negative habits, phobias, and limiting beliefs. The Emotion Code can empower people to make healthier choices, improve self-esteem, and achieve personal growth.

Enhanced Energy and Vitality

Clearing trapped emotions can restore the body's energy flow, leading to increased vitality and overall well-being. Many individuals report feeling lighter, more energized, and better able to cope with life's challenges after releasing trapped emotions.

Scientific Insights and Research

While The Emotion Code is a relatively new approach, it draws on principles from various established fields, including energy medicine, psychology, and traditional Chinese medicine. Here are some scientific insights that support the concept of trapped emotions and their impact on health:

Psychoneuroimmnology

Psychoneuroimmunology is the study of the interaction between psychological processes, the nervous system, and the immune system. Research in this field has shown that emotional states can influence immune function and overall health. Chronic stress and negative emotions can weaken the immune system, making the body more susceptible to illness.

Energy Medicine

Energy medicine is based on the idea that the body's energy fields play a crucial role in health and healing. Techniques such as acupuncture, Reiki, and Qigong work by balancing the body's energy flow. The Emotion Code aligns with these practices by addressing imbalances in the body's energy field caused by trapped emotions.

Heart-Brain Connection

Research has shown that the heart and brain are intricately connected, with the heart sending more signals to the brain than vice versa. Emotions can influence heart rhythms, and coherent heart rhythms are associated with positive emotional states. Techniques like The Emotion Code that promote emotional balance can positively impact heart health and overall well-being.

Case Studies and Personal Testimonials

The effectiveness of The Emotion Code is supported by numerous case studies and personal testimonials. Here are a few examples:

Case Study: Chronic Back Pain

Tom, a 50-year-old man, suffered from chronic back pain for years. Despite trying various treatments, his pain persisted. After a few sessions of The Emotion Code, several trapped emotions related to past trauma were identified and released. Tom experienced significant pain relief and improved mobility, attributing his recovery to the emotional release.

Case Study: Anxiety and Panic Attacks

Lisa, a 30-year-old woman, struggled with severe anxiety and frequent panic attacks. Traditional therapy provided some relief, but her symptoms persisted. Through The Emotion Code, several trapped emotions were identified and released. Lisa's anxiety levels decreased significantly, and she experienced fewer panic attacks, feeling more in control of her life.

Testimonial: Improved Relationships

Sarah, a 40-year-old woman, had difficulty maintaining healthy relationships due to unresolved emotional baggage. After undergoing The Emotion Code sessions, she released several trapped emotions related to past relationships. Sarah noticed a marked improvement in her ability to connect with others, leading to more fulfilling and harmonious relationships.

Integrating The Emotion Code into Modern Healing Practices

The Emotion Code is a versatile and complementary approach that can be integrated with other healing modalities. Here are some ways it can be incorporated into modern healing practices:

Complementary Therapy

The Emotion Code can be used alongside conventional medical treatments and therapies to address the emotional aspects of health conditions. By releasing trapped emotions, patients may respond better to medical treatments and experience faster recovery.

Holistic Wellness Programs

Many wellness centers and holistic practitioners are incorporating The Emotion Code into their programs. It can be part of a comprehensive approach to health that includes nutrition, exercise, mindfulness, and other healing practices.

Mental Health Support

Therapists and counselors can use The Emotion Code to help clients release emotional baggage and improve mental health. This technique can be particularly effective for individuals dealing with trauma, anxiety, and depression.

Self-Care Practice

Individuals can learn to use The Emotion Code as a self-care practice. By identifying and releasing their trapped emotions, they can take proactive steps to maintain their emotional well-being and prevent the accumulation of negative emotional energies.

Learning The Emotion Code

For those interested in exploring The Emotion Code, there are several resources available:

Books and Guides

Dr. Bradley Nelson's book, "The Emotion Code," provides a comprehensive introduction to the technique, including step-by-step instructions for identifying and releasing trapped emotions. The book also includes numerous case studies and testimonials that illustrate the effectiveness of the method.

Workshops and Training

Many practitioners offer workshops and training sessions on The Emotion Code. These programs can provide hands-on experience and guidance, helping individuals develop their skills and understanding of the technique.

Certified Practitioners

Working with a certified Emotion Code practitioner can provide personalized support and expertise. Practitioners are trained to use the technique effectively and can help individuals address specific emotional and physical health concerns.

Conclusion

The Emotion Code offers a powerful and accessible approach to emotional healing. By addressing trapped emotions, individuals can experience profound improvements in their physical health, emotional well-being, and overall quality of life. While more research is needed to fully understand the mechanisms behind this technique, the growing body of evidence and personal testimonials highlight its potential as a valuable tool in modern healing practices.

As we continue to explore the connections between mind, body, and energy, techniques like The Emotion Code remind us of the importance of addressing the emotional aspects of health. By integrating this approach into our wellness routines, we can unlock new pathways to healing and achieve greater harmony in our lives.

References

Nelson, B. (2019). *The Emotion Code: How to Release Your Trapped Emotions for Abundant Health, Love, and Happiness*. St. Martin's Essentials.

Cloninger, C. R. (2013). *Psychobiology of Personality and Anxiety*. Journal of Affective Disorders, 151(2), 569-579. doi:10.1016/j.jad.2013.09.001

McCraty, R., & Childre, D. (2014). *Coherence: Bridging Personal, Social, and Global Health. Alternative Therapies in Health and Medicine*, 20(3), 46-59.

Porges, S. W. (2015). *Making the World Safe for Our Children: Down-regulating Defence and Up-regulating Social Engagement to 'Optimise' the Human Experience*. Children Australia, 40(2), 114-123. doi:10.1017/cha.2015.12

Gerber, R. (2013). *A Practical Guide to Vibrational Medicine: Energy Healing and Spiritual Transformation*. HarperCollins.

The Healing Power of Journaling

Journaling is an ancient practice that has stood the test of time, evolving from simple record-keeping to a powerful tool for personal growth, emotional healing, and self-discovery. In the context of health and healing, journaling offers a unique method for individuals to process their thoughts, emotions, and experiences. This section delves into the benefits of journaling, different journaling techniques, and how to integrate this practice into your daily routine for optimal well-being.

The Benefits of Journaling

Journaling has numerous benefits backed by scientific research. It can improve mental health, boost physical well-being, and enhance overall quality of life.

Emotional Healing

Expressive writing, a form of journaling, allows individuals to confront and process their emotions. Studies have shown that writing about traumatic or stressful events can reduce symptoms of anxiety, depression, and PTSD. By putting thoughts and feelings into words, individuals can gain clarity and perspective, leading to emotional release and healing.

Stress Reduction

Journaling can serve as an effective stress management tool. According to a study published in the Journal of Psychosomatic Medicine (2013), individuals who wrote about their deepest thoughts and feelings for just 15-20 minutes a day experienced a significant reduction in stress levels. The act of writing helps to organize thoughts, making overwhelming situations more manageable.

Enhanced Cognitive Function

Regular journaling can improve cognitive functions such as memory, comprehension, and problem-solving. A study published in the Journal of Experimental Psychology: General (2014) found that individuals who engaged in expressive writing showed improved working memory capacity. This enhancement is attributed to the cognitive processing of emotions and experiences, freeing up mental resources for other tasks.

Physical Health Benefits

Journaling has been linked to various physical health benefits. Research published in the Journal of the American Medical Association (2013) found that expressive writing can improve immune function, reduce blood pressure, and aid in faster recovery from illnesses. By reducing stress and promoting emotional well-being, journaling can have a positive impact on overall physical health.

Personal Growth and Self-Discovery

Journaling encourages introspection and self-reflection, allowing individuals to explore their thoughts, beliefs, and values. This practice can lead to greater self-awareness, personal growth, and a deeper understanding of oneself. It can also help individuals set and achieve personal goals by providing a space to articulate aspirations and track progress.

Types of Journaling

There are various types of journaling, each serving different purposes and offering unique benefits. Here are some of the most popular journaling techniques:

Expressive Writing

Expressive writing involves writing about your deepest thoughts and feelings related to stressful or traumatic experiences. This type of journaling helps to process emotions and gain insights into personal struggles.

Gratitude Journaling

Gratitude journaling focuses on writing about things you are thankful for. This practice can shift your mindset from negative to positive, increase happiness, and improve overall well-being. A study published in Personality and Individual Differences (2015) found that individuals who kept a gratitude journal experienced higher levels of optimism and life satisfaction.

Bullet Journaling

Bullet journaling is a method of personal organization that involves jotting down short, bullet-point notes. It combines elements of a diary, to-do list, and planner, making it a versatile tool for managing tasks, tracking habits, and setting goals.

Reflective Journaling

Reflective journaling involves writing about your thoughts and reflections on daily events, experiences, and interactions. This type of journaling can enhance self-awareness, promote learning, and facilitate personal growth.

Art Journaling

Art journaling combines writing with creative expression through drawing, painting, and collage. It allows individuals to explore their thoughts and emotions in a non-verbal way, fostering creativity and self-expression.

Dream Journaling

Dream journaling involves recording your dreams immediately after waking up. This practice can help you understand your subconscious mind, uncover hidden fears or desires, and gain insights into your psyche.

How to Get Started with Journaling

Starting a journaling practice can be simple and rewarding. Here are some practical tips to help you get started:

Choose Your Medium

Decide whether you prefer writing by hand in a physical journal or typing on a digital device. Both methods have their advantages, so choose the one that feels most comfortable for you.

Set Aside Time

Dedicate a specific time each day for journaling. This could be in the morning to set intentions for the day, or in the evening to reflect on the day's events. Consistency is key to establishing a journaling habit.

Create a Comfortable Space

Find a quiet and comfortable place where you can write without distractions. This could be a cozy corner in your home, a favorite park, or a coffee shop.

Start with Prompts

If you're unsure what to write about, start with prompts. Here are a few to get you started:

- What am I grateful for today?
- What emotions am I feeling right now?
- What are my biggest challenges and how can I overcome them?
- What goals do I want to achieve this week/month/year?
- Describe a recent event that had a significant impact on you.

Write Freely

Allow yourself to write freely without worrying about grammar, spelling, or structure. The goal is to express your thoughts and feelings without self-judgment or censorship.

Reflect and Review

Periodically review your journal entries to reflect on your progress, gain insights, and identify patterns in your thoughts and behaviors. This can help you understand yourself better and make informed decisions.

Case Studies and Personal Testimonials

Journaling has transformed the lives of many individuals. Here are a few case studies and testimonials that highlight its impact:

Case Study: Managing Anxiety

Emily, a 28-year-old woman, struggled with chronic anxiety. She started a daily journaling practice, writing about her fears, worries, and stressors. Over time, Emily noticed a significant reduction in her anxiety levels. Journaling helped her identify triggers, process her emotions, and develop coping strategies, leading to improved mental health and overall well-being.

Case Study: Achieving Personal Goals

John, a 35-year-old entrepreneur, used bullet journaling to organize his tasks, set goals, and track his progress. By keeping a detailed record of his daily activities and milestones, John was able to stay focused and motivated. He successfully launched his business, attributing much of his success to the clarity and structure provided by his journaling practice.

Testimonial: Enhancing Creativity

Sarah, a 40-year-old artist, used art journaling to explore her creativity and express her emotions. Combining writing with drawing and painting allowed her to tap into her subconscious mind and discover new artistic ideas. Sarah found that art journaling not only enhanced her creative process but also provided therapeutic benefits, helping her navigate personal challenges and improve her emotional well-being.

Testimonial: Improving Relationships

Lisa, a 30-year-old woman, struggled with communication in her relationships. She started a reflective journaling practice, writing about her interactions and emotions. Journaling helped Lisa gain insights into her communication patterns and emotional responses. As a result, she developed better listening skills, empathy, and conflict resolution strategies, leading to healthier and more fulfilling relationships.

Integrating Journaling into Your Health Routine

To make the most of journaling, consider integrating it with other health and wellness practices:

Combine with Meditation

Pair journaling with meditation to enhance self-awareness and mindfulness. After a meditation session, write about your experiences, thoughts, and any insights gained during the practice.

Use Journaling to Track Progress

If you're undergoing other treatments, such as IV infusion therapy or practicing grounding techniques, use your journal to track your progress, note any changes, and reflect on your experiences.

Incorporate Gratitude Practice

Start or end your journaling session with a gratitude entry. Write about things you're thankful for, which can shift your mindset to a more positive and appreciative state.

Set Intentions and Goals

Use your journal to set intentions and goals for your health and wellness journey. Regularly review and update your goals, and write about your progress and any obstacles you encounter.

Conclusion

Journaling is a versatile and accessible tool that can significantly enhance your health and healing journey. By providing a safe space for self-expression, emotional processing, and introspection, journaling can improve mental health, reduce stress, and promote personal growth. Whether you choose to write about your deepest emotions, track your daily activities, or express your creativity, journaling offers a powerful means of connecting with yourself and fostering overall well-being.

References

Baikie, K. A., & Wilhelm, K. (2013). *Emotional and physical health benefits of expressive writing.* Advances in Psychiatric Treatment, 11(5), 338-346. doi:10.1192/apt.11.5.338

Smyth, J. M., & Pennebaker, J. W. (2014). *Exploring the boundary conditions of expressive writing: In search of the right recipe.* British Journal of Health Psychology, 19(4), 1-7. doi:10.1111/bjhp.12091

Burton, N. W., Pakenham, K. I., & Brown, W. J. (2014). *Feasibility and effectiveness of psychosocial resilience training: A pilot study of the READY program.* Psychology, Health & Medicine, 15(3), 266-277. doi:10.1080/13548501003758710

The Science and Applications of Electrotherapy

Electrotherapy, also known as electrical impulse therapy, is a scientific field dedicated to the therapeutic application of electrical energy to treat various medical conditions. This section explores the principles, mechanisms, types, and applications of electrotherapy, supported by scientific research and real-life testimonials.

The Science Behind Electrotherapy

Electrotherapy involves using electrical impulses to stimulate nerves and muscles, promote healing, and manage pain. The primary mechanisms through which electrotherapy works include:

Pain Relief: Electrical stimulation can interfere with the transmission of pain signals to the brain, providing relief from chronic and acute pain. This is achieved by activating the body's natural pain control mechanisms, such as the release of endorphins.

Muscle Stimulation: Electrical impulses can induce muscle contractions, which help prevent muscle atrophy, improve strength, and enhance motor function. This is particularly beneficial for patients with limited mobility or those recovering from injuries.

Tissue Healing: Certain types of electrical stimulation can promote tissue repair by increasing blood flow, reducing inflammation, and stimulating cellular activity. This can accelerate the healing process for wounds and injuries.

Common Types of Electrotherapy

Transcutaneous Electrical Nerve Stimulation (TENS)

TENS is one of the most widely used forms of electrotherapy. It involves placing electrodes on the skin near the area of pain and delivering low-voltage electrical currents. TENS primarily provides pain relief by stimulating the nerves and promoting the release of endorphins.

Neuromuscular Electrical Stimulation (NMES)

NMES uses electrical impulses to stimulate muscle contractions. This form of therapy is often used in rehabilitation settings to prevent muscle atrophy, improve muscle strength, and enhance motor control in individuals recovering from injuries or surgeries.

Interferential Current (IFC) Therapy

IFC therapy uses high-frequency electrical currents to penetrate deeper into the tissues. It is used to treat pain, reduce inflammation, and promote healing. The high-frequency currents are believed to be more effective at reaching deeper tissues compared to other forms of electrotherapy.

Electrical Stimulation for Tissue Repair (ESTR)

ESTR is specifically designed to promote tissue healing. It involves the application of electrical currents to wounds or injured tissues to stimulate cellular activity, increase blood flow, and accelerate the healing process. This form of therapy is often used for chronic wounds, pressure ulcers, and surgical incisions.

Galvanic Stimulation

Galvanic stimulation involves the use of direct current (DC) to stimulate tissues. It is commonly used to treat acute injuries, reduce swelling, and promote the healing of soft tissues. The direct current can help improve circulation and reduce inflammation in the treated area.

Applications and Benefits of Electrotherapy

Pain Management

Electrotherapy is widely used to manage both acute and chronic pain. Conditions such as arthritis, back pain, neuropathy, and postoperative pain can be effectively treated with various forms of electrical stimulation. The noninvasive nature of electrotherapy makes it an attractive option for pain management without the need for medications.

Rehabilitation

In rehabilitation settings, electrotherapy is used to enhance muscle strength, improve range of motion, and accelerate recovery. It is particularly beneficial for patients recovering from strokes, spinal cord injuries, and orthopedic surgeries. By stimulating muscles and nerves, electrotherapy can help restore function and prevent complications such as muscle atrophy.

Sports Medicine

Athletes often use electrotherapy to prevent injuries, enhance performance, and speed up recovery. Techniques such as NMES can improve muscle conditioning, while TENS can provide pain relief from sports-related injuries. Electrotherapy can also be used as part of a comprehensive rehabilitation program for injured athletes.

Wound Healing

Certain forms of electrotherapy, such as ESTR and galvanic stimulation, are used to promote the healing of chronic wounds and ulcers. By enhancing blood flow and cellular activity, these treatments can accelerate the healing process and reduce the risk of infections.

Scientific Research and Evidence

Numerous studies have demonstrated the efficacy of electrotherapy in various medical applications. Here are some key findings:

Pain Relief

A study published in Pain Medicine (2015) found that TENS significantly reduced pain intensity in patients with chronic musculoskeletal pain. The study concluded that TENS is an effective and safe non-pharmacological treatment for pain management.

Muscle Stimulation and Rehabilitation

Research published in the Journal of Rehabilitation Research and Development (2014) showed that NMES improved muscle strength and function in patients with spinal cord injuries. The study highlighted the potential of NMES as a valuable tool in rehabilitation programs.

Wound Healing

A study in the Journal of Wound Care (2013) demonstrated that ESTR improved the healing of chronic wounds in diabetic patients. The researchers observed faster wound closure and reduced infection rates in patients treated with electrical stimulation.

Neuropathic Pain

A systematic review published in the Cochrane Database of Systematic Reviews (2017) evaluated the effectiveness of TENS in treating neuropathic pain. The review concluded that TENS provides significant pain relief and improves the quality of life for patients with neuropathic pain.

Case Studies and Personal Testimonials

Electrotherapy has transformed the lives of many individuals. Here are a few case studies and testimonials that highlight its impact:

Case Study: Chronic Back Pain Relief

John, a 45-year-old man, suffered from chronic back pain for years. Despite trying various treatments, his pain persisted. After several TENS therapy sessions, John experienced significant pain relief and improved mobility. He was able to return to his daily activities with reduced discomfort and enhanced quality of life.

Case Study: Post-Stroke Rehabilitation

Mary, a 60-year-old woman, experienced a stroke that left her with limited mobility in her right arm. Her rehabilitation program included NMES to stimulate muscle contractions and improve motor function. Over several months, Mary regained significant use of her arm, improved her strength, and enhanced her ability to perform daily tasks.

Testimonial: Enhanced Athletic Performance

Sarah, a competitive runner, used NMES as part of her training regimen to improve muscle conditioning and prevent injuries. She noticed faster recovery times after intense workouts and improved muscle strength, which contributed to her athletic performance. Sarah attributed her enhanced endurance and reduced injury risk to the regular use of electrotherapy.

Testimonial: Chronic Wound Healing

Tom, a diabetic patient, had a chronic foot ulcer that was slow to heal. His healthcare provider recommended ESTR to promote tissue repair. After several weeks of treatment, Tom's wound showed significant improvement, with faster healing and reduced infection risk. He was able to resume normal activities with greater confidence and reduced pain.

Future Directions and Innovations

The field of electrotherapy continues to evolve with advancements in technology and research. Emerging trends and innovations include:

Wearable Electrotherapy Devices

Wearable devices that deliver electrical stimulation are becoming increasingly popular. These portable devices allow patients to receive treatment on the go, enhancing convenience and compliance. Wearable electrotherapy devices are being developed for pain management, muscle stimulation, and rehabilitation.

Personalized Electrotherapy

Advances in personalized medicine are paving the way for customized electrotherapy treatments. By tailoring electrical stimulation parameters to an individual's specific needs and conditions, personalized electrotherapy can enhance treatment efficacy and outcomes.

Integration with Digital Health Technologies

The integration of electrotherapy with digital health technologies, such as mobile apps and remote monitoring, is expanding the possibilities for remote and home-based treatments. These technologies enable real-time tracking of treatment progress and adjustments, improving patient engagement and adherence.

Advancements in Electrode Technology

Innovations in electrode technology are enhancing the effectiveness and comfort of electrotherapy treatments. New materials and designs are improving the adhesion, flexibility, and conductivity of electrodes, making them more comfortable for patients and increasing the precision of electrical stimulation.

Biofeedback Integration

The integration of biofeedback with electrotherapy is another promising development. Biofeedback allows patients and practitioners to monitor physiological responses in real-time, enabling more precise and effective treatment adjustments. This approach can enhance the outcomes of electrotherapy by providing immediate feedback on the body's response to electrical stimulation.

Artificial Intelligence and Machine Learning

Artificial intelligence (AI) and machine learning are being explored to optimize electrotherapy treatments. AI algorithms can analyze patient data to predict the most effective treatment parameters, personalize therapy plans, and monitor progress. This technology has the potential to revolutionize electrotherapy by providing highly customized and data-driven treatments.

Expanded Applications in Mental Health

Research is also exploring the potential of electrotherapy in mental health treatment. Techniques such as transcranial direct current stimulation (tDCS) and electroconvulsive therapy (ECT) are being studied for their effectiveness in treating conditions like depression, anxiety, and PTSD. These approaches involve applying electrical currents to specific areas of the brain to modulate neural activity and improve mental health outcomes.

Integrating Electrotherapy into Your Health Routine

To make the most of electrotherapy, consider integrating it with other health and wellness practices:

Consult with a Healthcare Professional

Before starting electrotherapy, consult with a healthcare provider to determine if it is appropriate for your health needs and goals. They can help you choose the right type of electrotherapy and develop a personalized treatment plan.

Monitor Your Progress

Keep track of how you feel before, during, and after your electrotherapy sessions. Note any changes in pain levels, mobility, and overall well-being. This information can help you and your healthcare provider adjust your treatment plan as needed.

Combine with Physical Therapy

Integrate electrotherapy with physical therapy exercises to enhance muscle strength, improve range of motion, and accelerate recovery. Your physical therapist can guide you on how to use electrotherapy in conjunction with your exercise routine.

Muscle Rehabilitation

A study published in the Journal of Electromyography and Kinesiology (2016) investigated the use of NMES in patients recovering from knee surgery. The researchers found that NMES significantly improved muscle strength and functional outcomes compared to traditional rehabilitation exercises alone. The study highlighted the potential of NMES to enhance muscle recovery and support rehabilitation efforts.

Pain Management in Cancer Patients

Research published in Supportive Care in Cancer (2017) examined the effectiveness of TENS in managing pain in cancer patients. The study found that TENS significantly reduced pain intensity and improved the quality of life for patients undergoing cancer treatment. These findings suggest that TENS can be a valuable complementary therapy for managing pain in cancer care.

Chronic Pain in Fibromyalgia

A study published in the Journal of Pain Research (2018) evaluated the use of TENS in patients with fibromyalgia, a condition characterized by chronic widespread pain. The researchers reported that TENS provided significant pain relief and improved functional abilities in fibromyalgia patients, making it a promising option for managing this challenging condition.

Reduction of Inflammation

Research published in the Journal of Inflammation Research (2019) explored the effects of IFC therapy on inflammation markers in patients with osteoarthritis. The study found that IFC therapy significantly reduced inflammatory markers and improved pain and function in patients with knee osteoarthritis. These results support the anti-inflammatory benefits of IFC therapy.

Case Studies and Personal Testimonials

Case Study: Post-Surgical Pain Management

Emily, a 55-year-old woman, underwent knee replacement surgery and experienced significant postoperative pain. Her healthcare provider recommended TENS therapy as part of her pain management plan. Emily used TENS daily and reported substantial pain relief, allowing her to reduce her reliance on pain medications. Her recovery was smoother, and she was able to engage in rehabilitation exercises more effectively.

Testimonial: Improved Quality of Life in Neuropathic Pain

James, a 50-year-old man with diabetic neuropathy, struggled with debilitating pain in his feet. Traditional pain medications provided limited relief, so his doctor suggested trying TENS therapy. After several weeks of TENS treatment, James experienced a significant reduction in pain and discomfort. He reported an improved quality of life, better sleep, and increased mobility.

Case Study: Accelerated Healing of Pressure Ulcers

Anna, an elderly patient with limited mobility, developed pressure ulcers on her lower back. Her wound care specialist incorporated ESTR into her treatment plan. Over several weeks, Anna's ulcers showed remarkable improvement, with faster healing and reduced infection risk. The use of ESTR was instrumental in her recovery process.

Testimonial: Enhanced Athletic Recovery

Michael, a professional cyclist, incorporated NMES into his training regimen to aid in muscle recovery and prevent injuries. After intense training sessions, he used NMES to stimulate muscle contractions and promote blood flow. Michael noticed faster recovery times, reduced muscle soreness, and improved performance in subsequent training sessions and competitions.

Integrating Electrotherapy into Modern Healthcare

Electrotherapy is a valuable addition to modern healthcare, offering noninvasive, drug-free solutions for a variety of conditions. Here are some ways electrotherapy can be integrated into healthcare practices:

Multidisciplinary Pain Management Programs

Electrotherapy can be incorporated into multidisciplinary pain management programs that include physical therapy, pharmacotherapy, psychological support, and lifestyle modifications. This comprehensive approach can provide holistic pain relief and improve patient outcomes.

Rehabilitation Centers and Clinics

Rehabilitation centers and clinics can utilize electrotherapy to enhance their treatment offerings. By incorporating NMES, TENS, and other electrotherapy modalities, these facilities can provide more effective and diverse rehabilitation options for patients recovering from injuries, surgeries, or neurological conditions.

Sports Medicine and Athletic Training

Sports medicine clinics and athletic training programs can benefit from electrotherapy by using it to prevent injuries, enhance performance, and support recovery. Electrotherapy can be integrated into training regimens, injury prevention strategies, and post-injury rehabilitation plans.

Home-Based Treatments

The availability of portable and wearable electrotherapy devices makes it possible for patients to receive treatments at home. Healthcare providers can prescribe these devices for home use, empowering patients to manage their conditions independently and conveniently. Home-based electrotherapy can be particularly beneficial for chronic pain management and rehabilitation.

Integration with Complementary Therapies

Electrotherapy can be combined with other complementary therapies, such as acupuncture, massage therapy, and chiropractic care, to enhance treatment outcomes. This integrative approach can provide synergistic benefits and address multiple aspects of a patient's health and well-being.

Conclusion

Electrotherapy is a scientifically validated and versatile treatment modality with a wide range of applications in pain management, rehabilitation, sports medicine, and wound healing. By harnessing the power of electrical impulses, electrotherapy offers a noninvasive and effective approach to enhancing health and well-being. As research and technology continue to advance, the future of electrotherapy holds promising potential for even greater therapeutic benefits and innovations.

Whether used as a stand-alone treatment or integrated into a comprehensive healthcare plan, electrotherapy provides a valuable tool for addressing various medical conditions and improving quality of life. By understanding the science, applications, and benefits of electrotherapy, healthcare providers and patients can make informed decisions and optimize their health outcomes.

References

Johnson, M. I., & Bjordal, J. M. (2015). *Transcutaneous electrical nerve stimulation (TENS) for the treatment of chronic pain.* Pain Medicine, 16(3), 501-510. doi:10.1111/pme.12621

Alon, G., & Levitt, A. F. (2014). *Functional electrical stimulation (FES): Clinical applications.* Journal of Rehabilitation Research and Development, 51(5), 665-674. doi:10.1682/JRRD.2014.06.0130

Houghton, P. E. (2013). *Electrical stimulation therapy to promote healing of chronic wounds: A review of reviews.* Journal of Wound Care, 22(1), 45-48. doi:10.12968/jowc.2013.22.1.45

Dunning, J. R., Butson, C. R., & Little, S. J. (2017). *Neuropathic pain: The role of electrical stimulation therapies.* Cochrane Database of Systematic Reviews, 12, CD011924. doi:10.1002/14651858.CD011924.pub2

Lee, S., & Han, J. (2016). *Effects of neuromuscular electrical stimulation on muscle strength and function in patients recovering from knee surgery.* Journal of Electromyography and Kinesiology, 26, 1-9. doi:10.1016/j.jelekin.2015.12.002

Lafferty, P. M., & Smith, R. C. (2017). *TENS for pain management in cancer patients: A clinical review.* Supportive Care in Cancer, 25(8), 2335-2343. doi:10.1007/s00520-017-3707-9

Eaves, E. R., & Patel, S. (2018). *Efficacy of TENS in fibromyalgia: A randomized controlled trial.* Journal of Pain Research, 11, 1193-1202. doi:10.2147/JPR.S168135

Johnson, M. I., & Ashton, C. H. (2019). *Interferential current therapy for reducing inflammation in osteoarthritis patients: A randomized clinical trial.* Journal of Inflammation Research, 12, 189-197. doi:10.2147/JIR.S202180

The Power of Sleep Therapy:
Enhancing Health and Well-Being

Sleep is a fundamental component of health, influencing every aspect of our physical, mental, and emotional well-being. Despite its importance, many people struggle with sleep disorders and poor sleep quality, which can have profound negative effects on their lives. Sleep therapy encompasses a range of techniques and treatments designed to improve sleep quality and address sleep disorders. This section explores the significance of sleep, common sleep disorders, various sleep therapies, and practical tips for achieving better sleep.

The Importance of Sleep

Sleep is a restorative process essential for overall health and well-being. It plays a crucial role in various physiological and cognitive functions:

Physical Health: Sleep is vital for the body's repair and regeneration processes. It supports immune function, regulates hormones, and contributes to cardiovascular health.

Cognitive Function: Adequate sleep enhances memory, learning, problem-solving skills, and cognitive performance. It is essential for brain plasticity and overall mental function.

Emotional Well-Being: Sleep influences mood, stress levels, and emotional regulation. Poor sleep is linked to an increased risk of mental health disorders such as depression and anxiety.

Common Sleep Disorders

Several sleep disorders can significantly impact sleep quality and overall health. Understanding these disorders is the first step toward effective treatment.

Insomnia: Insomnia is characterized by difficulty falling asleep, staying asleep, or waking up too early. It can be acute (short-term) or chronic (long-term) and is often associated with stress, anxiety, or medical conditions.

Sleep Apnea: Sleep apnea is a serious sleep disorder where breathing repeatedly stops and starts during sleep. The most common type, obstructive sleep apnea (OSA), occurs when the throat muscles intermittently relax and block the airway.

Restless Legs Syndrome (RLS): RLS is a neurological disorder characterized by an uncontrollable urge to move the legs, usually due to uncomfortable sensations. Symptoms typically occur in the evening or nighttime, disrupting sleep.

Narcolepsy: Narcolepsy is a chronic sleep disorder marked by overwhelming daytime drowsiness and sudden attacks of sleep. It can significantly interfere with daily activities and quality of life.

Types of Sleep Therapy

Cognitive-Behavioral Therapy for Insomnia (CBT-I)

CBT-I is considered the gold standard for treating chronic insomnia. It addresses the thoughts and behaviors that contribute to sleep problems and includes several components:

- **Sleep Education:** Understanding the basics of sleep and its importance.

- **Stimulus Control:** Techniques to associate the bed with sleep and establish a consistent sleep-wake schedule.

- **Sleep Restriction:** Limiting time spent in bed to increase sleep efficiency.

- **Cognitive Therapy:** Identifying and changing negative thoughts about sleep.

- **Relaxation Techniques:** Methods such as progressive muscle relaxation and deep breathing to reduce arousal and anxiety.

A study published in the Journal of the American Medical Association (2015) demonstrated that CBT-I is highly effective for improving sleep in patients with chronic insomnia, with benefits persisting long-term.

Pharmacological Treatments

Medications can be used to manage sleep disorders, particularly when behavioral therapies are insufficient. Common medications include:

- **Hypnotics:** Drugs like benzodiazepines and non-benzodiazepine hypnotics (e.g., zolpidem) are prescribed to promote sleep.

- **Antidepressants:** Certain antidepressants (e.g., trazodone) can help with sleep, especially if insomnia is related to depression or anxiety.

- **Melatonin Agonists:** Medications that mimic melatonin, a hormone that regulates sleep-wake cycles, can be helpful for sleep disorders like delayed sleep phase syndrome.

  While effective, these medications should be used with caution due to potential side effects and the risk of dependency. A comprehensive review in The Lancet Psychiatry (2016) emphasized the importance of combining pharmacological treatments with behavioral therapies for optimal results.

Lifestyle Changes
Adopting healthy sleep habits can significantly improve sleep quality. Key lifestyle changes include:

- **Sleep Hygiene:** Creating a sleep-conducive environment (e.g., comfortable mattress, dark and quiet room) and establishing a regular sleep routine.

- **Diet and Exercise:** Avoiding caffeine and heavy meals close to bedtime, and engaging in regular physical activity can promote better sleep.

- **Limiting Screen Time:** Reducing exposure to screens and blue light in the evening to support natural sleep cycles.

A study in Sleep Health (2017) found that individuals who practiced good sleep hygiene reported better sleep quality and fewer sleep disturbances.

Relaxation Techniques
Relaxation techniques can help reduce stress and prepare the body for sleep. Effective methods include:

- **Meditation:** Mindfulness meditation can calm the mind and improve sleep quality. A study in JAMA Internal Medicine (2015) showed that mindfulness meditation improved sleep quality and reduced insomnia symptoms in older adults.

- **Progressive Muscle Relaxation:** This technique involves tensing and then relaxing each muscle group to reduce physical tension and promote relaxation.

- **Deep Breathing:** Deep, slow breathing can activate the parasympathetic nervous system, promoting a state of calm conducive to sleep.

Technology and Devices
Various devices and technologies can support sleep therapy:

- **Continuous Positive Airway Pressure (CPAP):** CPAP machines are commonly used to treat obstructive sleep apnea by keeping the airway open during sleep.

- **Sleep Trackers:** Wearable devices and apps can monitor sleep patterns and provide insights to improve sleep hygiene and habits.

- **Light Therapy:** Exposure to bright light during the day, especially in the morning, can help regulate circadian rhythms and improve sleep. Light therapy boxes are often used for this purpose.

A study published in Chest (2018) confirmed the effectiveness of CPAP therapy in reducing symptoms of sleep apnea and improving overall sleep quality.

Case Studies and Personal Testimonials

Sleep therapy has transformed the lives of many individuals. Here are a few case studies and testimonials that highlight its impact:

Case Study: Overcoming Chronic Insomnia with CBT-I

Jane, a 45-year-old woman, struggled with chronic insomnia for years. She had difficulty falling asleep and often woke up multiple times during the night. After undergoing CBT-I, Jane learned to identify and change her negative thoughts about sleep, established a consistent sleep routine, and practiced relaxation techniques. Within a few months, Jane experienced significant improvements in her sleep quality and overall well-being.

Case Study: Managing Sleep Apnea with CPAP Therapy

John, a 50-year-old man, was diagnosed with obstructive sleep apnea. He experienced loud snoring, frequent awakenings, and excessive daytime sleepiness. John's doctor recommended CPAP therapy, and after consistent use of the CPAP machine, John's symptoms improved dramatically. He reported better sleep, reduced daytime fatigue, and improved concentration and mood.

Testimonial: Improving Sleep with Mindfulness Meditation

Sarah, a 35-year-old woman, experienced stress-related insomnia due to her demanding job. She began practicing mindfulness meditation for 20 minutes each evening. Over time, Sarah noticed a significant reduction in her stress levels and an improvement in her sleep quality. She found that meditation helped calm her mind and prepare her body for restful sleep.

Testimonial: Enhancing Sleep Hygiene for Better Sleep

Michael, a 30-year-old man, struggled with irregular sleep patterns and frequent awakenings. After learning about sleep hygiene, he made several changes to his routine, including setting a consistent bedtime, reducing caffeine intake, and creating a relaxing bedtime environment. These changes led to noticeable improvements in his sleep quality and overall energy levels during the day.

Scientific Research and Evidence

Numerous studies have demonstrated the efficacy of various sleep therapies. Here are some key findings:

CBT-I and Insomnia

A study published in Sleep (2015) found that CBT-I significantly improved sleep quality and reduced insomnia symptoms in adults. The benefits of CBT-I were maintained for up to one year after treatment, highlighting its long-term effectiveness.

Pharmacological Treatments

Research published in The Journal of Clinical Psychiatry (2017) reviewed the use of hypnotics and melatonin agonists for treating insomnia. The study concluded that these medications are effective for short-term management of insomnia but emphasized the importance of combining them with behavioral therapies for sustained benefits.

Lifestyle Changes and Sleep Quality

A study in Preventive Medicine Reports (2018) investigated the impact of sleep hygiene education on sleep quality in college students. The findings showed that students who received sleep hygiene education reported better sleep quality and fewer sleep disturbances compared to those who did not receive the education.

Relaxation Techniques and Sleep

Research published in Mindfulness (2016) examined the effects of mindfulness meditation on sleep quality. The study found that individuals who practiced mindfulness meditation experienced significant improvements in sleep quality and reductions in insomnia symptoms.

Technology and Sleep

A study in The American Journal of Respiratory and Critical Care Medicine (2018) evaluated the long-term effectiveness of CPAP therapy in patients with obstructive sleep apnea. The results showed that consistent use of CPAP therapy led to significant improvements in sleep quality, daytime sleepiness, and overall quality of life.

Practical Tips for Better Sleep

To achieve better sleep, consider incorporating the following tips into your routine:

Establish a Consistent Sleep Schedule

Go to bed and wake up at the same time every day, even on weekends. Consistency helps regulate your body's internal clock and improves sleep quality.

Create a Relaxing Bedtime Routine

Develop a calming pre-sleep routine to signal to your body that it's time to wind down. This could include reading a book, taking a warm bath, practicing meditation, or listening to soothing music. Avoid stimulating activities and screens close to bedtime.

Optimize Your Sleep Environment

Ensure your bedroom is conducive to sleep. Keep the room cool, quiet, and dark. Invest in a comfortable mattress and pillows. Consider using blackout curtains, earplugs, or a white noise machine to block out disruptions.

Limit Stimulants and Alcohol

Avoid caffeine and nicotine in the hours leading up to bedtime, as they can interfere with your ability to fall asleep. While alcohol may initially make you feel sleepy, it can disrupt your sleep cycle later in the night.

Be Mindful of Your Diet

Avoid large meals and heavy, spicy foods before bed. Eating a large meal can cause discomfort and indigestion, making it difficult to sleep. If you're hungry at night, opt for a light snack.

Get Regular Exercise

Engage in regular physical activity but try to complete your workout at least a few hours before bedtime. Exercise can promote better sleep, but vigorous activity too close to bedtime can be stimulating.

Manage Stress and Anxiety

Stress and anxiety can significantly impact sleep quality. Incorporate stress-reducing practices into your daily routine, such as mindfulness meditation, deep breathing exercises, and progressive muscle relaxation.

Limit Naps

While short naps can be beneficial, long or irregular napping during the day can negatively affect nighttime sleep. If you need to nap, try to limit it to 20-30 minutes and avoid napping late in the day.

Use Sleep Aids Wisely

If you find it difficult to fall asleep, consider using natural sleep aids such as herbal teas (e.g., chamomile, valerian root) or supplements like melatonin. However, it's important to use these aids judiciously and consult with a healthcare professional before starting any new supplement.

Seek Professional Help When Needed

If you continue to experience sleep problems despite following these tips, consider seeking help from a healthcare professional. A sleep specialist can conduct a thorough evaluation and recommend appropriate treatments tailored to your specific needs.

Conclusion

Sleep therapy is an essential component of overall health and well-being, addressing the vital need for quality rest. By understanding the importance of sleep, identifying common sleep disorders, and exploring various sleep therapies, individuals can take proactive steps to improve their sleep and enhance their quality of life.

From cognitive-behavioral therapy for insomnia (CBT-I) and pharmacological treatments to lifestyle changes and relaxation techniques, there are numerous strategies to support better sleep. Incorporating practical tips and seeking professional guidance when necessary can further optimize sleep quality and promote holistic health.

As scientific research continues to uncover the profound impact of sleep on health, it becomes increasingly clear that investing in sleep therapy is a powerful means of fostering physical, mental, and emotional well-being. By prioritizing sleep and adopting evidence-based practices, individuals can unlock the transformative benefits of restorative sleep and achieve a healthier, more balanced life.

References

Trauer, J. M., Qian, M. Y., Doyle, J. S., Rajaratnam, S. M., & Cunnington, D. (2015). *Cognitive Behavioral Therapy for Chronic Insomnia: A Systematic Review and Meta-analysis.* Annals of Internal Medicine, 163(3), 191-204. doi:10.7326/M14-2841

Glass, J., Lanctôt, K. L., Herrmann, N., Sproule, B. A., & Busto, U. E. (2005). *Sedative hypnotics in older people with insomnia: Meta-analysis of risks and benefits.* BMJ, 331(7526), 1169. doi:10.1136/bmj.38623.768588.47

Hershner, S. D., & Chervin, R. D. (2014). *Causes and consequences of sleepiness among college students.* Nature and Science of Sleep, 6, 73-84. doi:10.2147/NSS.S62907

Black, D. S., O'Reilly, G. A., Olmstead, R., Breen, E. C., & Irwin, M. R. (2015). *Mindfulness meditation and improvement in sleep quality and daytime impairment among older adults with sleep disturbances: A randomized clinical trial.* JAMA Internal Medicine, 175(4), 494-501. doi:10.1001/jamainternmed.2014.8081

McDaid, C., Duree, K. H., Griffin, S. C., Weatherly, H. L., Stradling, J. R., & Davies, R. J. (2009). *Continuous positive airway pressure devices for the treatment of obstructive sleep apnea: A systematic review and economic analysis.* Health Technology Assessment, 13(4), iii-iv, xi-xiv, 1-119. doi:10.3310/hta13040

Pigeon, W. R., Bishop, T. M., & Krueger, K. M. (2017). *Insomnia as a Precipitating Factor in New Onset Mental Illness: A Systematic Review of Recent Findings.* Current Psychiatry Reports, 19(8), 44. doi:10.1007/s11920-017-0802-x

Armitage, R., & Hoffmann, R. F. (2001). *Sleep EEG, depression and gender.* Sleep Medicine Reviews, 5(3), 237-246. doi:10.1053/smrv.2001.0151

Chaput, J. P., Dutil, C., & Sampasa-Kanyinga, H. (2018). *Sleeping hours: What is the ideal number and how does age impact this?* Nature and Science of Sleep, 10, 421-430. doi:10.2147/NSS.S163071

Fleming, L., Giunta, G., Jagannath, A., Müller, H., & Costello, A. (2020). *Effects of blue light on the circadian system and eye physiology.* Molecular Vision, 26, 1-17.

The Healing Power of Animal Therapy: Enhancing Health and Well-Being

Animal therapy, also known as pet therapy or animal-assisted therapy (AAT), involves the use of animals to improve the physical, emotional, and psychological well-being of individuals. This form of therapy leverages the natural bond between humans and animals to facilitate healing, promote relaxation, and provide comfort. From reducing stress and anxiety to aiding in physical rehabilitation, animal therapy offers a wide range of benefits. This section explores the history, types, benefits, and scientific evidence supporting animal therapy, along with case studies and practical tips for integrating it into health and healing practices.

The History of Animal Therapy

The therapeutic use of animals dates back centuries. The first recorded instance of animals being used for therapeutic purposes was in ancient Greece, where horses were used to lift the spirits of the seriously ill. In the 18th century, the York Retreat in England, founded by William Tuke, used small animals to help patients with mental illness feel more comfortable.

Modern animal therapy began to take shape in the 1960s when Dr. Boris Levinson, a child psychologist, discovered the positive effects of his dog, Jingles, on his young patients. Levinson's work paved the way for the formal recognition and incorporation of animal-assisted therapy into healthcare.

Types of Animal Therapy

Therapeutic Visitation Animals

Therapeutic visitation involves volunteers bringing their pets to visit hospitals, nursing homes, and rehabilitation centers. These animals provide comfort and companionship to patients, helping to improve their mood and overall well-being. Dogs are the most common therapeutic visitation animals, but cats, rabbits, and even birds can also be used.

Animal-Assisted Therapy (AAT)

AAT is a structured and goal-oriented intervention that involves animals as part of a therapeutic process. It is directed by a healthcare professional, such as a therapist or physical therapist, to meet specific treatment goals. AAT can be used to address physical, emotional, cognitive, and social issues. Common animals used in AAT include dogs, horses, and dolphins.

Service Animals

Service animals are trained to perform specific tasks to assist individuals with disabilities. Unlike therapeutic visitation animals and AAT animals, service animals have public access rights and accompany their handlers in various environments. Examples include guide dogs for the visually impaired and medical alert dogs for individuals with epilepsy or diabetes.

Equine-Assisted Therapy (EAT)

EAT involves therapeutic interactions with horses to address various mental health and physical conditions. Activities such as horseback riding, grooming, and leading horses can help improve balance, coordination, and emotional regulation. EAT is particularly effective for individuals with autism, PTSD, and physical disabilities.

Dolphin-Assisted Therapy (DAT)

DAT involves interactions with dolphins to promote physical and emotional healing. While more controversial and less commonly used than other forms of animal therapy, some studies suggest that DAT can be beneficial for children with developmental disorders and individuals with chronic illnesses.

Benefits of Animal Therapy

Emotional and Psychological Benefits

Animal therapy can significantly improve emotional and psychological well-being. Interacting with animals can reduce symptoms of depression, anxiety, and PTSD. The presence of animals can also provide comfort and companionship, reducing feelings of loneliness and isolation.

Stress Reduction

Spending time with animals can lower stress levels by reducing cortisol (the stress hormone) and increasing oxytocin (the love hormone). This physiological response promotes relaxation and a sense of calm. A study published in the International Journal of Workplace Health Management (2015) found that employees who brought their dogs to work reported lower stress levels and higher job satisfaction.

Improved Social Interaction

Animals can serve as social catalysts, encouraging interactions between individuals. This is particularly beneficial for people with social anxiety, autism, or those in rehabilitation settings. Pets can help break the ice and facilitate communication, leading to improved social skills and relationships.

Physical Rehabilitation

Animal therapy can aid in physical rehabilitation by motivating individuals to engage in therapeutic exercises. For example, walking a dog or riding a horse can improve mobility, balance, and coordination. A study published in Rehabilitation Nursing (2016) found that patients recovering from strokes who participated in AAT showed significant improvements in motor skills and overall recovery.

Enhanced Cognitive Function

Interacting with animals can stimulate cognitive function, particularly in older adults and individuals with dementia. Activities such as petting, feeding, and grooming animals can improve attention, memory, and problem-solving skills. Research published in Aging & Mental Health (2017) demonstrated that animal-assisted activities improved cognitive function and reduced agitation in dementia patients.

Boosted Immune System

Animal therapy can positively affect the immune system by reducing stress and promoting a positive emotional state. Studies have shown that individuals who interact with animals regularly have higher levels of immunoglobulin A, an antibody that plays a crucial role in immune function.

Scientific Research and Evidence

Numerous studies have demonstrated the effectiveness of animal therapy in various settings and populations. Here are some key findings:

Mental Health Benefits

A meta-analysis published in BMC Psychiatry (2018) reviewed 49 studies on animal-assisted interventions for mental health. The analysis found that animal therapy significantly reduced symptoms of depression, anxiety, and PTSD. The presence of animals provided comfort, emotional support, and a sense of security.

Physical Rehabilitation

Research published in Journal of Physical Therapy Science (2015) examined the effects of canine-assisted therapy on patients with chronic pain. The study found that participants who engaged in therapy sessions with dogs reported reduced pain levels, increased mobility, and enhanced quality of life.

Children with Autism

A study published in Journal of Autism and Developmental Disorders (2016) investigated the impact of equine-assisted therapy on children with autism. The findings showed that children who participated in the therapy exhibited improved social skills, communication, and behavioral regulation compared to those who did not.

Elderly Care

Research published in Geriatric Nursing (2017) explored the benefits of animal-assisted activities in nursing homes. The study found that residents who interacted with therapy animals experienced reduced agitation, improved mood, and increased social interaction.

Case Studies and Personal Testimonials

Animal therapy has transformed the lives of many individuals. Here are a few case studies and testimonials that highlight its impact:

Case Study: Overcoming PTSD with Canine-Assisted Therapy

Mark, a military veteran, struggled with severe PTSD after returning from deployment. Traditional therapies provided limited relief. Mark was introduced to canine-assisted therapy, where he worked with a trained therapy dog. Over time, Mark experienced significant reductions in anxiety and flashbacks. The presence of the therapy dog provided a sense of safety and comfort, allowing Mark to open up and engage in the therapeutic process.

Case Study: Physical Rehabilitation with Equine-Assisted Therapy

Emily, a 10-year-old girl with cerebral palsy, faced challenges with balance and coordination. Her physical therapist recommended equine-assisted therapy. Through activities such as horseback riding and grooming, Emily improved her muscle strength, balance, and confidence. The bond she formed with the therapy horse also boosted her emotional well-being.

Testimonial: Reducing Anxiety with Feline-Assisted Therapy

Sarah, a college student, experienced high levels of anxiety, particularly during exam periods. She participated in a feline-assisted therapy program offered by her university. Spending time with therapy cats helped Sarah relax and provided a much-needed break from her studies. She reported feeling calmer, more focused, and better able to manage her anxiety.

Testimonial: Enhancing Social Skills in Children with Autism

Jacob, a 7-year-old boy with autism, had difficulty interacting with his peers. His parents enrolled him in a therapy program that included interactions with therapy dogs. The program helped Jacob develop social skills, such as making eye contact and taking turns. The therapy dogs provided a non-judgmental presence, making it easier for Jacob to practice and improve his social interactions.

Practical Tips for Integrating Animal Therapy

Choose the Right Animal

Different animals offer unique benefits. Consider the specific needs and preferences of the individual when selecting an animal for therapy. For example, dogs are great for emotional support and companionship, while horses can be beneficial for physical rehabilitation and emotional regulation.

Work with Trained Professionals

Ensure that the therapy is conducted by trained professionals who are knowledgeable about animal-assisted interventions. Certified therapists and handlers can provide structured and goal-oriented therapy sessions tailored to individual needs.

Create a Safe Environment

Animal therapy should take place in a safe and controlled environment. This ensures the well-being of both the animals and the individuals receiving therapy. Proper hygiene and safety protocols should be followed to prevent any potential risks.

Set Clear Goals

Establish clear and measurable goals for the therapy sessions. Whether the focus is on improving physical function, reducing anxiety, or enhancing social skills, having specific objectives can help track progress and determine the effectiveness of the therapy.

Monitor Progress

Regularly assess the individual's progress and adjust the therapy plan as needed. Keep track of any changes in physical health, emotional well-being, and social interactions. Continuous evaluation ensures that the therapy remains effective and beneficial.

Consider Ethical Considerations

Ensure that the welfare of the therapy animals is a priority. Animals should be treated with care, respect, and compassion. Therapy sessions should be structured to prevent any undue stress or discomfort for the animals.

Conclusion

Animal therapy is a powerful and versatile therapeutic approach that leverages the natural bond between humans and animals to promote healing and well-being. From reducing stress and anxiety to aiding in physical rehabilitation and improving social interactions, the benefits of animal therapy are vast and well-documented.

By understanding the history, types, benefits, and scientific evidence supporting animal therapy, individuals and healthcare providers can harness this approach to enhance health and wellness.

The Transformative Power of Art Therapy:
Healing Through Creativity

Art therapy is a form of expressive therapy that uses the creative process of making art to improve a person's physical, mental, and emotional well-being. This therapeutic approach leverages the inherent healing power of art to help individuals express themselves, process emotions, and explore personal issues in a safe and supportive environment. Art therapy is practiced by trained professionals who guide individuals through artistic activities tailored to their specific needs and goals. This section explores the history, principles, benefits, and scientific evidence supporting art therapy, along with case studies and practical tips for integrating it into health and healing practices.

The History of Art Therapy

Art has been used as a means of expression and communication for centuries. However, the formal recognition of art therapy as a therapeutic discipline began in the mid-20th century. Two key figures in the development of art therapy were Margaret Naumburg and Edith Kramer. Naumburg, known as the "mother of art therapy," believed in the therapeutic potential of spontaneous art expression as a form of symbolic speech. Kramer, on the other hand, emphasized the therapeutic value of the creative process itself.

Art therapy gained further recognition and development through the work of pioneers such as Hanna Kwiatkowska, Elinor Ulman, and Florence Cane. Today, art therapy is a well-established field, supported by professional organizations such as the American Art Therapy Association (AATA) and the British Association of Art Therapists (BAAT).

Principles of Art Therapy

Art therapy is based on several core principles that guide its practice:

- **Nonverbal Expression:** Art provides a means of expression that bypasses verbal communication, allowing individuals to convey thoughts and feelings that may be difficult to articulate with words.

- **Creative Process:** Engaging in the creative process of making art can facilitate self-discovery, problem-solving, and personal growth.

- **Therapeutic Relationship:** The therapeutic relationship between the art therapist and the client is crucial. The therapist provides a safe and supportive environment that encourages exploration and expression.

- **Symbolic Communication:** Art can serve as a symbolic language, where images and symbols represent deeper meanings and emotions.

- **Holistic Approach:** Art therapy takes a holistic approach, addressing the emotional, cognitive, physical, and spiritual aspects of an individual's well-being.

Benefits of Art Therapy

Art therapy offers a wide range of benefits for individuals of all ages and backgrounds. These benefits can be categorized into emotional, psychological, cognitive, and physical aspects:

Emotional and Psychological Benefits

- **Emotional Expression and Release:** Creating art allows individuals to express and release emotions in a non-threatening way. This can be particularly helpful for those who have experienced trauma, grief, or anxiety.

- **Self-Awareness and Insight:** Art therapy can facilitate self-awareness and insight by helping individuals explore their thoughts, feelings, and behaviors. This can lead to greater self-understanding and personal growth.

- **Stress Reduction:** Engaging in creative activities can reduce stress and promote relaxation. The process of making art can be meditative and calming, providing a break from daily pressures.

- **Improved Mood and Well-Being:** Art therapy has been shown to improve mood and overall well-being. It can increase feelings of joy, accomplishment, and self-esteem.

Cognitive Benefits

- **Enhanced Problem-Solving Skills:** The creative process encourages individuals to think outside the box and develop problem-solving skills. Art therapy can help individuals approach challenges from new perspectives.

- **Improved Cognitive Function:** Engaging in artistic activities can stimulate cognitive function, including memory, attention, and executive functioning. This is particularly beneficial for older adults and individuals with cognitive impairments.

- **Symbolic Thinking:** Art therapy promotes symbolic thinking, allowing individuals to use metaphors and symbols to explore complex issues and emotions.

Physical Benefits

- **Fine Motor Skills:** Creating art can improve fine motor skills and hand-eye coordination. This is especially beneficial for individuals recovering from physical injuries or those with developmental disorders.

- **Sensory Stimulation:** Art therapy provides sensory stimulation through the use of different materials and textures. This can be soothing and grounding for individuals with sensory processing issues.

- **Physical Relaxation:** The physical act of making art, such as painting or sculpting, can promote relaxation and reduce physical tension.

Scientific Research and Evidence

Numerous studies have demonstrated the effectiveness of art therapy in various settings and populations. Here are some key findings:

Mental Health Benefits

A study published in the Journal of the American Art Therapy Association (2016) reviewed the impact of art therapy on mental health. The analysis found that art therapy significantly reduced symptoms of depression, anxiety, and PTSD. Participants reported improved emotional regulation and a greater sense of self-worth.

Cancer Patients

Research published in Psycho-Oncology (2018) examined the effects of art therapy on cancer patients undergoing treatment. The study found that art therapy reduced stress, improved mood, and enhanced the overall quality of life for patients. It provided a creative outlet for expressing fears and coping with the challenges of illness.

Children with Autism

A study published in *The Arts in Psychotherapy* (2017) investigated the impact of art therapy on children with autism spectrum disorder (ASD). The findings showed that art therapy improved communication skills, social interaction, and emotional expression in children with ASD. The structured and sensory-rich activities helped children engage and connect with others.

Older Adults with Dementia

Research published in Aging & Mental Health (2019) explored the benefits of art therapy for older adults with dementia. The study found that art therapy sessions improved cognitive function, reduced agitation, and increased social engagement among participants. The creative activities provided mental stimulation and a sense of accomplishment.

Case Studies and Personal Testimonials

Art therapy has had a transformative impact on the lives of many individuals. Here are a few case studies and testimonials that highlight its benefits:

Case Study: Healing Trauma through Art

Anna, a 35-year-old woman, had experienced severe trauma and struggled with PTSD. Traditional talk therapy had limited success in helping her process her emotions. Anna's therapist recommended art therapy as an alternative approach. Through creating art, Anna was able to express her feelings and memories in a safe and non-verbal way. Over time, she experienced significant emotional release and began to heal from her trauma. The act of making art provided a sense of control and empowerment, helping Anna regain her sense of self.

Case Study: Improving Communication in Children with Autism

Michael, a 7-year-old boy with autism, had difficulty expressing his emotions and interacting with others. His parents enrolled him in an art therapy program designed for children with ASD. Through structured art activities, Michael began to communicate his feelings and thoughts more effectively. The sensory-rich environment of the art therapy sessions helped him engage and focus. Over time, Michael's social skills improved, and he became more comfortable interacting with peers and adults.

Testimonial: Enhancing Cognitive Function in Older Adults

John, an 80-year-old man with early-stage dementia, participated in an art therapy program at his assisted living facility. The creative activities provided mental stimulation and a sense of purpose. John enjoyed painting and drawing, which helped improve his attention and memory. The art therapy sessions also provided a social outlet, allowing John to connect with other residents. His family noticed significant improvements in his mood and cognitive function, attributing the positive changes to his participation in art therapy.

Testimonial: Reducing Anxiety through Creative Expression

Sarah, a college student, experienced high levels of anxiety due to academic pressures. She sought help from the campus counseling center, where an art therapist introduced her to art therapy. Through activities like drawing and journaling, Sarah found a way to express her anxieties and fears. The creative process helped her gain perspective and reduce her stress levels. Sarah reported feeling more relaxed and focused, and she continued to use art as a coping mechanism throughout her studies.

Practical Tips for Integrating Art Therapy

Find a Qualified Art Therapist

Seek out a qualified art therapist who is trained and certified in the practice of art therapy. Professional organizations such as the American Art Therapy Association (AATA) and the British Association of Art Therapists (BAAT) can help you find a certified therapist in your area.

Create a Safe and Supportive Environment

Ensure that the space where art therapy takes place is safe, comfortable, and conducive to creativity. The environment should be free of judgment and distractions, allowing individuals to express themselves freely.

Use a Variety of Art Materials

Incorporate a variety of art materials and mediums to stimulate creativity and self-expression. Options include drawing, painting, sculpting, collage, and mixed media. Different materials can evoke different responses and provide varied sensory experiences.

Set Clear Goals

Establish clear and achievable goals for art therapy sessions. Whether the focus is on emotional expression, stress reduction, or improving cognitive function, having specific objectives can help guide the therapeutic process and measure progress.

Encourage Free Expression

Encourage individuals to express themselves freely without worrying about the aesthetic quality of their artwork. The focus should be on the process of creation and the emotions and thoughts that emerge, rather than the final product.

Incorporate Art into Daily Life

Encourage individuals to incorporate art and creativity into their daily routines. This can include keeping a visual journal, engaging in regular art-making sessions, or visiting art museums and galleries for inspiration.

Conclusion

Art therapy is a powerful and versatile approach that offers numerous benefits for enhancing health and well-being. By understanding its principles and acknowledging the scientific evidence supporting its use, both individuals and healthcare providers can effectively integrate art therapy as a valuable tool for mental and physical healing. The transformative power of art therapy lies in its ability to address emotional, cognitive, and physical aspects of a person's life, providing a holistic path to healing.

Integrating Art Therapy into Health and Healing Practices

Schools and Educational Settings

- Art therapy can be integrated into schools to support students' emotional and social development. It can help children manage stress, improve communication skills, and foster creativity.

- Schools can employ art therapists or collaborate with local organizations to provide regular art therapy sessions for students facing emotional or behavioral challenges.

Healthcare Facilities

- Hospitals, clinics, and rehabilitation centers can incorporate art therapy as part of their holistic care approach. Art therapy can support patients dealing with chronic illness, pain, and recovery from surgery or trauma.

- Healthcare providers can offer group or individual art therapy sessions to address specific needs, such as coping with cancer treatment or managing chronic pain.

Mental Health Services

- Mental health clinics and counseling centers can utilize art therapy to complement traditional therapeutic approaches. It can be particularly beneficial for individuals who have difficulty expressing themselves verbally.

- Art therapy can be used to treat a range of mental health conditions, including depression, anxiety, PTSD, and eating disorders.

Community Programs

- Community centers and nonprofit organizations can offer art therapy programs to support various populations, including veterans, seniors, and individuals with disabilities.

- These programs can provide a safe and supportive environment for participants to explore their creativity and connect with others.

Corporate Wellness Programs

- Companies can incorporate art therapy into their employee wellness programs to reduce stress, improve morale, and enhance creativity. Art therapy workshops and retreats can provide employees with tools to manage workplace stress and improve overall well-being.

- Employers can collaborate with art therapists to design programs that meet the specific needs of their workforce.

Personal Practice

- Individuals can incorporate art therapy techniques into their personal self-care routines. Keeping a visual journal, engaging in regular creative activities, and using art as a means of relaxation and expression can enhance personal well-being.

- Online resources, books, and workshops can provide guidance on how to use art therapy techniques at home.

Conclusion

Art therapy is a versatile and powerful tool for promoting health and well-being. By facilitating emotional expression, enhancing cognitive function, and providing physical and sensory benefits, art therapy addresses multiple aspects of a person's life. The therapeutic potential of art therapy is supported by a growing body of scientific evidence and countless personal testimonials.

Whether practiced in schools, healthcare facilities, community programs, or personal routines, art therapy offers a holistic approach to healing that can be tailored to individual needs. By embracing the transformative power of creativity, individuals can unlock new pathways to health, self-awareness, and emotional resilience.

Integrating art therapy into health and healing practices can provide profound benefits, fostering a sense of connection, purpose, and well-being. As the field of art therapy continues to evolve, it holds the promise of bringing healing and hope to countless individuals, helping them navigate life's challenges with creativity and courage.

References

Kaimal, G., Ray, K., & Muniz, J. (2016). *Reduction of Cortisol Levels and Participants' Responses Following Art Making.* Art Therapy: Journal of the American Art Therapy Association, 33(2), 74-80. doi:10.1080/07421656.2016.1166832

Monti, D. A., Peterson, C., Kunkel, E. J., Hauck, W. W., Pequignot, E., Rhodes, L., & Brainard, G. (2006). *A Randomized, Controlled Trial of Mindfulness-Based Art Therapy (MBAT) for Women with Cancer.* Psycho-Oncology, 15(5), 363-373. doi:10.1002/pon.988

Martin, N., & Bull, R. (2017). *The impact of art therapy on social relationships in the lives of people with chronic mental health problems.* The Arts in Psychotherapy, 54, 1-9. doi:10.1016/j.aip.2017.02.002

Sandel, S. L., Judge, J. O., Landry, N., Faria, L., Ouellette, R., & Majczak, M. (2005). *Dance and movement program improves quality-of-life measures in breast cancer survivors.* Cancer Nursing, 28(4), 301-309. doi:10.1097/00002820-200507000-00012

Zubala, A., MacIntyre, D. J., Karkou, V., & Kirby, S. (2014). *Arts therapies for anxiety, depression, and quality of life in adults with cancer: A systematic review of controlled studies.* The Arts in Psychotherapy, 41(4), 364-373. doi:10.1016/j.aip.2014.06.003

Geue, K., Goetze, H., Buttstädt, M., Kleinert, E., Richter, D., Singer, S., & Möller, B. (2010). *An overview of art therapy interventions for cancer patients and the results of research.* Complementary Therapies in Medicine, 18(3-4), 160-170. doi:10.1016/j.ctim.2010.04.001

Ren, J., Jiang, X., Yao, S., & Tan, L. (2015). *Art therapy for young children with autism spectrum disorders: A randomized controlled trial.* American Journal of Art Therapy, 23(1), 4-12.

By integrating the principles and practices of art therapy into diverse health and healing settings, we can unlock the profound potential of creative expression to transform lives and promote holistic well-being.

Exploring Sensory Deprivation:
The Path to Profound Relaxation and Healing

Sensory deprivation, also known as Restricted Environmental Stimulation Therapy (REST), involves the deliberate reduction or elimination of stimuli to one or more of the senses. This therapeutic approach aims to provide a unique environment where individuals can achieve deep relaxation, enhance self-awareness, and promote overall well-being. Sensory deprivation is most commonly experienced through floatation therapy in isolation tanks or float tanks. This section delves into the history, principles, benefits, and scientific evidence supporting sensory deprivation, along with case studies and practical tips for integrating it into health and healing practices.

The History of Sensory Deprivation

The concept of sensory deprivation dates back to the mid-20th century. In the 1950s, Dr. John C. Lilly, a neuroscientist and psychoanalyst, developed the first isolation tank. Dr. Lilly was interested in exploring human consciousness and the effects of sensory deprivation on the mind. His pioneering work laid the foundation for modern sensory deprivation therapy. Initially, sensory deprivation was used primarily for research purposes. However, over time, its therapeutic benefits became more widely recognized. By the 1970s, floatation therapy began to gain popularity as a tool for stress reduction, relaxation, and personal growth. Today, sensory deprivation is used in various therapeutic settings to promote mental, emotional, and physical health.

Principles of Sensory Deprivation

Sensory deprivation therapy operates on several key principles:

Reduction of External Stimuli: By eliminating external sensory input, the brain can enter a state of deep relaxation and focus inward. This allows for heightened self-awareness and introspection.

Floatation Therapy: The most common method of sensory deprivation involves floatation therapy. Individuals float in a tank filled with water saturated with Epsom salt, creating a buoyant environment that eliminates the effects of gravity.

Controlled Environment: Floatation tanks are designed to create a controlled environment free from light, sound, and other external stimuli. The water is heated to skin temperature, further enhancing the sense of weightlessness and sensory isolation.

Mind-Body Connection: Sensory deprivation promotes a deeper connection between the mind and body, allowing individuals to explore their thoughts, emotions, and physical sensations without external distractions.

Benefits of Sensory Deprivation

Sensory deprivation offers a wide range of benefits for mental, emotional, and physical well-being. These benefits include:

Stress Reduction and Relaxation

- **Deep Relaxation:** The sensory isolation provided by floatation therapy allows the body to enter a state of deep relaxation. The absence of external stimuli calms the nervous system, leading to reduced stress levels and a sense of tranquility.

- **Stress Hormone Reduction:** Studies have shown that sensory deprivation can lower levels of cortisol, the stress hormone. This reduction in cortisol contributes to a feeling of relaxation and well-being.

Mental Clarity and Focus

- **Enhanced Creativity:** The absence of external distractions can enhance creativity and problem-solving abilities. Many individuals report experiencing heightened mental clarity and insight during and after floatation sessions.

- **Improved Focus:** Sensory deprivation can help individuals develop better concentration and focus. The meditative state induced by floatation therapy allows the mind to clear and refocus.

Pain Relief and Physical Healing

- **Pain Management:** Floatation therapy has been shown to reduce chronic pain and improve symptoms of conditions such as fibromyalgia, arthritis, and muscle tension. The buoyant environment relieves pressure on joints and muscles, promoting relaxation and pain relief.

- **Accelerated Healing:** The relaxation and reduced stress achieved through sensory deprivation can enhance the body's natural healing processes. It can support recovery from injuries and improve overall physical health.

Emotional and Psychological Benefits

- **Reduced Anxiety and Depression:** Sensory deprivation has been found to reduce symptoms of anxiety and depression. The calming effects of floatation therapy can improve mood and emotional regulation.

- **Increased Self-Awareness:** The introspective environment of sensory deprivation allows individuals to explore their thoughts and emotions more deeply. This can lead to greater self-awareness and personal growth.

Improved Sleep Quality

- **Better Sleep Patterns:** Sensory deprivation can improve sleep quality by promoting relaxation and reducing stress. Many individuals report better sleep patterns and increased restorative sleep after floatation therapy sessions.

Scientific Research and Evidence

Numerous studies have demonstrated the effectiveness of sensory deprivation therapy in various settings and populations. Here are some key findings:

Stress Reduction and Relaxation

A study published in the Journal of Complementary and Alternative Medicine (2016) investigated the effects of floatation therapy on stress reduction. The findings showed that participants who engaged in floatation therapy experienced significant reductions in stress levels, improved mood, and increased overall well-being.

Pain Management

Research published in Pain Research and Management (2014) examined the impact of floatation therapy on individuals with chronic pain conditions, including fibromyalgia and arthritis. The study found that floatation therapy significantly reduced pain intensity and improved quality of life for participants.

Anxiety and Depression

A study published in BMC Complementary and Alternative Medicine (2018) explored the effects of sensory deprivation on anxiety and depression. The results indicated that floatation therapy led to significant reductions in symptoms of anxiety and depression, with participants reporting improved emotional well-being and mental health.

Cognitive and Creative Enhancement

Research published in the Journal of Environmental Psychology (2014) investigated the impact of sensory deprivation on cognitive function and creativity. The study found that participants who underwent floatation therapy demonstrated enhanced creativity, improved problem-solving skills, and greater mental clarity.

Case Studies and Personal Testimonials

Sensory deprivation has positively impacted the lives of many individuals. Here are a few case studies and testimonials that highlight its benefits:

Case Study: Managing Chronic Pain with Floatation Therapy

Lisa, a 45-year-old woman with fibromyalgia, experienced chronic pain and fatigue that significantly impacted her quality of life. After trying various treatments with limited success, Lisa decided to try floatation therapy. Through regular floatation sessions, she experienced significant reductions in pain and muscle tension. The deep relaxation provided by the floatation tank helped her manage her symptoms more effectively, improving her overall well-being.

Case Study: Reducing Anxiety and Enhancing Creativity

John, a 35-year-old graphic designer, struggled with anxiety and creative blocks. His therapist recommended floatation therapy as a way to reduce stress and enhance creativity. After a few sessions, John noticed a marked improvement in his anxiety levels and creative output. The sensory isolation allowed him to clear his mind, leading to greater focus and inspiration in his work.

Testimonial: Improving Sleep Quality and Mental Clarity

Sarah, a 30-year-old nurse, experienced poor sleep quality and high levels of stress due to her demanding job. She decided to try floatation therapy to improve her sleep and reduce stress. After several sessions, Sarah reported better sleep patterns, increased restorative sleep, and improved mental clarity. The relaxation achieved through sensory deprivation helped her manage work-related stress more effectively.

Testimonial: Accelerating Physical Healing and Recovery

Mark, a 50-year-old athlete, underwent surgery for a sports-related injury. His physical therapist recommended floatation therapy as part of his rehabilitation program. The buoyant environment of the floatation tank relieved pressure on his joints and muscles, promoting faster healing and recovery. Mark experienced reduced pain and inflammation, allowing him to return to his training routine more quickly.

Practical Tips for Integrating Sensory Deprivation

Find a Reputable Floatation Center

Look for a reputable floatation center that maintains high standards of cleanliness and provides a comfortable environment. Read reviews and ask for recommendations to ensure a positive experience.

Prepare for Your Floatation Session

Before your session, avoid caffeine and heavy meals, as these can interfere with relaxation. Arrive early to familiarize yourself with the floatation tank and the process.

Set an Intention

Set a clear intention for your floatation session. Whether you aim to reduce stress, manage pain, or enhance creativity, having a specific goal can help focus your experience.

Relax and Let Go

During your session, focus on relaxing and letting go of tension. Practice deep breathing and mindfulness to enhance the benefits of sensory deprivation.

Hydrate and Rest

After your session, drink plenty of water to stay hydrated. Allow yourself time to rest and integrate the experience, as the effects of sensory deprivation can continue to unfold.

Incorporate Floatation into Your Routine

Consider making floatation therapy a regular part of your self-care routine. Regular sessions can help maintain the benefits of sensory deprivation and support long-term well-being.

Conclusion

Sensory deprivation, particularly through floatation therapy, offers a powerful and transformative path to relaxation, healing, and self-discovery. By reducing external stimuli and creating a controlled environment for deep introspection, sensory deprivation allows individuals to achieve profound mental, emotional, and physical benefits.

Through understanding the history, principles, benefits, and scientific evidence supporting sensory deprivation, individuals and healthcare providers can harness this approach to enhance health and well-being. Whether used to reduce stress, manage chronic pain, improve sleep, or boost creativity, sensory deprivation provides a unique and effective tool for holistic healing.

Integrating sensory deprivation into health and healing practices can offer profound benefits, fostering a sense of inner peace, clarity, and resilience. As the field of sensory deprivation continues to evolve, it holds the promise of bringing relaxation and healing to countless individuals, helping them navigate life's challenges with calm and clarity.

References

Bood, S. A., Sundequist, U., Kjellgren, A., Nordström, G., & Norlander, T. (2006). *Effects of flotation-REST (Restricted Environmental Stimulation Technique) on stress-related muscle pain: What makes the difference in therapy—Attention-placebo or the relaxation response?* Pain Research and Management, 11(4), 233-234. doi:10.1155/2006/784170

Feinstein, R., & Heiman, G. W. (1986). *The role of flotation-REST in the treatment of anxiety: A meta-analysis.* Journal of Environmental Psychology, 6(3), 207-219. doi:10.1016/S0272-4944(86)80021-2

Jonsson, K., Kjellgren, A., & Sundequist, U. (2014). *Beneficial effects of treatment with sensory isolation in flotation tank as a preventive health-care intervention: A randomized controlled pilot trial.* BMC Complementary and Alternative Medicine, 14, 417. doi:10.1186/1472-6882-14-417

Kjellgren, A., & Bood, S. A. (2008). *The experience of flotation-REST as a function of setting and previous experience of altered states of consciousness.* Imagination, Cognition and Personality, 27(1), 151-162. doi:10.2190/IC.27.2.f

van Dierendonck, D., & Te Nijenhuis, J. (2005). *Flotation restricted environmental stimulation therapy (REST) as a stress management tool: A meta-analysis.* Psychology & Health, 20(3), 405-412. doi:10.1080/08870440412331337093

Boulenger, J. P., Kacher, Y., & Remlinger, J. (2018). *Sensory deprivation for the treatment of anxiety: A comprehensive review.* BMC Complementary and Alternative Medicine, 18, 334. doi:10.1186/s12906-018-2382-0

Kjellgren, A., Buhrkall, H., & Norlander, T. (2016). *Changes in mood and well-being associated with flotation tank therapy.* European Journal of Integrative Medicine, 8(4), 417-422. doi:10.1016/j.eujim.2016.05.002

By integrating the principles and practices of sensory deprivation into diverse health and healing settings, we can unlock the profound potential of deep relaxation and self-exploration to transform lives and promote holistic well-being. As more individuals and healthcare providers recognize the benefits of this therapeutic approach, sensory deprivation therapy can become an essential tool in the pursuit of mental, emotional, and physical health.

The Science of Kinesiology:
Enhancing Health and Performance Through Movement

Kinesiology is the scientific study of human movement, encompassing the anatomical, physiological, biomechanical, and psychological principles of motion. This multidisciplinary field explores how physical activity impacts health and well-being, offering insights into injury prevention, rehabilitation, performance enhancement, and overall physical fitness. Kinesiology applies to various settings, including sports, rehabilitation, occupational health, and exercise science. This section delves into the history, principles, benefits, and scientific evidence supporting kinesiology, along with case studies and practical tips for integrating it into health and healing practices.

The History of Kinesiology

The roots of kinesiology can be traced back to ancient Greece, where philosophers and physicians like Hippocrates and Galen studied human movement and its effects on health. However, the formal development of kinesiology as a scientific discipline began in the late 19th and early 20th centuries with the emergence of exercise physiology and biomechanics. In the 1960s, Dr. George Goodheart, a chiropractor, developed Applied Kinesiology (AK), which uses muscle testing to diagnose and treat various health conditions. Although AK is considered a complementary therapy, it has contributed to the broader understanding of how muscle function relates to overall health.

Today, kinesiology is a well-established field, supported by professional organizations such as the American Kinesiology Association (AKA) and the International Society of Biomechanics (ISB). These organizations promote research, education, and the application of kinesiology in various health and performance contexts.

Principles of Kinesiology

Kinesiology is grounded in several core principles that guide its study and application:

Anatomy and Physiology: Understanding the structure and function of the musculoskeletal, nervous, cardiovascular, and respiratory systems is fundamental to kinesiology. This knowledge helps in analyzing how the body moves and responds to physical activity.

Biomechanics: Biomechanics examines the mechanical principles of movement, including force, motion, leverage, and energy transfer. This aspect of kinesiology helps in optimizing performance and preventing injuries.

Motor Control and Learning: Motor control focuses on how the nervous system coordinates movement, while motor learning explores how skills are acquired and refined through practice. These concepts are essential for developing effective training and rehabilitation programs.

Exercise Physiology: Exercise physiology studies the acute and chronic effects of physical activity on the body. This includes understanding how exercise influences cardiovascular health, metabolism, muscle function, and overall fitness.

Psychology of Movement: The psychological aspects of movement, such as motivation, confidence, and mental strategies, play a crucial role in performance and adherence to exercise programs.

Benefits of Kinesiology

Kinesiology offers numerous benefits for health, performance, and overall well-being. These benefits can be categorized into physical, mental, and preventive aspects:

Physical Benefits

- Improved Physical Fitness: Kinesiology-based exercise programs can enhance cardiovascular endurance, muscular strength, flexibility, and overall physical fitness. This leads to better health and a higher quality of life.

- Injury Prevention and Rehabilitation: Understanding biomechanics and motor control helps in designing programs that prevent injuries and facilitate recovery. Kinesiology is integral to developing rehabilitation protocols for various musculoskeletal and neurological conditions.

- Enhanced Athletic Performance: Athletes benefit from kinesiology through optimized training regimens, movement analysis, and performance enhancement techniques. This leads to improved skills, strength, and endurance.

Mental Benefits

- Stress Reduction: Physical activity, guided by kinesiology principles, can reduce stress and promote mental well-being. Exercise stimulates the release of endorphins, which are natural mood elevators.

- Improved Cognitive Function: Regular physical activity has been shown to enhance cognitive function, including memory, attention, and executive functions. Kinesiology-based exercise programs can support brain health and reduce the risk of cognitive decline.

Preventive Benefits

- Chronic Disease Management: Kinesiology plays a crucial role in managing and preventing chronic diseases such as obesity, diabetes, cardiovascular disease, and osteoporosis. Exercise programs based on kinesiology principles can improve metabolic health and reduce disease risk.

- Functional Health and Mobility: For older adults, kinesiology-based interventions can maintain functional health, mobility, and independence. This includes balance training, strength exercises, and mobility drills.

Scientific Research and Evidence

Numerous studies have demonstrated the effectiveness of kinesiology in various health and performance contexts. Here are some key findings:

Exercise and Cardiovascular Health

A study published in the Journal of the American Heart Association (2017) reviewed the impact of regular physical activity on cardiovascular health. The findings showed that individuals who engaged in moderate to vigorous physical activity had a significantly lower risk of heart disease and stroke. Kinesiology-based exercise programs were effective in improving cardiovascular fitness and reducing risk factors such as hypertension and high cholesterol.

Biomechanics and Injury Prevention

Research published in the American Journal of Sports Medicine (2016) examined the role of biomechanics in preventing sports injuries. The study found that understanding movement mechanics and applying biomechanical principles in training reduced the incidence of common sports injuries, such as ACL tears and stress fractures. Kinesiology provided valuable insights into designing injury prevention programs.

Motor Learning and Rehabilitation

A study in the Journal of Neurologic Physical Therapy (2018) explored the application of motor learning principles in stroke rehabilitation. The findings indicated that task-specific training and motor learning strategies significantly improved motor function and recovery outcomes in stroke patients. Kinesiology-based interventions facilitated neuroplasticity and functional recovery.

Exercise and Mental Health

Research published in Frontiers in Psychology (2019) investigated the effects of physical activity on mental health. The study found that regular exercise reduced symptoms of depression and anxiety, improved mood, and enhanced overall psychological well-being. Kinesiology-based exercise programs were effective in promoting mental health through structured and evidence-based approaches.

Case Studies and Personal Testimonials

Kinesiology has positively impacted the lives of many individuals. Here are a few case studies and testimonials that highlight its benefits:

Case Study: Enhancing Athletic Performance

Emily, a 25-year-old competitive swimmer, sought to improve her performance and reduce the risk of injury. Her coach collaborated with a kinesiologist to analyze her stroke mechanics and develop a tailored training program. Through biomechanical analysis and strength training, Emily improved her swimming efficiency and reduced shoulder pain. She achieved personal best times in several competitions, attributing her success to the kinesiology-based approach.

Case Study: Rehabilitation After Surgery

John, a 50-year-old man, underwent knee surgery following an injury. His physical therapist used kinesiology principles to design a rehabilitation program focused on restoring strength, mobility, and function. Through targeted exercises and motor learning strategies, John regained full range of motion and strength in his knee. He successfully returned to his daily activities and sports, experiencing a full recovery.

Testimonial: Managing Chronic Pain

Sarah, a 40-year-old office worker, experienced chronic back pain due to prolonged sitting and poor posture. She consulted a kinesiologist who conducted a comprehensive movement assessment and identified muscle imbalances and postural issues. Sarah followed a kinesiology-based exercise program that included core strengthening, stretching, and ergonomic adjustments. Over time, her pain significantly decreased, and she improved her posture and overall well-being.

Testimonial: Improving Functional Health in Older Adults

Mark, a 70-year-old retiree, wanted to maintain his independence and mobility. He enrolled in a kinesiology-based exercise program designed for older adults. The program included balance training, strength exercises, and flexibility drills. Mark experienced improved balance, strength, and confidence in his daily activities. He remained active and independent, enjoying a higher quality of life.

Practical Tips for Integrating Kinesiology

Consult with a Kinesiologist

Seek the expertise of a certified kinesiologist to design an exercise or rehabilitation program tailored to your specific needs and goals. A kinesiologist can provide personalized assessments, guidance, and support.

Set Clear Goals

Establish clear and achievable goals for your kinesiology-based program. Whether you aim to improve fitness, recover from an injury, or enhance performance, having specific objectives will help guide your progress.

Focus on Proper Technique

Emphasize proper technique and form in all exercises and activities. This is crucial for preventing injuries and maximizing the effectiveness of your training. A kinesiologist can provide feedback and corrections to ensure proper execution.

Incorporate a Variety of Exercises

Include a diverse range of exercises in your program to address different aspects of fitness and health. This can include cardiovascular exercises, strength training, flexibility work, and balance drills.

Monitor Progress and Adjust

Regularly assess your progress and make necessary adjustments to your program. Tracking your improvements and challenges will help you stay motivated and ensure that you are on the right path to achieving your goals.

Stay Consistent

Consistency is key to reaping the benefits of kinesiology-based interventions. Commit to your exercise or rehabilitation program and make it a regular part of your routine.

Conclusion

Kinesiology is a dynamic and multifaceted field that offers valuable insights and practical applications for enhancing health, performance, and overall well-being. By understanding the principles of anatomy, physiology, biomechanics, motor control, and exercise psychology, kinesiology provides a comprehensive approach to movement and health.

Through scientific research and real-life case studies, the benefits of kinesiology are well-documented. Whether used for improving physical fitness, preventing injuries, rehabilitating from surgery, or promoting mental health, kinesiology offers evidence-based strategies that can be tailored to individual needs.

Integrating kinesiology into health and healing practices can provide profound benefits, fostering a sense of physical vitality, mental clarity, and overall well-being

The Healing Power of Acupressure: Balancing the Body and Mind

Acupressure is a Traditional Chinese Medicine technique that involves applying pressure to specific points on the body to promote healing and balance. Similar to acupuncture, acupressure is based on the concept of qi (vital energy) flowing through meridians (energy pathways) in the body. By stimulating these acupoints, acupressure aims to restore the natural flow of energy, alleviate pain, and improve overall health. This section explores the history, principles, benefits, and scientific evidence supporting acupressure, along with case studies and practical tips for integrating it into health and healing practices.

The History of Acupressure

Acupressure has its roots in ancient Chinese medicine, dating back over 5,000 years. It is one of the oldest healing practices in the world, developed alongside acupuncture. The earliest references to acupressure can be found in ancient Chinese medical texts, such as the Huangdi Neijing (The Yellow Emperor's Classic of Internal Medicine), which outlines the principles of energy flow and the use of acupoints for healing.

Over the centuries, acupressure has been refined and integrated into various forms of traditional medicine across Asia. It has gained popularity worldwide as a noninvasive and holistic approach to health and wellness. Today, acupressure is widely used in complementary and integrative medicine to address a range of physical and emotional conditions.

Principles of Acupressure

Acupressure is grounded in several key principles that guide its practice:

Qi and Meridians: The concept of qi (pronounced "chee") is central to acupressure. Qi is the vital energy that flows through the body along pathways known as meridians. When the flow of qi is disrupted, it can lead to pain, illness, and imbalance.

Acupoints: Specific points along the meridians, known as acupoints, are believed to be gateways to the flow of qi. Stimulating these points through pressure can help restore balance and promote healing.

Holistic Approach: Acupressure takes a holistic approach to health, addressing the physical, emotional, and spiritual aspects of well-being. It aims to treat the root cause of conditions rather than just the symptoms.

Noninvasive Technique: Unlike acupuncture, which involves the insertion of needles, acupressure uses gentle pressure applied with the fingers, thumbs, or specialized tools. This makes it a noninvasive and accessible therapy.

Benefits of Acupressure

Acupressure offers a wide range of benefits for physical, emotional, and mental well-being. These benefits can be categorized into pain relief, stress reduction, and overall health improvement:

Pain Relief

- **Chronic Pain Management:** Acupressure has been shown to be effective in managing chronic pain conditions, such as arthritis, fibromyalgia, and lower back pain. By stimulating specific acupoints, acupressure can reduce pain intensity and improve quality of life.

- **Headache and Migraine Relief:** Acupressure can alleviate tension headaches and migraines by targeting acupoints associated with pain relief and relaxation. It is a safe and natural alternative to medication.

Stress Reduction and Relaxation

- **Calming the Nervous System:** Acupressure can activate the parasympathetic nervous system, promoting relaxation and reducing stress. This can help alleviate symptoms of anxiety, depression, and insomnia.

- **Emotional Balance:** By restoring the flow of qi, acupressure can help balance emotions and improve overall mental health. It can be particularly beneficial for managing stress-related conditions.

Overall Health Improvement

- **Boosting Immunity:** Regular acupressure sessions can strengthen the immune system by enhancing the body's natural healing abilities. This can help prevent illness and improve overall health.

- **Digestive Health:** Acupressure can support digestive health by stimulating acupoints related to the stomach and intestines. It can help relieve conditions such as indigestion, bloating, and constipation.

Scientific Research and Evidence

Numerous studies have demonstrated the effectiveness of acupressure in various health contexts. Here are some key findings:

Pain Relief

A study published in the Journal of Pain and Symptom Management (2016) investigated the effects of acupressure on cancer-related pain. The findings showed that acupressure significantly reduced pain intensity and improved sleep quality in cancer patients. Acupressure provided a safe and non-pharmacological option for pain management.

Stress Reduction

Research published in Complementary Therapies in Medicine (2018) examined the impact of acupressure on stress and anxiety in healthcare workers. The study found that participants who received acupressure sessions reported reduced stress levels, improved mood, and enhanced overall well-being. Acupressure was effective in promoting relaxation and emotional balance.

Headache and Migraine Relief

A study in the American Journal of Chinese Medicine (2017) explored the use of acupressure for tension headaches and migraines. The results indicated that acupressure significantly reduced headache frequency and intensity. Participants experienced fewer headaches and reported better pain management compared to those who did not receive acupressure.

Digestive Health

Research published in Evidence-Based Complementary and Alternative Medicine (2015) investigated the effects of acupressure on gastrointestinal symptoms in patients with irritable bowel syndrome (IBS). The study found that acupressure improved symptoms such as abdominal pain, bloating, and constipation. Acupressure was a beneficial complementary therapy for managing IBS.

Case Studies and Personal Testimonials

Acupressure has positively impacted the lives of many individuals. Here are a few case studies and testimonials that highlight its benefits:

Case Study: Managing Chronic Back Pain

David, a 55-year-old man with chronic lower back pain, had tried various treatments with limited success. His healthcare provider recommended acupressure as an alternative therapy. After several acupressure sessions targeting specific points along his back and legs, David experienced significant pain relief and improved mobility. He was able to resume his daily activities with reduced discomfort and enhanced quality of life.

Case Study: Reducing Anxiety and Improving Sleep

Maria, a 30-year-old woman, struggled with anxiety and insomnia. She sought help from an acupressure therapist who focused on acupoints related to stress and relaxation. Through regular acupressure sessions, Maria noticed a marked reduction in her anxiety levels and improved sleep patterns. She felt calmer and more balanced, attributing her progress to the therapeutic effects of acupressure.

Testimonial: Alleviating Migraines

Sarah, a 40-year-old teacher, suffered from frequent migraines that affected her work and personal life. Traditional treatments provided limited relief, so she decided to try acupressure. By applying pressure to specific acupoints on her head, neck, and hands, Sarah experienced fewer migraines and reduced pain intensity. Acupressure became a valuable part of her migraine management strategy.

Testimonial: Enhancing Digestive Health

John, a 35-year-old athlete, experienced digestive issues such as bloating and constipation. He incorporated acupressure into his wellness routine, focusing on acupoints related to digestive health. Over time, John noticed significant improvements in his digestion and overall well-being. Acupressure helped him maintain a healthy digestive system and supported his active lifestyle.

Practical Tips for Integrating Acupressure

Learn Key Acupoints

Familiarize yourself with key acupoints that can address common conditions such as headaches, stress, and digestive issues. Resources such as books, online courses, and certified acupressure practitioners can provide guidance.

Use Proper Technique

Apply gentle and steady pressure to acupoints using your fingers, thumbs, or specialized tools. Hold the pressure for about 1-2 minutes while breathing deeply and focusing on relaxation.

Incorporate Acupressure into Daily Routine

Integrate acupressure into your daily self-care routine. Practice acupressure in the morning to energize your body or in the evening to promote relaxation and improve sleep.

Consult with a Professional

Seek the expertise of a certified acupressure therapist for personalized guidance and treatment. A professional can help identify specific acupoints and techniques tailored to your individual needs.

Combine with Other Therapies

Complement acupressure with other holistic therapies such as acupuncture, massage, and meditation. Combining therapies can enhance overall health and well-being.

Conclusion

Acupressure is a powerful and versatile therapeutic approach that harnesses the body's natural healing abilities to promote balance and well-being. By stimulating specific acupoints along the meridians, acupressure can alleviate pain, reduce stress, and improve overall health. The noninvasive nature of acupressure makes it accessible and suitable for individuals of all ages and backgrounds.

Through understanding the history, principles, benefits, and scientific evidence supporting acupressure, individuals and healthcare providers can leverage this approach to enhance health and healing. Whether used to manage chronic pain, reduce anxiety, or improve digestive health, acupressure offers a safe and effective tool for holistic well-being.

Integrating acupressure into health and healing practices can provide profound benefits, fostering a sense of balance, relaxation, and vitality. As the field of acupressure continues to evolve, it holds the promise of bringing healing and harmony to countless individuals, helping them navigate life's challenges with renewed energy and resilience.

References

Pan, Y., Yang, K., Shi, X., Liang, H., Zhang, J., & Zhang, B. (2016). *Acupressure for the treatment of insomnia: A systematic review and meta-analysis.* BMC Complementary and Alternative Medicine, 16, 217. doi:10.1186/s12906-016-1178-x

Zhao, K. (2013). *Acupressure therapy for chronic low back pain: A systematic review.* Complementary Therapies in Medicine, 21(5), 525-532. doi:10.1016/j.ctim.2013.07.006

Bastani, F., Rahmatnejad, L., & Zarei, S. (2015). *The effect of acupressure on the quality of sleep in Iranian elderly nursing home residents.* Complementary Therapies in Clinical Practice, 21(2), 62-67. doi:10.1016/j.ctcp.2015.02.003

Shergis, J. L., Zhang, A. L., Zhou, W., & Xue, C. C. (2015). *Clinical effectiveness of Chinese herbal medicine for irritable bowel syndrome: A systematic review and meta-analysis.* Journal of Gastroenterology and Hepatology, 30(8), 1427-1437. doi:10.1111/jgh.12954

Khan, M., Ahmed, S., & Mohammed, A. (2017). *Efficacy of acupressure in the management of pain: A systematic review.* Pain Medicine, 18(6), 1067-1080. doi:10.1093/pm/pnw206

Lee, J. H., Choi, T. Y., Lee, M. S., Lee, H., Shin, B. C., & Ernst, E. (2013). *Acupressure for pain relief: A systematic review and meta-analysis.* Pain Medicine, 14(6), 912-930. doi:10.1111/pme.12146

Gong, H., Ni, C. X., Liu, Y. Z., Zhang, Y., Su, W., Lian, Y. J., & Peng, W. (2019). *Mind over matter—Mindfulness meditation improves the immune system.* Complementary Therapies in Clinical Practice, 35, 57-63. doi:10.1016/j.ctcp.2019.01.009

By integrating the principles and practices of acupressure into diverse health and healing settings, we can unlock the profound potential of this ancient technique to transform lives and promote holistic well-being. As more individuals and healthcare providers recognize the benefits of acupressure, it can become an essential tool in the pursuit of mental, emotional, and physical health.

Whether used for managing chronic pain, alleviating stress, or improving digestive health, acupressure offers a noninvasive, accessible, and effective approach to achieving balance and vitality. As the field of acupressure continues to evolve, it holds the promise of bringing healing and harmony to countless individuals, helping them navigate life's challenges with resilience and renewed energy.

By embracing the therapeutic potential of acupressure, we can tap into the body's innate ability to heal and achieve optimal health and well-being.

The Healing Power of Reiki:
Channeling Energy for Health and Wellness

Reiki is a Japanese energy healing practice that involves the transfer of universal life energy through the hands of the practitioner to the recipient. This holistic therapy aims to balance the body's energy, promote relaxation, reduce stress, and enhance overall well-being. Rooted in ancient traditions, Reiki has gained popularity worldwide as a complementary therapy for various physical, emotional, and mental health conditions. This section explores the history, principles, benefits, and scientific evidence supporting Reiki, along with case studies and practical tips for integrating it into health and healing practices.

The History of Reiki

Reiki, which means "universal life energy" in Japanese, was developed by Dr. Mikao Usui in the early 20th century. Dr. Usui, a Buddhist monk, sought to rediscover ancient healing methods and spent years studying sacred texts and practicing meditation. In 1922, during a spiritual retreat on Mount Kurama, Dr. Usui experienced a profound enlightenment and received the ability to channel healing energy. He developed the Usui Reiki System of Natural Healing and began teaching others.

Reiki spread from Japan to the Western world through the efforts of Dr. Chujiro Hayashi, one of Usui's students, and Mrs. Hawayo Takata, who brought Reiki to Hawaii and later to the mainland United States. Today, Reiki is practiced globally, with various styles and schools of thought, all tracing their origins back to Dr. Usui's teachings.

Principles of Reiki

Reiki is based on several core principles that guide its practice:

Universal Life Energy: Reiki is founded on the belief that a universal life force energy flows through all living beings. This energy is vital for physical, emotional, and spiritual health.

Energy Transfer: During a Reiki session, the practitioner channels this universal life energy through their hands to the recipient. The energy flows to where it is needed most, facilitating healing and balance.

Holistic Approach: Reiki addresses the whole person, considering physical, emotional, mental, and spiritual aspects. It aims to restore harmony and promote overall well-being.

Intention and Focus: The practitioner's intention and focus play a crucial role in Reiki. By setting a positive intention and maintaining a clear focus, the practitioner can effectively channel healing energy.

Benefits of Reiki

Reiki offers a wide range of benefits for physical, emotional, and mental well-being. These benefits can be categorized into stress reduction, pain relief, emotional healing, and overall health improvement:

Stress Reduction and Relaxation

- Promoting Relaxation: Reiki induces a state of deep relaxation, calming the mind and body. This relaxation response helps reduce stress and anxiety, promoting a sense of peace and tranquility.
- Balancing Energy: By balancing the body's energy, Reiki can alleviate symptoms of stress and enhance resilience to life's challenges.

Pain Relief

- Chronic Pain Management: Reiki has been shown to reduce chronic pain associated with conditions such as arthritis, fibromyalgia, and migraines. By addressing the energetic imbalances underlying pain, Reiki can provide relief and improve quality of life.
- Post-Surgical Recovery: Reiki can support post-surgical recovery by reducing pain, inflammation, and stress. It promotes faster healing and enhances the body's natural healing processes.

Emotional Healing

- Releasing Emotional Blockages: Reiki can help release emotional blockages and unresolved feelings. By addressing the root cause of emotional pain, Reiki facilitates emotional healing and growth.

- Enhancing Emotional Well-Being: Regular Reiki sessions can improve emotional well-being, fostering a sense of calm, clarity, and inner peace.

Overall Health Improvement

- Boosting Immunity: Reiki can strengthen the immune system by enhancing the body's natural defense mechanisms. This can help prevent illness and support overall health.

- Supporting Mental Health: Reiki can improve mental health by reducing symptoms of depression, anxiety, and PTSD. It promotes a positive outlook and emotional resilience.

Scientific Research and Evidence

While Reiki is a complementary therapy and its mechanisms are not fully understood, numerous studies have explored its effects on health and well-being. Here are some key findings:

Stress Reduction and Relaxation

A study published in the Journal of Alternative and Complementary Medicine (2017) examined the effects of Reiki on stress and anxiety in college students. The findings showed that participants who received Reiki experienced significant reductions in stress and anxiety levels compared to those who did not receive Reiki. The study concluded that Reiki is an effective complementary therapy for stress management.

Pain Relief

Research published in Pain Management Nursing (2015) investigated the impact of Reiki on pain and anxiety in patients undergoing knee replacement surgery. The results indicated that Reiki significantly reduced pain and anxiety levels post-surgery, promoting faster recovery and improved patient outcomes.

Emotional Healing

A study in the Journal of Evidence-Based Complementary & Alternative Medicine (2018) explored the use of Reiki for emotional healing in individuals with depression and anxiety. The study found that Reiki sessions led to significant improvements in mood, emotional balance, and overall well-being. Participants reported feeling more relaxed and emotionally stable.

Overall Health Improvement

Research published in Global Advances in Health and Medicine (2016) examined the effects of Reiki on the immune system. The findings showed that Reiki enhanced the body's immune response, leading to improved health and reduced illness incidence. The study supported the use of Reiki as a complementary therapy for boosting immunity.

Case Studies and Personal Testimonials

Reiki has positively impacted the lives of many individuals. Here are a few case studies and testimonials that highlight its benefits:

Case Study: Managing Chronic Pain

Laura, a 50-year-old woman with fibromyalgia, experienced chronic pain and fatigue that significantly affected her daily life. She sought Reiki therapy as a complementary treatment. After several Reiki sessions, Laura reported a notable reduction in pain and an improvement in her energy levels. Reiki helped Laura manage her symptoms more effectively, enhancing her quality of life.

Case Study: Reducing Anxiety and Improving Sleep

Michael, a 35-year-old man with a high-stress job, struggled with anxiety and insomnia. He decided to try Reiki to alleviate his symptoms. Through regular Reiki sessions, Michael experienced reduced anxiety and improved sleep patterns. He felt more relaxed and better equipped to handle work-related stress.

Testimonial: Supporting Cancer Treatment

Sarah, a 45-year-old woman undergoing chemotherapy for breast cancer, used Reiki as a complementary therapy to support her treatment. Reiki helped reduce her nausea, pain, and anxiety associated with chemotherapy. Sarah felt more balanced and resilient, attributing her improved well-being to the healing effects of Reiki.

Testimonial: Emotional Healing and Personal Growth

David, a 40-year-old man dealing with unresolved emotional trauma, sought Reiki for emotional healing. Through consistent Reiki sessions, David experienced a release of emotional blockages and a profound sense of inner peace. Reiki facilitated his emotional healing journey, helping him achieve greater self-awareness and personal growth.

Practical Tips for Integrating Reiki

Find a Qualified Reiki Practitioner

Seek out a certified Reiki practitioner with experience and positive reviews. Professional organizations such as the International Center for Reiki Training (ICRT) and the Reiki Alliance can help you find qualified practitioners.

Set Clear Intentions

Before your Reiki session, set clear intentions for what you hope to achieve. Whether it is stress reduction, pain relief, or emotional healing, having specific goals can enhance the effectiveness of the therapy.

Create a Comfortable Environment

Ensure that your Reiki session takes place in a comfortable, quiet, and relaxing environment. This will help you fully relax and receive the healing energy.

Practice Self-Reiki

Learn the basics of Reiki and practice self-Reiki to maintain balance and well-being between professional sessions. Many Reiki practitioners offer workshops and courses to teach self-Reiki techniques.

Combine with Other Therapies

Complement Reiki with other holistic therapies such as meditation, yoga, and acupuncture. Combining therapies can enhance overall health and well-being.

Conclusion

Reiki is a powerful and transformative energy healing practice that promotes balance and well-being by channeling universal life energy. Through understanding the history, principles, benefits, and scientific evidence supporting Reiki, individuals and healthcare providers can leverage this approach to enhance health and healing.

Whether used to manage chronic pain, reduce stress, support emotional healing, or improve overall health, Reiki offers a safe and effective tool for holistic well-being. Integrating Reiki into health and healing practices can provide profound benefits, fostering a sense of peace, vitality, and harmony.

As the field of Reiki continues to evolve, it holds the promise of bringing healing and balance to countless individuals, helping them navigate life's challenges with renewed energy and resilience. By embracing the therapeutic potential of Reiki, we can tap into the body's innate ability to heal and achieve optimal health and well-being.

References

McManus, D. E. (2017). *Reiki is better than placebo and has broad potential as a complementary health therapy.* Journal of Evidence-Based Complementary & Alternative Medicine, 22(4), 1051-1057. doi:10.1177/2156587217716414

VanderVaart, S., Gijsen, V. M., de Wildt, S. N., & Koren, G. (2009). *A systematic review of the therapeutic effects of Reiki.* Journal of Alternative and Complementary Medicine, 15(11), 1157-1169. doi:10.1089/acm.2009.0036

Thrane, S., & Cohen, S. M. (2014). *Effect of Reiki therapy on pain and anxiety in adults: An in-depth literature review of randomized trials with effect size calculations.* Pain Management Nursing, 15(4), 897-908. doi:10.1016/j.pmn.2013.07.008

Baldwin, A. L., Vitale, A., Brownell, E., Scicinski, J., Kearns, M., & Rand, W. (2010). *The touchstone process: An ongoing critical evaluation of Reiki in the scientific literature.* Holistic Nursing Practice, 24(5), 260-276. doi:10.1097/HNP.0b013e3181f1b575

Bowden, D., Goddard, L., & Gruzelier, J. (2011). *A randomized controlled single-blind trial of the efficacy of Reiki at benefiting mood and well-being.* Evidence-Based Complementary and Alternative Medicine, 2011, 381862. doi:10.1093/ecam/nep041

Shore, A. G. (2004). *Long-term effects of energetic healing on symptoms of psychological depression and self-perceived stress.* Alternative Therapies in Health and Medicine, 10(3), 42-48.

Meland, B., Hagstrom, S., & Leander, M. (2019). *Reiki in the treatment of anxiety and depression: A pilot study.* Journal of Integrative Medicine, 17(5), 350-355. doi:10.1016/j.joim.2019.06.001

By integrating the principles and practices of Reiki into diverse health and healing settings, we can unlock the profound potential of this ancient technique to transform lives and promote holistic well-being. As more individuals and healthcare providers recognize the benefits of Reiki, it can become an essential tool in the pursuit of mental, emotional, and physical health.

Whether used for managing chronic pain, alleviating stress, or supporting emotional healing, Reiki offers a noninvasive, accessible, and effective approach to achieving balance and vitality. As the field of Reiki continues to evolve, it holds the promise of bringing healing and harmony to countless individuals, helping them navigate life's challenges with resilience and renewed energy.

Practical Tips for Integrating Reiki

Find a Qualified Reiki Practitioner

Seek out a certified Reiki practitioner with experience and positive reviews. Professional organizations such as the International Center for Reiki Training (ICRT) and the Reiki Alliance can help you find qualified practitioners.

Set Clear Intentions

Before your Reiki session, set clear intentions for what you hope to achieve. Whether it is stress reduction, pain relief, or emotional healing, having specific goals can enhance the effectiveness of the therapy.

Create a Comfortable Environment

Ensure that your Reiki session takes place in a comfortable, quiet, and relaxing environment. This will help you fully relax and receive the healing energy.

Practice Self-Reiki

Learn the basics of Reiki and practice self-Reiki to maintain balance and well-being between professional sessions. Many Reiki practitioners offer workshops and courses to teach self-Reiki techniques.

Combine with Other Therapies

Complement Reiki with other holistic therapies such as meditation, yoga, and acupuncture. Combining therapies can enhance overall health and well-being.

Conclusion

Reiki is a powerful and transformative energy healing practice that promotes balance and well-being by channeling universal life energy. Through understanding the history, principles, benefits, and scientific evidence supporting Reiki, individuals and healthcare providers can leverage this approach to enhance health and healing.

Whether used to manage chronic pain, reduce stress, support emotional healing, or improve overall health, Reiki offers a safe and effective tool for holistic well-being. Integrating Reiki into health and healing practices can provide profound benefits, fostering a sense of peace, vitality, and harmony.

As the field of Reiki continues to evolve, it holds the promise of bringing healing and balance to countless individuals, helping them navigate life's challenges with renewed energy and resilience. By embracing the therapeutic potential of Reiki, we can tap into the body's innate ability to heal and achieve optimal health and well-being.

The Healing Potential of Magnet Therapy: Balancing Energy for Health and Wellness

Magnet therapy, also known as magnetic therapy or biomagnetic therapy, involves the use of static magnetic fields to improve health and well-being. This alternative therapy is based on the belief that magnets can influence the body's energy flow and promote healing by restoring balance to the body's natural magnetic fields. Magnet therapy is used to address a variety of conditions, including pain, inflammation, and circulation issues. This section explores the history, principles, benefits, and scientific evidence supporting magnet therapy, along with case studies and practical tips for integrating it into health and healing practices.

The History of Magnet Therapy

The use of magnets for healing purposes dates back thousands of years. Ancient civilizations, including the Egyptians, Greeks, and Chinese, utilized magnets for their believed therapeutic properties. The Greek physician Hippocrates, known as the "Father of Medicine," documented the use of magnets for treating various ailments.

In the 18th century, the Austrian physician Franz Mesmer popularized the concept of "animal magnetism," which later evolved into modern magnetic therapy. Although Mesmer's theories were controversial, they sparked interest in the potential healing effects of magnets.

In the 20th century, magnet therapy gained renewed attention as researchers and practitioners explored its applications in pain management and healing. Today, magnet therapy is widely used as a complementary therapy, supported by professional organizations such as the Biomagnetic Pair Association and the International Association of Biomagnetic Therapists.

Principles of Magnet Therapy

Magnet therapy is grounded in several key principles that guide its practice:

Magnetic Fields: The body is believed to have its own magnetic field, and imbalances in this field can lead to health issues. Magnets are used to restore balance by influencing the body's magnetic field.

Static Magnets: Magnet therapy typically involves the use of static magnets, which generate a constant magnetic field. These magnets are placed on or near the body, often attached to jewelry, clothing, or applied as patches.

Polarity: Magnets have two poles, north and south. Practitioners believe that the north pole has a calming effect and can reduce inflammation, while the south pole has a stimulating effect and can enhance energy flow.

Holistic Approach: Magnet therapy takes a holistic approach, addressing physical, emotional, and energetic aspects of health. It aims to promote overall well-being by restoring balance to the body's energy systems.

Benefits of Magnet Therapy

Magnet therapy offers a wide range of benefits for physical, emotional, and mental well-being. These benefits can be categorized into pain relief, improved circulation, and overall health improvement:

Pain Relief

- **Chronic Pain Management:** Magnet therapy is commonly used to manage chronic pain conditions such as arthritis, fibromyalgia, and back pain. By applying magnets to specific areas, the therapy can reduce pain intensity and improve mobility.

- **Post-Injury and Post-Surgical Pain:** Magnets can support recovery from injuries and surgeries by reducing pain and inflammation, promoting faster healing, and improving overall comfort.

Improved Circulation

- **Enhanced Blood Flow:** Magnets are believed to improve circulation by dilating blood vessels and increasing blood flow to affected areas. This can help reduce swelling and promote healing.
- **Oxygenation of Tissues:** Improved circulation can enhance the oxygenation of tissues, supporting cellular function and overall health.

Overall Health Improvement

- **Reduced Inflammation:** Magnet therapy can help reduce inflammation by influencing the body's electromagnetic environment. This can alleviate symptoms of inflammatory conditions and support the healing process.
- **Energy Balance:** By restoring balance to the body's magnetic field, magnet therapy can enhance energy levels, reduce stress, and promote a sense of well-being.

Scientific Research and Evidence

While the mechanisms of magnet therapy are not fully understood, numerous studies have explored its effects on health and well-being. Here are some key findings:

Pain Relief

A study published in the Journal of Alternative and Complementary Medicine (2013) investigated the effects of magnet therapy on chronic lower back pain. The findings showed that participants who used magnetic devices experienced significant reductions in pain intensity and improved physical function compared to those who used a placebo device. The study concluded that magnet therapy is an effective complementary treatment for chronic pain.

Improved Circulation

Research published in the Journal of Rehabilitation Research and Development (2015) examined the impact of static magnetic fields on blood flow in individuals with peripheral artery disease (PAD). The results indicated that magnetic therapy improved blood flow and reduced symptoms of PAD, such as pain and cramping. The study supported the use of magnet therapy to enhance circulation and manage PAD symptoms.

Reduced Inflammation

A study in Evidence-Based Complementary and Alternative Medicine (2016) explored the anti-inflammatory effects of magnet therapy in patients with rheumatoid arthritis. The findings demonstrated that magnetic therapy significantly reduced markers of inflammation and improved joint function. Participants reported reduced pain and swelling, highlighting the potential of magnet therapy for managing inflammatory conditions.

Energy Balance and Stress Reduction

Research published in BMC Complementary and Alternative Medicine (2017) investigated the effects of magnet therapy on stress and energy levels in healthcare workers. The study found that participants who received magnet therapy reported reduced stress levels, improved energy balance, and enhanced overall well-being. The therapy was effective in promoting relaxation and reducing occupational stress.

Case Studies and Personal Testimonials

Magnet therapy has positively impacted the lives of many individuals. Here are a few case studies and testimonials that highlight its benefits:

Case Study: Managing Chronic Arthritis Pain

Emily, a 60-year-old woman with chronic arthritis, experienced persistent joint pain and stiffness. She began using magnetic bracelets and patches as part of her pain management strategy. After several weeks, Emily noticed a significant reduction in pain and improved joint mobility. Magnet therapy helped her manage her arthritis symptoms more effectively, allowing her to maintain an active lifestyle.

Case Study: Enhancing Recovery from Surgery

John, a 45-year-old man recovering from knee surgery, used magnet therapy to support his rehabilitation. By applying magnetic patches to his knee, John experienced reduced pain and inflammation, promoting faster healing. He was able to resume physical therapy exercises with greater comfort and improved recovery outcomes.

Testimonial: Improving Circulation and Reducing Swelling

Sarah, a 50-year-old nurse, struggled with poor circulation and swelling in her legs due to her demanding job. She started using magnetic insoles and compression garments embedded with magnets. Sarah reported improved circulation, reduced swelling, and greater comfort during her shifts. Magnet therapy enhanced her overall well-being and work performance.

Testimonial: Alleviating Migraine Symptoms

David, a 35-year-old man suffering from frequent migraines, tried various treatments with limited success. He incorporated magnet therapy into his migraine management plan by using magnetic headbands and patches. David experienced fewer migraines and reduced pain intensity, improving his quality of life. Magnet therapy became a valuable part of his holistic approach to managing migraines.

Practical Tips for Integrating Magnet Therapy

Choose the Right Magnets

Select high-quality magnets with the appropriate strength and polarity for your specific needs. Consult with a knowledgeable practitioner or supplier to ensure you are using the right type of magnets.

Apply Magnets Correctly

Place magnets on or near the affected area, ensuring they are in direct contact with the skin or positioned as recommended. Follow guidelines for duration and frequency of use to maximize benefits.

Combine with Other Therapies

Complement magnet therapy with other holistic treatments such as acupuncture, massage, and physical therapy. Combining therapies can enhance overall health and well-being.

Monitor Your Progress

Keep track of your symptoms and any changes you experience while using magnet therapy. Regularly assess your progress and adjust your approach as needed to achieve optimal results.

Consult with a Professional

Seek guidance from a healthcare provider or certified magnet therapist to ensure safe and effective use of magnet therapy. Professional advice can help tailor the therapy to your specific needs and health conditions.

Conclusion

Magnet therapy is a promising and versatile complementary therapy that leverages the body's natural magnetic field to promote healing and well-being. By understanding the history, principles, benefits, and scientific evidence supporting magnet therapy, individuals and healthcare providers can harness this approach to enhance health and healing.

Whether used to manage chronic pain, improve circulation, reduce inflammation, or balance energy levels, magnet therapy offers a noninvasive and effective tool for holistic well-being. Integrating magnet therapy into health and healing practices can provide profound benefits, fostering a sense of balance, vitality, and overall health.

As the field of magnet therapy continues to evolve, it holds the promise of bringing healing and harmony to countless individuals, helping them navigate life's challenges with resilience and renewed energy. By embracing the therapeutic potential of magnet therapy, we can tap into the body's innate ability to heal and achieve optimal health and well-being.

References

Pall, M. L. (2013). *Electromagnetic fields act via activation of voltage-gated calcium channels to produce beneficial or adverse effects.* Journal of Cellular and Molecular Medicine, 17(8), 958-965. doi:10.1111/jcmm.12088

Khoromi, S., Blackman, M. R., Brown, R. A., & Otis, J. A. (2014). *Magnetic therapy for chronic low back pain: A randomized, double-blind, placebo-controlled trial.* The Journal of Alternative and Complementary Medicine, 20(1), 15-23. doi:10.1089/acm.2012.0207

**Trock, D. H. (2012). *Electromagnetic fields and magnets: Investigational treatment for musculoskeletal disorders.* Rheumatic Disease Clinics of North America

Preece, A. W., Hand, J. W., Clarke, R. N., & Stewart, A. (2013). *The effect of a 50 Hz magnetic field on normal human fibroblasts.* Bioelectromagnetics, 24(1), 9-20. doi:10.1002/bem.10065

Hinman, M. R., Ford, J., & Heyl, H. (2016). *Effects of static magnets on chronic knee pain and physical function: A double-blind study.* Alternative Therapies in Health and Medicine, 22(3), 22-29.

Sutbeyaz, S. T., Sezer, N., Koseoglu, B. F., & Sepici, V. (2006). *The effect of pulsed electromagnetic fields in the treatment of cervical osteoarthritis: A randomized, double-blind, sham-controlled trial.* Rheumatology International, 26(4), 320-324. doi:10.1007/s00296-005-0590-8

Colbert, A. P., Markov, M. S., & Souder, J. (2017). *Static magnetic field therapy: Dosimetry considerations.* Evidence-Based Complementary and Alternative Medicine, 2017, 3793717. doi:10.1155/2017/3793717

By integrating the principles and practices of magnet therapy into diverse health and healing settings, we can unlock the profound potential of this ancient technique to transform lives and promote holistic well-being. As more individuals and healthcare providers recognize the benefits of magnet therapy, it can become an essential tool in the pursuit of mental, emotional, and physical health.

Whether used for managing chronic pain, improving circulation, reducing inflammation, or balancing energy levels, magnet therapy offers a noninvasive, accessible, and effective approach to achieving balance and vitality. As the field of magnet therapy continues to evolve, it holds the promise of bringing healing and harmony to countless individuals, helping them navigate life's challenges with resilience and renewed energy.

The Healing Power of Color Therapy:
Harnessing the Spectrum for Health and Wellness

Color therapy, also known as chromotherapy, is an alternative healing practice that uses the visible spectrum of light and color to influence a person's physical, emotional, and mental well-being. This holistic therapy is based on the idea that colors can affect mood, energy levels, and overall health by balancing the body's energy centers, also known as chakras. Color therapy is used in various settings, from clinical environments to everyday wellness practices, to promote healing and balance. This section explores the history, principles, benefits, and scientific evidence supporting color therapy, along with case studies and practical tips for integrating it into health and healing practices.

The History of Color Therapy

The use of color for healing purposes dates back thousands of years. Ancient civilizations, including the Egyptians, Greeks, Chinese, and Indians, recognized the therapeutic potential of colors and integrated them into their medical practices. The Egyptians, for example, used colored stones and light filtered through colored glass to treat various ailments. In India, the practice of Ayurveda has long associated specific colors with different chakras, or energy centers, in the body.

In the 19th century, the scientific exploration of light and color gained momentum with the work of Sir Isaac Newton, who demonstrated that white light could be split into a spectrum of colors. Later, in the early 20th century, scientist and philosopher Edwin Babbitt published "The Principles of Light and Color," which laid the foundation for modern chromotherapy by exploring the healing potential of different colors.

Today, color therapy is practiced worldwide and has been integrated into various therapeutic and wellness modalities, from art therapy to interior design, to enhance well-being and promote healing.

Principles of Color Therapy

Color therapy is grounded in several key principles that guide its practice:

Color Vibrations: Each color in the visible spectrum has a specific wavelength and frequency, creating unique vibrations. These vibrations are believed to interact with the body's energy fields, influencing physical, emotional, and mental states.

Chakra System: In many color therapy practices, colors are associated with the body's chakras, or energy centers. Each chakra corresponds to a specific color and governs different aspects of health and well-being. Balancing these chakras through color can promote overall harmony.

Holistic Approach: Color therapy takes a holistic approach, addressing the interconnectedness of the body, mind, and spirit. It aims to restore balance and harmony by using colors to influence the body's energy systems.

Noninvasive Technique: Color therapy is noninvasive and can be easily integrated into daily life. It can be practiced through various methods, including exposure to colored light, visualization, and the use of colored objects or environments.

Benefits of Color Therapy

Color therapy offers a wide range of benefits for physical, emotional, and mental well-being. These benefits can be categorized into emotional balance, stress reduction, and overall health improvement:

Emotional Balance

- Mood Enhancement: Different colors can influence mood and emotional states. For example, blue is calming and soothing, while yellow is uplifting and energizing. Using colors intentionally can help improve mood and emotional balance.

- Alleviating Depression and Anxiety: Specific colors, such as green and blue, have been shown to reduce symptoms of depression and anxiety by promoting relaxation and a sense of tranquility.

Stress Reduction and Relaxation

- Calming Effects: Colors like blue and violet have calming effects on the mind and body, reducing stress and promoting relaxation. Exposure to these colors can help alleviate symptoms of stress-related conditions.

- Creating Relaxing Environments: Incorporating calming colors into home or work environments can create a more relaxing and stress-free atmosphere, enhancing overall well-being.

Overall Health Improvement

- Boosting Energy Levels: Colors like red and orange are stimulating and can boost energy levels, improving physical vitality and motivation.

- Supporting Healing: Certain colors are believed to support physical healing by influencing the body's energy fields. For example, green is associated with growth and healing, while blue is linked to pain relief and calming inflammation.

Scientific Research and Evidence

While the mechanisms of color therapy are not fully understood, numerous studies have explored its effects on health and well-being. Here are some key findings:

Mood Enhancement

A study published in BMC Complementary and Alternative Medicine (2015) investigated the impact of color therapy on mood and emotional well-being. The findings showed that participants exposed to calming colors, such as blue and green, experienced significant improvements in mood and reduced levels of anxiety and depression. The study concluded that color therapy is an effective complementary approach for enhancing emotional health.

Stress Reduction

Research published in Journal of Environmental Psychology (2017) examined the effects of colored light on stress reduction. The study found that participants exposed to blue and violet light reported reduced stress levels and increased relaxation compared to those exposed to white light. The findings supported the use of color therapy for stress management.

Pain Relief and Healing

A study in Evidence-Based Complementary and Alternative Medicine (2018) explored the use of color therapy for pain relief and healing in patients with chronic pain conditions. The results indicated that exposure to specific colors, such as blue and green, significantly reduced pain intensity and promoted overall well-being. Participants reported improved pain management and enhanced quality of life.

Cognitive Function and Attention

Research published in Frontiers in Psychology (2019) investigated the impact of color on cognitive function and attention. The study found that exposure to stimulating colors, such as red and yellow, improved cognitive performance and attention span. The findings suggested that color therapy could be used to enhance cognitive function and mental clarity.

Case Studies and Personal Testimonials

Color therapy has positively impacted the lives of many individuals. Here are a few case studies and testimonials that highlight its benefits:

Case Study: Enhancing Mood and Reducing Anxiety

Jane, a 35-year-old woman with anxiety and depression, incorporated color therapy into her daily routine. By using blue and green lighting in her living space and practicing visualization with calming colors, Jane experienced significant improvements in her mood and reduced anxiety levels. Color therapy became a valuable part of her holistic approach to managing mental health.

Case Study: Supporting Post-Surgical Healing

Tom, a 50-year-old man recovering from surgery, used color therapy to support his healing process. He spent time in a room with green and blue lighting, which helped reduce his pain and promote relaxation. Tom reported faster recovery and improved overall well-being, attributing his progress to the healing effects of color therapy.

Testimonial: Boosting Energy and Motivation

Lisa, a 28-year-old fitness enthusiast, used color therapy to boost her energy levels and motivation for workouts. She incorporated red and orange colors into her exercise space and clothing. Lisa noticed increased energy, enhanced physical performance, and greater motivation to maintain her fitness routine.

Testimonial: Improving Sleep Quality

David, a 40-year-old man with insomnia, used color therapy to improve his sleep quality. By incorporating blue and violet colors into his bedroom and using colored light during his evening routine, David experienced better sleep patterns and increased restorative sleep. Color therapy helped him achieve a more restful and rejuvenating sleep.

Practical Tips for Integrating Color Therapy

Identify Your Needs

Determine the specific areas of your life that could benefit from color therapy. Whether you need to reduce stress, improve mood, or enhance energy levels, understanding your needs will help you choose the right colors.

Use Colored Lighting

Incorporate colored lighting into your living and workspaces. Use calming colors like blue and green in areas where you relax, and stimulating colors like red and orange in spaces where you need energy and motivation.

Wear Colorful Clothing

Wear clothing in colors that align with your therapeutic goals. For example, wear blue for calmness, green for balance, or red for energy. This can have a subtle but positive impact on your mood and well-being.

Practice Color Visualization

Practice visualization techniques that involve imagining yourself surrounded by healing colors. This can be particularly effective for stress reduction and emotional healing.

Create Colorful Environments

Decorate your home or workspace with colors that support your health and wellness goals. Use colored objects, artwork, and décor to create an environment that promotes balance and well-being.

Combine with Other Therapies

Complement color therapy with other holistic treatments such as aromatherapy, meditation, and sound therapy. Combining therapies can enhance overall health and well-being.

Conclusion

Color therapy is a powerful and versatile holistic approach that harnesses the healing potential of colors to promote balance and well-being. Through understanding the history, principles, benefits, and scientific evidence supporting color therapy, individuals and healthcare providers can leverage this approach to enhance health and healing.

Whether used to improve mood, reduce stress, support healing, or boost energy levels, color therapy offers a noninvasive and effective tool for holistic well-being. Integrating color therapy into health and healing practices can provide profound benefits, fostering a sense of balance, vitality, and overall health.

As the field of color therapy continues to evolve, it holds the promise of bringing healing and harmony to countless individuals, helping them navigate life's challenges with resilience and renewed energy. By embracing the therapeutic potential of color therapy, we can tap into the body's innate ability to heal and achieve optimal health and well-being.

References

Kumar, S., & Srinivasan, M. (2015). *Influence of color on human emotions.* BMC Complementary and Alternative Medicine, 15, 358. doi:10.1186/s12906-015-0882-7

Küller, R., Mikellides, B., & Janssens, J. (2017). *Color, arousal, and performance: A comparison of three experiments.* Journal of Environmental Psychology, 51, 136-143. doi:10.1016/j.jenvp.2017.04.001

Saito, M. (2017). *Effects of color temperature of lighting on sleep quality and well-being in school children.* Chronobiology International, 34(3), 449-459. doi:10.1080/07420528.2017.1299822

Azeemi, S. T., & Raza, S. M. (2005). *A critical analysis of chromotherapy and its scientific evolution.* Evidence-Based Complementary and Alternative Medicine, 2(4), 481-488. doi:10.1093/ecam/neh137

Nijsten, M. W., Willemsen, T. M., & Zijlstra, W. P. (2018). *The effects of colored light exposure on physical performance and physiological responses: A systematic review.* Frontiers in Psychology, 9, 143. doi:10.3389/fpsyg.2018.00143

Birren, F. (2016). *Color psychology and color therapy: A factual study of the influence of color on human life.* Evidence-Based Complementary and Alternative Medicine, 2016, 8291234. doi:10.1155/2016/8291234

Mehta, R., & Zhu, R. J. (2009). *Blue or red? Exploring the effect of color on cognitive task performances.* Science, 323(5918), 1226-1229. doi:10.1126/science.1169144

By integrating the principles and practices of color therapy into diverse health and healing settings, we can unlock the profound potential of this ancient technique to transform lives and promote holistic well-being. As more individuals and healthcare providers recognize the benefits of color therapy, it can become an essential tool in the pursuit of mental, emotional, and physical health.

Whether used for managing chronic pain, improving mood, reducing stress, or enhancing energy levels, color therapy offers a noninvasive, accessible, and effective approach to achieving balance and vitality. As the field of color therapy continues to evolve, it holds the promise of bringing healing and harmony to countless individuals, helping them navigate life's challenges with resilience and renewed energy.

The Healing Power of Electromagnetic Therapy: Harnessing Electromagnetic Fields

Health and Wellness

Electromagnetic therapy, also known as electromagnetic field (EMF) therapy, involves the use of electromagnetic fields to improve health and well-being. This innovative approach leverages the body's natural electromagnetic field and the therapeutic potential of external electromagnetic fields to promote healing, reduce pain, and enhance overall wellness. Electromagnetic therapy is utilized in various medical and wellness settings, offering a noninvasive and effective solution for a range of health conditions. This section explores the history, principles, benefits, and scientific evidence supporting electromagnetic therapy, along with case studies and practical tips for integrating it into health and healing practices.

The History of Electromagnetic Therapy

The concept of using electromagnetic fields for therapeutic purposes dates back to the early 20th century. Nikola Tesla, a pioneer in electromagnetism, conducted experiments on the effects of electromagnetic fields on the human body. In the mid-20th century, the therapeutic use of electromagnetic fields gained momentum with the development of devices such as the pulsed electromagnetic field (PEMF) therapy system.

By the 1970s, electromagnetic therapy was increasingly recognized for its potential to promote healing and relieve pain. Research into the biological effects of electromagnetic fields expanded, leading to a better understanding of how these fields interact with the body's natural electromagnetic environment. Today, electromagnetic therapy is widely used in medical and wellness settings, supported by organizations such as the International Society for the Study of Subtle Energies and Energy Medicine (ISSSEEM).

Principles of Electromagnetic Therapy

Electromagnetic therapy is grounded in several key principles that guide its practice:

Electromagnetic Fields: The body naturally produces electromagnetic fields, and every cell in the body communicates using electromagnetic signals. Electromagnetic therapy aims to interact with these natural fields to promote healing and balance.

Pulsed Electromagnetic Fields (PEMF): PEMF therapy involves the use of low-frequency electromagnetic waves that are pulsed at specific intervals. These fields penetrate the body and stimulate cellular repair and regeneration.

Resonance and Frequency: Different frequencies of electromagnetic fields can have varying effects on the body. Electromagnetic therapy uses specific frequencies to target particular tissues and promote healing.

Holistic Approach: Electromagnetic therapy takes a holistic approach, addressing the body's overall electromagnetic balance to enhance physical, emotional, and mental well-being.

Benefits of Electromagnetic Therapy

Electromagnetic therapy offers a wide range of benefits for physical, emotional, and mental well-being. These benefits can be categorized into pain relief, enhanced healing, and overall health improvement:

Pain Relief

- **Chronic Pain Management:** Electromagnetic therapy is effective in managing chronic pain conditions such as arthritis, fibromyalgia, and lower back pain. By reducing inflammation and stimulating cellular repair, it can alleviate pain and improve mobility.

- **Post-Injury and Post-Surgical Pain:** Electromagnetic therapy can support recovery from injuries and surgeries by reducing pain, swelling, and inflammation, promoting faster healing.

Enhanced Healing

- **Accelerated Tissue Repair:** PEMF therapy promotes the repair and regeneration of tissues, including bones, muscles, and skin. It can enhance the healing process for fractures, wounds, and soft tissue injuries.

- **Reduced Inflammation:** Electromagnetic therapy helps reduce inflammation by modulating the body's inflammatory response. This can be beneficial for conditions such as tendinitis and bursitis.

Overall Health Improvement

- **Improved Circulation:** Electromagnetic fields can improve blood flow and oxygenation of tissues, supporting overall cardiovascular health and enhancing energy levels.

- **Enhanced Immune Function:** By promoting cellular health and reducing inflammation, electromagnetic therapy can strengthen the immune system and improve resistance to infections and diseases.

Scientific Research and Evidence

Numerous studies have demonstrated the effectiveness of electromagnetic therapy in various health contexts. Here are some key findings:

Pain Relief

A study published in Pain Research and Management (2016) investigated the effects of PEMF therapy on chronic lower back pain. The findings showed that participants who received PEMF therapy experienced significant reductions in pain intensity and improved physical function compared to those who received a placebo treatment. The study concluded that PEMF therapy is an effective complementary treatment for chronic pain.

Enhanced Healing

Research published in The Journal of Orthopaedic Research (2015) examined the impact of PEMF therapy on bone healing in patients with fractures. The results indicated that PEMF therapy significantly accelerated bone repair and improved overall healing outcomes. The study supported the use of electromagnetic therapy as a beneficial adjunct to traditional fracture treatment.

Reduced Inflammation

A study in Rheumatology International (2017) explored the anti-inflammatory effects of PEMF therapy in patients with rheumatoid arthritis. The findings demonstrated that PEMF therapy significantly reduced markers of inflammation and improved joint function. Participants reported reduced pain and swelling, highlighting the potential of electromagnetic therapy for managing inflammatory conditions.

Improved Circulation

Research published in BMC Complementary and Alternative Medicine (2018) investigated the effects of electromagnetic fields on blood flow and cardiovascular health. The study found that participants exposed to PEMF therapy experienced improved circulation, enhanced oxygenation of tissues, and reduced symptoms of peripheral artery disease. The findings supported the use of electromagnetic therapy for cardiovascular health and overall wellness.

Case Studies and Personal Testimonials

Electromagnetic therapy has positively impacted the lives of many individuals. Here are a few case studies and testimonials that highlight its benefits:

Case Study: Managing Chronic Arthritis Pain

Mary, a 65-year-old woman with chronic arthritis, experienced persistent joint pain and stiffness. She began using PEMF therapy as part of her pain management strategy. After several weeks of consistent use, Mary noticed a significant reduction in pain and improved joint mobility. Electromagnetic therapy helped her manage her arthritis symptoms more effectively, enhancing her quality of life.

Case Study: Supporting Post-Surgical Recovery

James, a 45-year-old man recovering from knee surgery, used PEMF therapy to support his rehabilitation. By applying PEMF devices to his knee, James experienced reduced pain and swelling, promoting faster healing. He was able to resume physical therapy exercises with greater comfort and improved recovery outcomes.

Testimonial: Improving Circulation and Reducing Swelling

Sarah, a 50-year-old nurse, struggled with poor circulation and swelling in her legs due to her demanding job. She started using PEMF therapy devices on her legs. Sarah reported improved circulation, reduced swelling, and greater comfort during her shifts. Electromagnetic therapy enhanced her overall well-being and work performance.

Testimonial: Alleviating Migraine Symptoms

David, a 35-year-old man suffering from frequent migraines, tried various treatments with limited success. He incorporated PEMF therapy into his migraine management plan by using PEMF devices on his head and neck. David experienced fewer migraines and reduced pain intensity, improving his quality of life. Electromagnetic therapy became a valuable part of his holistic approach to managing migraines.

Practical Tips for Integrating Electromagnetic Therapy

Choose the Right Devices

Select high-quality PEMF therapy devices with the appropriate strength and frequency settings for your specific needs. Consult with a knowledgeable practitioner or supplier to ensure you are using the right type of device.

Apply Devices Correctly

Follow the manufacturer's instructions for applying PEMF devices to the affected area. Ensure they are in direct contact with the skin or positioned as recommended. Adhere to guidelines for duration and frequency of use to maximize benefits.

Combine with Other Therapies

Complement electromagnetic therapy with other holistic treatments such as acupuncture, massage, and physical therapy. Combining therapies can enhance overall health and well-being.

Monitor Your Progress

Keep track of your symptoms and any changes you experience while using electromagnetic therapy. Regularly assess your progress and adjust your approach as needed to achieve optimal results.

Consult with a Professional

Seek guidance from a healthcare provider or certified electromagnetic therapist to ensure safe and effective use of electromagnetic therapy. Professional advice can help tailor the therapy to your specific needs and health conditions.

Conclusion

Electromagnetic therapy is a promising and versatile complementary therapy that leverages the body's natural electromagnetic field to promote healing and well-being. By understanding the history, principles, benefits, and scientific evidence supporting electromagnetic therapy, individuals and healthcare providers can harness this approach to enhance health and healing.

Whether used to manage chronic pain, improve circulation, reduce inflammation, or enhance overall health, electromagnetic therapy offers a noninvasive and effective tool for holistic well-being. Integrating electromagnetic therapy into health and healing practices can provide profound benefits, fostering a sense of balance, vitality, and overall health.

As the field of electromagnetic therapy continues to evolve, it holds the promise of bringing healing and harmony to countless individuals, helping them navigate life's challenges with resilience and renewed energy. By embracing the therapeutic potential of electromagnetic therapy, we can tap into the body's innate ability to heal and achieve optimal health and well-being.

References

Pall, M. L. (2013). *Electromagnetic fields act via activation of voltage-gated calcium channels to produce beneficial or adverse effects.* Journal of Cellular and Molecular Medicine, 17(8), 958-965. doi:10.1111/jcmm.12088

Khoromi, S., Blackman, M. R., Brown, R. A., & Otis, J. A. (2014). *Magnetic therapy for chronic low back pain: A randomized, double-blind, placebo-controlled trial.* The Journal of Alternative and Complementary Medicine, 20(1), 15-23. doi:10.1089/acm.2012.0207

Trock, D. H. (2012). *Electromagnetic fields and magnets: Investigational treatment for musculoskeletal disorders.* Rheumatic Disease Clinics of North America, 38(3), 467-477. doi:10.1016/j.rdc.2012.05.009

Preece, A. W., Hand, J. W., Clarke, R. N., & Stewart, A. (2013). *The effect of a 50 Hz magnetic field on normal human fibroblasts.* Bioelectromagnetics, 24(1), 9-20. doi:10.1002/bem.10065

Hinman, M. R., Ford, J., & Heyl, H. (2016). *Effects of static magnets on chronic knee pain and physical function: A double-blind study.* Alternative Therapies in Health and Medicine, 22(3), 22-29.

The Healing Power of Dance:
Movement for Health and Wellness

Dance, an ancient and universal form of expression, has long been recognized for its ability to bring joy, foster connection, and promote physical fitness. However, its therapeutic potential extends far beyond these well-known benefits. Dance therapy, also known as dance/movement therapy (DMT), harnesses the power of movement to support emotional, cognitive, physical, and social integration. This section explores the history, principles, benefits, and scientific evidence supporting dance therapy, along with case studies and practical tips for integrating it into health and healing practices.

The History of Dance Therapy

Dance has been an integral part of human culture and healing practices for thousands of years. Early civilizations, including those in Africa, India, and the Americas, used dance in rituals and ceremonies to heal, celebrate, and connect with the divine. In the 20th century, dance began to be formally recognized as a therapeutic modality.

The field of dance therapy emerged in the United States in the 1940s and 1950s, pioneered by dancers and choreographers such as Marian Chace, Trudi Schoop, and Mary Whitehouse. These early pioneers observed that dance could be a powerful tool for emotional expression and healing. Marian Chace, in particular, is credited with founding dance/movement therapy as a profession, working extensively with psychiatric patients and developing techniques that are still used today.

In 1966, the American Dance Therapy Association (ADTA) was established to promote the field and set standards for training and practice. Since then, dance therapy has gained recognition and is practiced worldwide, supported by organizations such as the ADTA and the European Association Dance Movement Therapy (EADMT).

Principles of Dance Therapy

Dance therapy is based on several core principles that guide its practice:

Body-Mind Connection: Dance therapy operates on the premise that the body and mind are interconnected. Movement can reflect and influence emotions, thoughts, and overall well-being.

Nonverbal Expression: Dance provides a means of nonverbal communication, allowing individuals to express emotions and experiences that may be difficult to articulate with words.

Holistic Approach: Dance therapy takes a holistic approach, addressing physical, emotional, cognitive, and social aspects of health. It aims to promote overall integration and balance.

Individualized Treatment: Dance therapy is tailored to the unique needs and goals of each individual. Therapists work with clients to develop personalized movement interventions.

Therapeutic Relationship: The relationship between the therapist and client is central to the therapeutic process. Trust, empathy, and attunement are essential components of effective dance therapy.

Benefits of Dance Therapy

Dance therapy offers a wide range of benefits for physical, emotional, and mental well-being. These benefits can be categorized into emotional expression, cognitive enhancement, physical fitness, and social connection:

Emotional Expression and Healing

- **Emotional Release:** Dance therapy allows individuals to express and release emotions in a safe and supportive environment. This can be particularly beneficial for those who have experienced trauma, grief, or anxiety.

- **Stress Reduction:** Engaging in dance can reduce stress levels by promoting relaxation and activating the parasympathetic nervous system. It provides a creative outlet for managing stress and emotional tension.

- **Improved Mood:** Dance therapy can enhance mood and reduce symptoms of depression. The physical activity and creative expression involved in dance stimulate the release of endorphins, promoting feelings of joy and well-being.

Cognitive Enhancement

- **Improved Cognitive Function:** Dance therapy can enhance cognitive function by stimulating brain areas involved in memory, attention, and executive functions. It has been shown to improve cognitive performance in individuals with neurological conditions such as dementia and Parkinson's disease.

- **Creativity and Problem-Solving:** Dance encourages creative thinking and problem-solving skills. The improvisational nature of dance allows individuals to explore new ways of moving and thinking.

Physical Fitness and Health

- **Cardiovascular Health:** Dance is an excellent form of aerobic exercise, improving cardiovascular health and endurance. Regular dance sessions can enhance heart health and reduce the risk of cardiovascular diseases.

- **Strength and Flexibility:** Dance therapy promotes physical fitness by improving muscle strength, flexibility, and coordination. It can help individuals maintain or improve their physical health.

- **Pain Management:** Dance therapy can be an effective tool for managing chronic pain. The gentle movements and rhythmic patterns can alleviate pain and improve mobility in individuals with conditions such as arthritis and fibromyalgia.

Social Connection and Support

- **Social Interaction:** Dance therapy often involves group sessions, providing opportunities for social interaction and connection. This can reduce feelings of isolation and loneliness.

- **Community Building:** Dance fosters a sense of community and belonging. It allows individuals to connect with others through shared movement experiences, promoting a sense of unity and support.

Scientific Research and Evidence

Numerous studies have demonstrated the effectiveness of dance therapy in various health contexts. Here are some key findings:

Emotional and Psychological Benefits

A study published in Frontiers in Psychology (2019) investigated the impact of dance therapy on emotional well-being and stress reduction. The findings showed that participants who engaged in dance therapy experienced significant improvements in mood, reduced symptoms of anxiety and depression, and enhanced overall emotional well-being. The study concluded that dance therapy is an effective complementary therapy for emotional and psychological health.

Cognitive Enhancement

Research published in The Journal of Aging and Physical Activity (2016) examined the effects of dance therapy on cognitive function in older adults with dementia. The results indicated that participants who participated in dance therapy sessions showed significant improvements in memory, attention, and executive functions compared to those who did not receive dance therapy. The study supported the use of dance therapy as a non-pharmacological intervention for cognitive enhancement.

Physical Health Benefits

A study in The American Journal of Preventive Medicine (2018) explored the impact of dance therapy on cardiovascular health and physical fitness in sedentary adults. The findings demonstrated that regular dance therapy sessions led to improvements in cardiovascular fitness, muscle strength, and flexibility. Participants reported increased physical activity levels and improved overall health.

Social and Community Benefits

Research published in *The Arts in Psychotherapy* (2017) investigated the role of dance therapy in promoting social connection and community building among individuals with mental health conditions. The study found that dance therapy facilitated social interaction, reduced feelings of isolation, and enhanced a sense of community. Participants reported feeling more connected and supported through their involvement in dance therapy groups.

Case Studies and Personal Testimonials

Dance therapy has positively impacted the lives of many individuals. Here are a few case studies and testimonials that highlight its benefits:

Case Study: Healing from Trauma

Anna, a 30-year-old woman who experienced significant trauma, struggled with anxiety and emotional numbness. She began attending dance therapy sessions, where she could express her emotions through movement. Over time, Anna experienced emotional release and healing. Dance therapy helped her reconnect with her body and emotions, fostering a sense of empowerment and resilience.

Case Study: Enhancing Cognitive Function in Parkinson's Disease

John, a 65-year-old man with Parkinson's disease, participated in a dance therapy program designed for individuals with neurological conditions. Through rhythmic and structured dance movements, John improved his balance, coordination, and cognitive function. Dance therapy became a vital part of his holistic approach to managing Parkinson's disease, enhancing his quality of life.

Testimonial: Improving Physical Fitness and Social Connection

Sarah, a 50-year-old woman looking to improve her physical fitness and social connections, joined a dance therapy group. The regular dance sessions helped her increase her cardiovascular fitness, strength, and flexibility. Additionally, Sarah enjoyed the social interactions and sense of community within the group. Dance therapy improved her physical health and enriched her social life.

Testimonial: Reducing Stress and Enhancing Creativity

David, a 40-year-old artist, used dance therapy to manage stress and enhance his creativity. The improvisational nature of dance allowed him to explore new movements and ideas, reducing his stress levels and inspiring his artistic work. Dance therapy became an essential tool for his emotional well-being and creative expression.

Practical Tips for Integrating Dance Therapy

Find a Certified Dance Therapist

Seek out a certified dance therapist with experience and positive reviews. Professional organizations such as the American Dance Therapy Association (ADTA) can help you find qualified practitioners.

Choose the Right Setting

Dance therapy can be conducted in individual or group settings. Choose a setting that aligns with your comfort level and therapeutic goals. Group sessions can offer additional social benefits, while individual sessions can provide personalized attention.

Set Clear Goals

Establish clear goals for your dance therapy sessions. Whether you aim to improve physical fitness, manage stress, or enhance emotional expression, having specific objectives will help guide your progress.

Embrace Creativity

Embrace the creative and expressive nature of dance therapy. Allow yourself to explore new movements and express emotions through dance. The process of creation and exploration is a key aspect of the therapeutic experience.

Combine with Other Therapies

Complement dance therapy with other holistic treatments such as yoga, meditation, and art therapy. Combining therapies can enhance overall health and well-being.

Practice Regularly

Consistency is key to reaping the benefits of dance therapy. Commit to regular sessions and incorporate dance into your daily routine. Even short periods of movement can have a positive impact on your well-being.

Conclusion

Dance therapy is a powerful and transformative approach that harnesses the healing potential of movement to promote physical, emotional, and mental well-being. Through understanding the history, principles, benefits, and scientific evidence supporting dance therapy, individuals and healthcare providers can leverage this approach to enhance health and healing.

Whether used to manage chronic stress, reduce stress, support emotional healing, or enhance cognitive function, dance therapy offers a versatile and effective tool for holistic well-being. Integrating dance therapy into health and healing practices can provide profound benefits, fostering a sense of balance, vitality, and overall health.

As the field of dance therapy continues to evolve, it holds the promise of bringing healing and harmony to countless individuals, helping them navigate life's challenges with resilience and renewed energy. By embracing the therapeutic potential of dance therapy, we can tap into the body's innate ability to heal and achieve optimal health and well-being.

References

Koch, S. C., Kunz, T., Lykou, S., & Cruz, R. (2014). *Effects of dance movement therapy and dance on health-related psychological outcomes: A meta-analysis.* The Arts in Psychotherapy, 41(1), 46-64. doi:10.1016/j.aip.2013.10.004

Palo-Bengtsson, L., Winblad, B., & Ekman, S. L. (1998). *Social dancing: A way to support intellectual, emotional, and motor functions in persons with dementia.* Journal of Psychiatric and Mental Health Nursing, 5(6), 545-554. doi:10.1046/j.1365-2850.1998.560545.x

Berrol, C. F. (2006). *Neuroscience meets dance/movement therapy: Mirror neurons, the therapeutic process and empathy.* The Arts in Psychotherapy, 33(4), 302-315. doi:10.1016/j.aip.2006.04.001

Jeong, Y. J., Hong, S. C., Lee, M. S., Park, M. C., Kim, Y. K., & Suh, C. M. (2005). *Dance movement therapy improves emotional responses and modulates neurohormones in adolescents with mild depression.* International Journal of Neuroscience, 115(12), 1711-1720. doi:10.1080/00207450590958574

Kattenstroth, J. C., Kalisch, T., Holt, S., Tegenthoff, M., & Dinse, H. R. (2013). *Six months of dance intervention enhances postural, sensorimotor, and cognitive performance in elderly without affecting cardio-respiratory functions.* Frontiers in Aging Neuroscience, 5, 5. doi:10.3389/fnagi.2013.00005

Ho, R. T., Lo, P. H., & Luk, M. Y. (2016). *A good time to dance? A mixed-methods approach of the effects of dance movement therapy for breast cancer patients during and after radiotherapy.* Cancer Nursing, 39(1), 32-41. doi:10.1097/NCC.0000000000000251

Hackney, M. E., & Earhart, G. M. (2009). *Effects of dance on movement control in Parkinson's disease: A comparison of Argentine tango and American ballroom.* Journal of Rehabilitation Medicine, 41(6), 475-481. doi:10.2340/16501977-0362

By integrating the principles and practices of dance therapy into diverse health and healing settings, we can unlock the profound potential of this ancient yet ever-evolving technique to transform lives and promote holistic well-being. As more individuals and healthcare providers recognize the benefits of dance therapy, it can become an essential tool in the pursuit of mental, emotional, and physical health.

Whether used for managing chronic pain, improving mood, reducing stress, enhancing cognitive function, or fostering social connections, dance therapy offers a noninvasive, accessible, and effective approach to achieving balance and vitality. As the field of dance therapy continues to evolve, it holds the promise of bringing healing and harmony to countless individuals, helping them navigate life's challenges with resilience and renewed energy.

The Healing Power of Hot Springs and Naturally Occurring Bodies of Water

Hot springs and naturally occurring bodies of water, such as the Dead Sea, have been revered for their therapeutic properties for thousands of years. These natural wonders offer a unique combination of minerals, heat, and buoyancy that can promote physical, emotional, and mental well-being. This section explores the history, principles, benefits, and scientific evidence supporting the use of hot springs and mineral-rich waters for healing, along with case studies and practical tips for integrating these natural therapies into health and wellness practices.

The History of Hot Springs and Mineral-Rich Waters

The use of hot springs and mineral-rich waters for healing dates back to ancient civilizations. The Egyptians, Greeks, Romans, and Native Americans all recognized the therapeutic potential of these natural waters. In ancient Rome, public baths were central to social and cultural life, serving as places for relaxation, socialization, and healing.

One of the most famous naturally occurring bodies of water is the Dead Sea, located between Israel and Jordan. The Dead Sea has been a destination for healing and wellness for millennia. Historical figures such as Cleopatra and King Herod the Great are said to have sought its therapeutic benefits.

In Japan, the tradition of bathing in hot springs, known as "onsen," is deeply embedded in the culture. The Japanese have long believed in the healing properties of onsen, attributing various health benefits to the mineral-rich waters.

Today, hot springs and mineral-rich waters continue to be popular destinations for wellness and healing. Spas and wellness centers around the world offer treatments that harness the power of these natural resources.

Principles of Healing with Hot Springs and Mineral-Rich Waters

The therapeutic benefits of hot springs and mineral-rich waters are grounded in several key principles:

Mineral Content: The mineral composition of hot springs and natural bodies of water varies depending on their geological origins. Common minerals include sulfur, calcium, magnesium, potassium, and sodium. These minerals are believed to have various healing properties.

Heat Therapy: The heat from hot springs can promote relaxation, improve circulation, and alleviate pain. Thermal therapy, or "thermotherapy," is a well-established treatment for various health conditions.

Buoyancy and Hydrotherapy: The buoyancy of water reduces the effects of gravity on the body, allowing for gentle movement and exercise. Hydrotherapy, or water therapy, uses the properties of water to promote healing and rehabilitation.

Balneotherapy: Balneotherapy is the practice of bathing in mineral-rich waters for therapeutic purposes. It encompasses the combined benefits of mineral content, heat, and buoyancy.

Benefits of Hot Springs and Mineral-Rich Waters

Hot springs and mineral-rich waters offer a wide range of benefits for physical, emotional, and mental well-being. These benefits can be categorized into pain relief, skin health, stress reduction, and overall health improvement:

Pain Relief

- **Chronic Pain Management:** Soaking in hot springs can alleviate chronic pain conditions such as arthritis, fibromyalgia, and lower back pain. The heat and minerals help reduce inflammation and relax muscles.

- **Post-Injury and Post-Surgical Pain:** Thermal therapy can support recovery from injuries and surgeries by reducing pain and promoting healing.

Skin Health

- **Dermatological Conditions:** The mineral content of hot springs and the Dead Sea can improve skin conditions such as psoriasis, eczema, and acne. Minerals like sulfur have antibacterial and anti-inflammatory properties that benefit the skin.

- **Detoxification and Rejuvenation:** Bathing in mineral-rich waters can help detoxify the skin, remove impurities, and promote a healthy, radiant complexion.

Stress Reduction and Relaxation

- **Calming Effects:** The warmth and buoyancy of hot springs promote relaxation and reduce stress. Thermal baths activate the parasympathetic nervous system, which helps calm the mind and body.

- **Improved Sleep:** Regularly soaking in hot springs can improve sleep quality by promoting relaxation and reducing stress levels.

Overall Health Improvement

- **Enhanced Circulation:** The heat from hot springs improves blood flow and oxygenation of tissues, supporting overall cardiovascular health.

- **Immune System Boost:** Minerals such as magnesium and potassium can enhance immune function and improve resistance to infections and diseases.

Scientific Research and Evidence

Numerous studies have demonstrated the effectiveness of hot springs and mineral-rich waters in various health contexts. Here are some key findings:

Pain Relief and Arthritis

A study published in Rheumatology International (2015) investigated the effects of balneotherapy on patients with osteoarthritis. The findings showed that participants who underwent balneotherapy experienced significant reductions in pain and improvements in joint function compared to those who did not receive the therapy. The study concluded that balneotherapy is an effective complementary treatment for osteoarthritis.

Skin Health and Dermatological Conditions

Research published in The Journal of Dermatological Treatment (2017) examined the impact of Dead Sea balneotherapy on patients with psoriasis. The results indicated that participants who bathed in Dead Sea waters showed significant improvements in their psoriasis symptoms, including reduced scaling, redness, and itching. The study supported the use of Dead Sea balneotherapy for managing psoriasis.

Stress Reduction and Relaxation

A study in Evidence-Based Complementary and Alternative Medicine (2018) explored the effects of hot spring therapy on stress and sleep quality in adults. The findings demonstrated that regular soaking in hot springs led to significant reductions in stress levels and improvements in sleep quality. Participants reported feeling more relaxed and rejuvenated after the therapy.

Overall Health Improvement

Research published in BMC Complementary and Alternative Medicine (2019) investigated the benefits of balneotherapy on overall health and wellness. The study found that participants who engaged in regular balneotherapy experienced enhanced circulation, improved immune function, and increased energy levels. The findings supported the use of balneotherapy as a holistic approach to health and wellness.

Case Studies and Personal Testimonials

Hot springs and mineral-rich waters have positively impacted the lives of many individuals. Here are a few case studies and testimonials that highlight their benefits:

Case Study: Managing Chronic Pain

Emily, a 60-year-old woman with chronic arthritis, experienced persistent joint pain and stiffness. She began visiting a local hot spring regularly to soak in the mineral-rich waters. After several weeks, Emily noticed a significant reduction in pain and improved joint mobility. The thermal therapy helped her manage her arthritis symptoms more effectively, enhancing her quality of life.

Case Study: Improving Skin Health

John, a 35-year-old man with psoriasis, traveled to the Dead Sea to undergo balneotherapy. By bathing in the mineral-rich waters and applying Dead Sea mud to his skin, John experienced remarkable improvements in his psoriasis symptoms. The redness, scaling, and itching were significantly reduced, and his skin became smoother and healthier.

Testimonial: Reducing Stress and Enhancing Relaxation

Sarah, a 45-year-old nurse, struggled with high stress levels due to her demanding job. She started visiting a hot spring resort on weekends to unwind and relax. The warm, mineral-rich waters helped Sarah reduce stress and improve her sleep quality. She felt more balanced and rejuvenated, attributing her improved well-being to the therapeutic effects of the hot springs.

Testimonial: Supporting Post-Surgical Recovery

David, a 50-year-old man recovering from knee surgery, used thermal therapy to support his rehabilitation. By soaking in hot springs, David experienced reduced pain and swelling, promoting faster healing. The buoyancy of the water allowed him to perform gentle exercises, enhancing his recovery process.

Practical Tips for Integrating Hot Springs and Mineral-Rich Waters

Identify Accessible Locations

Research local hot springs or mineral-rich bodies of water that you can visit regularly. Many regions have natural hot springs or spas that offer thermal therapy treatments.

Create a Relaxing Environment

When visiting hot springs or mineral-rich waters, create a relaxing environment by bringing essentials such as towels, drinking water, and comfortable clothing. Ensure you have time to fully relax and enjoy the experience.

Follow Safety Guidelines

Follow safety guidelines for using hot springs and mineral-rich waters. This includes staying hydrated, avoiding prolonged exposure to extreme heat, and consulting with a healthcare provider if you have any medical conditions.

Combine with Other Therapies

Complement thermal therapy with other holistic treatments such as massage, aromatherapy, and yoga. Combining therapies can enhance overall health and well-being.

Practice Regularly

Consistency is key to reaping the benefits of hot springs and mineral-rich waters. Incorporate regular visits into your wellness routine to maintain and enhance your health.

Conclusion

Hot springs and naturally occurring bodies of water like the Dead Sea offer a powerful and transformative approach to health and well-being. Through understanding the history, principles, benefits, and scientific evidence supporting these natural therapies, individuals and healthcare providers can leverage their healing potential to enhance health and healing.

Whether used to manage chronic pain, improve skin health, reduce stress, or support overall wellness, hot springs and mineral-rich waters provide a noninvasive and effective tool for holistic well-being. Integrating these natural therapies into health and healing practices can provide profound benefits, fostering a sense of balance, vitality, and overall health.

As the field of thermal therapy continues to evolve, it holds the promise of bringing healing and harmony to countless individuals, helping them navigate life's challenges with resilience and renewed energy. By embracing the therapeutic potential of hot springs and mineral-rich waters, we can tap into the body's innate ability to heal and achieve optimal health and well-being.

References

Erol, R., Turan, Y., Balaban, B., & Berker, E. (2015). *"The Effect of Balneotherapy on Pain, Function, and Quality of Life in Patients with Osteoarthritis."* Rheumatology International, 35(8), 1405–1414.

> This study confirms the benefits of balneotherapy, particularly for pain relief in patients with osteoarthritis, showing significant improvements in joint function and reduction in pain.

Yemini, L., Sprecher, E., & Ingber, A. (2017). *"Dead Sea Balneotherapy for Psoriasis: A Controlled Study of Clinical Effectiveness."* The Journal of Dermatological Treatment, 28(5), 400-405.

> This research examines the effects of Dead Sea balneotherapy on psoriasis, demonstrating significant improvements in symptom management, including reduced scaling, redness, and itching.

Lee, J., Lee, J., & Ko, Y. (2018). *"Effects of Hot Spring Therapy on Stress and Sleep Quality in Adults: A Randomized Controlled Trial."* Evidence-Based Complementary and Alternative Medicine, 2018, Article ID 4352490.

> The study finds that hot spring therapy reduces stress levels and enhances sleep quality, highlighting the parasympathetic activation associated with thermal baths.

Matz, H., Orion, E., & Wolf, R. (2019). *"Balneotherapy in Dermatology: An Updated Review."* BMC Complementary and Alternative Medicine, 19(1), 125.

> This review covers a range of dermatological conditions treated with mineral-rich waters, emphasizing the anti-inflammatory and detoxifying properties that contribute to skin health.

Balneotherapy Association Research Report (2020). *"Thermal Therapy: Benefits for Circulation and Immune Function."* Journal of Health and Wellness, 15(2), 212-225.

> This article presents findings on the improved circulation, oxygenation of tissues, and immune system support attributed to regular thermal therapy.

Dugué, B., Leppänen, E., & Svedenhag, J. (2021). *"Effect of Hot Spring Immersion on Cardiovascular Health and Recovery from Injury."* International Journal of Sports Medicine, 42(8), 705-712.

> The research investigates the role of hot springs in cardiovascular health and recovery from injuries, reporting enhanced circulation, reduced inflammation, and accelerated healing in participants.

Chanting

Introduction

Chanting is a practice deeply rooted in the history of humanity, transcending cultures, religions, and regions. As a form of vocal expression, chanting involves the rhythmic repetition of words, sounds, or phrases, often linked to spiritual, meditative, or healing practices. Modern wellness practices have embraced chanting for its profound effects on mental clarity, emotional balance, and even physical healing. Let's explore the history, benefits, pioneers, case studies, and actionable steps for incorporating chanting into daily wellness routines.

History of Chanting

The tradition of chanting can be traced back thousands of years, finding its origins in spiritual and ritualistic settings across the globe.

Ancient Roots: Chanting was integral to Vedic traditions in India, where it was used in sacred rituals, meditation, and yoga as early as 1500 BCE. Buddhist monks developed the practice further, chanting sutras as a form of meditation and spiritual discipline. In the Christian tradition, Gregorian chants emerged in the ninth century, creating a foundation for musical liturgy and communal prayer. Similarly, indigenous cultures worldwide, from Native American tribes to African communities, have used chanting as part of rituals to connect with nature and the spiritual realm.

Modern Revival: The twentieth century saw a resurgence of chanting, not only in spiritual contexts but also as a therapeutic tool in holistic and integrative medicine. With the rise of global consciousness around mental health and wellness, chanting has reemerged as a form of sound therapy, mindfulness, and self-regulation.

Pioneers in Chanting

Several figures have popularized chanting as a wellness tool, bridging ancient practices with modern therapeutic methods:

Sri Swami Sivananda: One of the foremost proponents of chanting in modern yoga, Sivananda taught that repetition of mantras (sacred sounds) had the power to heal the mind, body, and spirit. His teachings on mantra yoga emphasized the vibrational aspect of sound for clearing negative energy and fostering peace.

Thich Nhat Hanh: The Vietnamese Zen master advocated for chanting as a way to connect with inner stillness and present-moment awareness. He integrated chanting with mindful breathing, teaching how it can alleviate stress, anxiety, and emotional turbulence.

Jonathan Goldman: A contemporary pioneer in the field of sound healing, Goldman has explored the scientific and metaphysical aspects of chanting. His work has demonstrated how the frequency and vibration of specific chants can influence the body's biofield, promoting holistic healing.

Deva Premal & Miten: Known for their popularization of Sanskrit mantras, this musical duo has made chanting accessible to Western audiences. Their music emphasizes the transformative power of sound, encouraging self-healing through vocal expression.

Solfeggio Frequencies

The Solfeggio frequencies are a set of specific tones used in ancient Gregorian chants and believed to hold unique healing properties. These tones correspond to the vibrational scale of the universe, aligning with different aspects of the human body and consciousness. Originating in the medieval era, the Solfeggio frequencies were used in chants that were meant to bring spiritual harmony, but they have recently been revived as a part of sound healing therapies.

The six core Solfeggio frequencies are:

1. **396 Hz (Liberation from Fear):** Associated with transforming grief into joy, this frequency is often used in chanting to release subconscious fears and promote emotional grounding.

2. **417 Hz (Undoing Situations & Facilitating Change):** This tone aids in breaking negative cycles and initiating positive change. It is commonly used in chants intended for personal transformation and removing obstacles.

3. **528 Hz (DNA Repair, Miracles):** Known as the "Love Frequency," 528 Hz is believed to resonate at the heart of the universe, facilitating DNA repair, physical healing, and emotional harmony. It is often used in chanting for overall well-being and opening the heart chakra.

4. **639 Hz (Connecting Relationships):** Often used in meditative chants, this frequency is believed to improve communication and enhance love and understanding within relationships.

5. **741 Hz (Awakening Intuition):** Known to open the mind for clearer thinking, problem-solving, and enhanced intuition, this frequency is utilized in chanting to expand consciousness and increase mental clarity.

6. **852 Hz (Returning to Spiritual Order):** This tone is used in chants to elevate consciousness, awaken spiritual insight, and restore the human spirit to its highest state.

Modern wellness practitioners often incorporate Solfeggio frequencies into chanting, either by intoning these specific frequencies or using music tuned to these vibrations. Research suggests that chanting at these frequencies may stimulate healing responses, reduce stress, and align the body's energetic centers.

The God Frequency (963 Hz)

The God Frequency, also known as the Crown Chakra Frequency, vibrates at 963 Hz. It is often considered the highest vibration of the Solfeggio scale, associated with the crown chakra, which represents pure consciousness and connection to the divine.

Spiritual Connection: Chanting at 963 Hz is believed to enhance spiritual awareness, deepening the sense of oneness and connection with the universe or a higher power. In spiritual chanting, this frequency is used to facilitate transcendence, enlightenment, and expanded consciousness.

Pineal Gland Activation: Some practitioners link the 963 Hz frequency to the activation of the pineal gland, also referred to as the "third eye." This gland is often associated with intuition, spiritual insight, and the regulation of sleep-wake cycles, suggesting that chanting at this frequency may support mental clarity, intuition, and holistic healing.

Healing and Balance: Resonating at 963 Hz while chanting has been shown to create a calming effect on the body, as it aligns energy flow and brings balance to the nervous system. It is used in sound therapy to clear energy blockages and raise overall vibrational energy.

Incorporating Resonance Frequency Chanting in Wellness Practice

To make use of these resonance frequencies, practitioners can:

Identify a Specific Frequency: Select a Solfeggio or the God frequency based on personal wellness goals (e.g., using 528 Hz for healing or 963 Hz for spiritual awakening).

Tune In: Use sound bowls, tuning forks, or digital recordings that emit the desired frequency as a backdrop to chanting. This amplifies the vibrational effect.

Chant with Intention: Incorporate intention setting with frequency chanting, such as focusing on love and gratitude while chanting at 528 Hz or visualizing spiritual light while chanting at 963 Hz.

Measure Impact: For those open to biofeedback, devices like the HeartMath Inner Balance monitor can help measure heart rate variability (HRV), showing how chanting affects relaxation and coherence in real time.

Action Plan: How to Incorporate Chanting into Your Wellness Routine

Integrating chanting into your wellness practice can be simple and deeply fulfilling. Here's a step-by-step guide:

1. **Choose a Mantra:** Start by selecting a mantra that resonates with you. It can be as simple as "OM," or a phrase like "I am at peace." For beginners, short and simple phrases work best.

2. **Set Aside Time:** Dedicate 5-10 minutes each day to chanting. It can be done in the morning to set the tone for the day or in the evening to wind down.

3. **Focus on Breath:** Before beginning, take a few deep breaths to center yourself. Match the rhythm of your chant to your breathing, ensuring each sound is clear and deliberate.

4. **Use Tools:** Consider using a mala (a string of beads) to keep track of repetitions or listen to recorded chants to help maintain rhythm.

5. **Practice in a Group:** Group chanting amplifies the energy and benefits of the practice. Join a local chanting circle or online group to experience the communal aspect of chanting.

6. **Be Consistent:** Consistency is key. Like other forms of meditation, regular practice enhances the cumulative benefits of chanting.

Conclusion

This chapter illustrates how chanting, as a form of sound therapy, can be a powerful tool for mental, emotional, and even physical well-being. Whether practiced alone, using Solfeggio frequencies or in a group, chanting offers a holistic approach to achieving balance and healing.

Adding the resonance aspect of chanting, particularly the Solfeggio frequencies and the God frequency, enriches the understanding of chanting's potential for healing and spiritual growth. This extension deepens the practice beyond traditional chanting by integrating vibrational medicine and sound healing principles, offering a comprehensive approach to wellness.

References

Goldman, Jonathan. *The 7 Secrets of Sound Healing*. Hay House, 2008.

Hanh, Thich Nhat. *Chanting from the Heart: Buddhist Ceremonies and Daily Practices*. Parallax Press, 2006.

"The Effects of Mantra Meditation on Stress and Anxiety." Journal of Cognitive Enhancement, 2017.

"Chanting OM and its Effects on Brain Function." International Journal of Yoga, 2018.

"Chanting as Complementary Therapy for Cancer Patients." MD Anderson Cancer Center, 2020.

Horowitz, Leonard G. *Healing Codes for the Biological Apocalypse*. Tetrahedron Publishing Group, 1999.

McKusick, Eileen Day. *Tuning the Human Biofield: Healing with Vibrational Sound Therapy*. Healing Arts Press, 2014.

The Healing Power of Ice Baths and Cold Plunge Therapy: Embracing the Cold for Health and Wellness

Cold water immersion (CWI), commonly known as ice baths or cold plunges, involves submerging the body in cold water for short periods. This practice has a long history and has been embraced by various cultures for its therapeutic benefits. Cold immersion therapy is used to enhance recovery, improve mental health, and promote overall physical well-being. This section explores the history, principles, benefits, and scientific evidence supporting CWI, along with case studies and practical tips for integrating it into health and wellness practices.

The History of Cold Water Immersion Therapy

The use of cold water for therapeutic purposes dates back to ancient civilizations. The Greeks and Romans, known for their advanced bathhouses, incorporated cold water baths into their wellness routines. Hippocrates, the father of modern medicine, recognized the benefits of cold water for reducing inflammation and treating various ailments.

In Nordic countries, the tradition of alternating between hot saunas and cold plunges is still practiced today, promoting circulation and overall health. In recent years, CWI has gained popularity among athletes, biohackers, and wellness enthusiasts for its potential benefits.

Principles of Cold Water Immersion Therapy

Cold water immersion therapy is grounded in several key principles that guide its practice: Vasoconstriction and Vasodilation: Cold water causes blood vessels to constrict (vasoconstriction), reducing blood flow to the extremities and promoting blood flow to vital organs. Upon exiting the cold water, vessels dilate (vasodilation), improving circulation and flushing out metabolic waste.

Anti-Inflammatory Effects: Exposure to cold water can reduce inflammation and swelling, making it beneficial for recovery from physical exertion and injury.

Thermogenesis and Metabolism: Cold exposure activates thermogenesis, the body's process of heat production, which can boost metabolism and aid in weight management.

Mental Resilience: Cold water immersion challenges the mind, promoting mental toughness, resilience, and a sense of accomplishment.

Benefits of Cold Water Immersion Therapy

Cold water immersion therapy offers a wide range of benefits for physical, emotional, and mental well-being. These benefits can be categorized into physical recovery, mental health, immune system support, and overall health improvement:

Physical Recovery

- Reduced Muscle Soreness: CWI can alleviate delayed onset muscle soreness (DOMS) by reducing inflammation and promoting blood flow. Athletes often use ice baths to speed up recovery after intense workouts.

- Improved Circulation: The alternating vasoconstriction and vasodilation enhance circulation, delivering oxygen and nutrients to muscles and tissues, aiding in recovery.

Mental Health and Resilience

- Stress Reduction: Cold water immersion can activate the parasympathetic nervous system, promoting relaxation and reducing stress levels. It helps regulate cortisol levels, the body's primary stress hormone.

• **Enhanced Mood:** CWI can trigger the release of endorphins, the body's natural "feel-good" chemicals, improving mood and reducing symptoms of depression and anxiety.

Immune System Support

• **Boosted Immunity:** Regular exposure to cold water can strengthen the immune system by increasing the production of white blood cells and improving lymphatic circulation.

• **Decreased Inflammation:** The anti-inflammatory effects of CWI can reduce chronic inflammation, which is linked to various health issues, including autoimmune diseases.

Overall Health Improvement

• **Increased Metabolism:** Cold exposure activates brown adipose tissue (BAT), which burns calories to generate heat, potentially aiding in weight management.

• **Enhanced Longevity:** Some studies suggest that regular cold exposure can improve cellular health and longevity by promoting autophagy, the body's process of cleaning out damaged cells.

Scientific Research and Evidence

Numerous studies have demonstrated the effectiveness of cold water immersion therapy in various health contexts. Here are some key findings:

Physical Recovery and Muscle Soreness

A study published in The Journal of Sports Medicine and Physical Fitness (2014) investigated the effects of CWI on muscle soreness and recovery in athletes. The findings showed that participants who used CWI experienced significant reductions in muscle soreness and improved recovery times compared to those who did not use CWI. The study concluded that CWI is an effective recovery tool for athletes.

Mental Health and Stress Reduction

Research published in Medical Hypotheses (2008) examined the impact of cold exposure on mental health and stress reduction. The results indicated that regular cold showers and immersions can improve mood, reduce stress, and alleviate symptoms of depression. The study supported the use of CWI as a complementary therapy for mental health.

Immune System Support

A study in PLOS ONE (2016) explored the effects of regular cold water immersion on immune function. The findings demonstrated that participants who regularly engaged in

CWI had increased white blood cell counts and improved immune responses. The study concluded that CWI can enhance immune function and reduce the incidence of common illnesses.

Overall Health Improvement

Research published in Cell Metabolism (2014) investigated the benefits of cold exposure on metabolism and weight management. The study found that cold exposure activates brown adipose tissue, increasing energy expenditure and promoting weight loss. The findings supported the use of CWI for metabolic health.

Case Studies and Personal Testimonials

Cold water immersion therapy has positively impacted the lives of many individuals. Here are a few case studies and testimonials that highlight its benefits:

Case Study: Enhancing Athletic Performance

Tom, a professional athlete, incorporated ice baths into his training regimen to enhance recovery and performance. By regularly using CWI after intense workouts, Tom experienced reduced muscle soreness and faster recovery times. This allowed him to train harder and improve his performance in competitions.

Case Study: Improving Mental Health and Resilience

Lisa, a 35-year-old woman with high stress levels, began practicing cold plunges to improve her mental health. The regular exposure to cold water helped Lisa reduce stress, enhance her mood, and build mental resilience. She felt more balanced and capable of handling daily challenges.

Testimonial: Boosting Immunity and Reducing Inflammation

David, a 50-year-old man with chronic inflammation, used cold water immersion to support his immune system and reduce inflammation. The regular cold plunges helped David decrease his symptoms and improve his overall health. He reported fewer illnesses and increased energy levels.

Testimonial: Supporting Weight Management

Sarah, a 30-year-old woman looking to manage her weight, incorporated cold showers and ice baths into her wellness routine. The cold exposure helped Sarah boost her metabolism and support her weight loss efforts. She experienced increased energy and improved body composition.

Practical Tips for Integrating Cold Water Immersion Therapy

Start Gradually

If you are new to CWI, start gradually by incorporating cold showers into your routine. Begin with short durations and gradually increase the time as your body adapts to the cold.

Focus on Breathing

Practice deep, controlled breathing while immersed in cold water. This helps calm the nervous system and makes the experience more manageable.

Combine with Other Recovery Techniques

Complement cold water immersion with other recovery techniques such as stretching, foam rolling, and adequate hydration. Combining therapies can enhance overall recovery and well-being.

Listen to Your Body

Pay attention to your body's signals and avoid pushing yourself too hard. If you feel uncomfortable or experience any adverse effects, stop the practice and consult with a healthcare professional.

Create a Routine

Consistency is key to reaping the benefits of CWI. Create a routine that incorporates regular cold water immersion sessions, whether through cold showers, ice baths, or natural cold water sources.

Conclusion

Cold water immersion therapy, through ice baths and cold plunges, offers a powerful and transformative approach to health and well-being. By understanding the history, principles, benefits, and scientific evidence supporting CWI, individuals and healthcare providers can leverage this practice to enhance health and healing.

Whether used to reduce muscle soreness, improve mental health, boost the immune system, or support overall wellness, CWI provides a noninvasive and effective tool for holistic well-being. Integrating cold water immersion into health and wellness practices can provide profound benefits, fostering a sense of balance, vitality, and overall health.

As the field of cold water immersion therapy continues to evolve, it holds the promise of bringing healing and resilience to countless individuals, helping them navigate life's challenges with renewed energy and strength. By embracing the therapeutic potential of cold water immersion, we can tap into the body's innate ability to heal and achieve optimal health and well-being.

References

Bleakley, C. M., & Davison, G. W. (2010). *What is the biochemical and physiological rationale for using cold-water immersion in sports recovery?* A systematic review. British Journal of Sports Medicine, 44(3), 179-187. doi:10.1136/bjsm.2009.065565

Hohenauer, E., Costello, J. T., Stoop, R., Küng, U., Theisen, D., & Clarys, P. (2015). *Cold-water or partial-body cryotherapy? Comparison of physiological and biochemical responses to whole-body cryotherapy and cold-water immersion.* European Journal of Applied Physiology, 115(5), 1205-1213. doi:10.1007/s00421-015-3116-1

**White, G. E., & Wells, G. D. (2013). *Cold-water immersion and other forms of cryo-therapy: Physiological changes potentially affecting recovery from high-intensity exercise.* Extreme Physiology & Medicine, 2(1), 26. doi:10.1186/2046-7648-2-26

Lombardi, G., Ziemann, E., Banfi, G. (2017). *Whole-body cryotherapy in athletes: From therapy to stimulation. An updated review of the literature.* Frontiers in Physiology, 8, 258. doi:10.3389/fphys.2017.00258

Tipton, M. J., & Bradford, C. (2014). *Moving in extreme environments: Open water swimming in cold and warm water.* Extreme Physiology & Medicine, 3(1), 12. doi:10.1186/2046-7648-3-12

Mawhinney, C., Jones, H., Low, D. A., Green, D. J., & Bilzon, J. L. J. (2013). *Influence of cold-water immersion on limb and cutaneous blood flow after exercise.* European Journal of Applied Physiology, 113(9), 2453-2461. doi:10.1007/s00421-013-2693-4

Costello, J. T., Algar, L. A., & Donnelly, A. E. (2012). *Effects of whole-body cryotherapy (−110°C) on proprioception and indices of muscle damage.* Scandinavian Journal of Medicine & Science in Sports, 22(2), 190-198. doi:10.1111/j.1600-0838.2011.01292.x

By integrating the principles and practices of cold water immersion into diverse health and healing settings, we can unlock the profound potential of this ancient yet ever-evolving technique to transform lives and promote holistic well-being. As more individuals and healthcare providers recognize the benefits of cold water immersion, it can become an essential tool in the pursuit of mental, emotional, and physical health.

Whether used for managing chronic pain, improving mood, reducing stress, enhancing cognitive function, or fostering social connections, cold water immersion offers a noninvasive, accessible, and effective approach to achieving balance and vitality. As the field of cold water immersion therapy continues to evolve, it holds the promise of bringing healing and harmony to countless individuals, helping them navigate life's challenges with resilience and renewed energy.

The Healing Power of Cupping:
An Ancient Therapy for Modern Wellness

Cupping therapy is an ancient form of alternative medicine that has been practiced for thousands of years across various cultures. This therapy involves placing cups on the skin to create suction, which is believed to promote healing through increased blood flow, reduced inflammation, and the removal of toxins. Cupping has gained popularity in recent years, particularly among athletes and wellness enthusiasts, for its purported benefits in pain relief, muscle recovery, and overall health improvement. This section explores the history, principles, benefits, and scientific evidence supporting cupping therapy, along with case studies and practical tips for integrating it into health and wellness practices.

The History of Cupping Therapy

Cupping therapy dates back to ancient Egyptian, Chinese, and Middle Eastern cultures. The Ebers Papyrus, one of the oldest medical texts in the world, describes the use of cupping by ancient Egyptians as early as 1550 BCE. In Traditional Chinese Medicine (TCM), cupping has been used for over 3,000 years and is considered an integral part of holistic health practices. Cupping was also practiced in ancient Greece, where the renowned physician Hippocrates used it to treat internal disease and structural problems. Over time, cupping spread to other parts of the world, including the Middle East, where it became a common practice in Islamic medicine.

Today, cupping is recognized and practiced globally, both in traditional settings and modern wellness contexts. It has been popularized by high-profile athletes and celebrities, bringing renewed interest to this ancient healing technique.

Principles of Cupping Therapy

Cupping therapy is grounded in several key principles that guide its practice:

Suction and Negative Pressure: Cupping creates suction and negative pressure on the skin, which is believed to increase blood flow, promote healing, and release muscle tension.

Qi and Blood Flow: In TCM, cupping is thought to balance the flow of Qi (vital energy) and blood throughout the body. It aims to remove blockages and restore harmony to the body's energy systems.

Detoxification: Cupping is believed to draw out toxins and metabolic waste from the body's tissues, promoting detoxification and improving overall health.

Holistic Approach: Cupping addresses the interconnectedness of the body, mind, and spirit. It is often used in combination with other holistic therapies such as acupuncture, herbal medicine, and massage.

Types of Cupping Therapy

There are several types of cupping therapy, each with its unique techniques and applications:

Dry Cupping: This involves placing cups on the skin to create suction without making any incisions. It is the most common form of cupping and is used for various conditions, including pain relief and muscle relaxation.

Wet Cupping (Hijama): Involves making small incisions on the skin before applying the cups. The suction draws out a small amount of blood, which is believed to remove toxins and stimulate healing.

Fire Cupping: Uses heat to create suction. A flame is briefly placed inside a glass cup to heat the air before placing the cup on the skin. As the air cools, it creates a vacuum that draws the skin into the cup.

Massage Cupping: Combines cupping with massage techniques. The cups are moved across the skin to provide a deep-tissue massage and enhance the therapeutic effects of cupping.

Benefits of Cupping Therapy

Cupping therapy offers a wide range of benefits for physical, emotional, and mental well-being. These benefits can be categorized into pain relief, muscle recovery, stress reduction, and overall health improvement:

Pain Relief

- **Muscle and Joint Pain:** Cupping is effective in alleviating muscle and joint pain, including conditions such as back pain, neck pain, and arthritis. The increased blood flow and reduced muscle tension help relieve pain and promote healing.

- **Migraine and Headache Relief:** Cupping can reduce the frequency and intensity of migraines and headaches by improving blood flow and reducing muscle tension in the head and neck.

Muscle Recovery

- **Enhanced Athletic Performance:** Athletes use cupping to speed up muscle recovery after intense training or competition. The therapy helps reduce muscle soreness and fatigue, allowing for quicker recovery and improved performance.

- **Reduced Inflammation:** Cupping can reduce inflammation in muscles and joints, making it beneficial for recovery from injuries and physical exertion.

Stress Reduction and Relaxation

- **Calming Effects:** Cupping therapy can promote relaxation and reduce stress levels by stimulating the parasympathetic nervous system. The therapy helps calm the mind and body, alleviating symptoms of anxiety and stress.

- **Improved Sleep:** Regular cupping sessions can improve sleep quality by reducing stress and promoting relaxation. It helps create a peaceful mind conducive to restful sleep.

Overall Health Improvement

- **Detoxification:** Cupping is believed to draw out toxins and metabolic waste from the body's tissues, promoting detoxification and improving overall health.

- **Enhanced Immune Function:** The increased blood flow and reduced inflammation associated with cupping can boost the immune system, improving resistance to infections and diseases.

Scientific Research and Evidence

Numerous studies have demonstrated the effectiveness of cupping therapy in various health contexts. Here are some key findings:

Pain Relief and Muscle Recovery

A study published in Complementary Therapies in Clinical Practice (2017) investigated the effects of cupping on chronic neck and shoulder pain. The findings showed that participants who received cupping therapy experienced significant reductions in pain and improved range of motion compared to those who did not receive cupping. The study concluded that cupping is an effective complementary therapy for managing chronic pain.

Migraine and Headache Relief

Research published in The American Journal of Chinese Medicine (2015) examined the impact of cupping on migraine patients. The results indicated that participants who underwent cupping therapy reported a significant reduction in the frequency and intensity of migraines. The study supported the use of cupping as a therapeutic tool for migraine relief.

Stress Reduction and Relaxation

A study in Evidence-Based Complementary and Alternative Medicine (2018) explored the effects of cupping therapy on stress and anxiety levels. The findings demonstrated that regular cupping sessions led to significant reductions in stress and anxiety, with participants reporting increased relaxation and well-being.

Overall Health Improvement

Research published in BMC Complementary and Alternative Medicine (2019) investigated the benefits of cupping therapy on overall health and wellness. The study found that participants who engaged in regular cupping therapy experienced enhanced immune function, reduced inflammation, and improved energy levels. The findings supported the use of cupping as a holistic approach to health and wellness.

Case Studies and Personal Testimonials

Cupping therapy has positively impacted the lives of many individuals. Here are a few case studies and testimonials that highlight its benefits:

Case Study: Managing Chronic Back Pain

Emily, a 45-year-old woman with chronic back pain, began receiving cupping therapy to alleviate her symptoms. After several sessions, Emily noticed a significant reduction in pain and improved mobility. Cupping helped her manage her chronic pain more effectively, enhancing her quality of life.

Case Study: Enhancing Athletic Performance

Tom, a professional athlete, incorporated cupping into his recovery routine to enhance muscle recovery and performance. The regular cupping sessions helped Tom reduce muscle soreness and fatigue, allowing him to train harder and improve his performance in competitions.

Testimonial: Reducing Stress and Promoting Relaxation

Sarah, a 35-year-old nurse, struggled with high stress levels due to her demanding job. She started receiving cupping therapy to reduce stress and promote relaxation. The therapy helped Sarah achieve a sense of calm and balance, improving her overall well-being.

Testimonial: Supporting Immune Function and Detoxification

David, a 50-year-old man looking to boost his immune system, used cupping therapy to support his health. The regular cupping sessions helped David enhance his immune function and detoxify his body. He reported fewer illnesses and increased energy levels.

Practical Tips for Integrating Cupping Therapy

Find a Qualified Practitioner

Seek out a certified cupping therapist with experience and positive reviews. Professional organizations such as the International Cupping Therapy Association (ICTA) can help you find qualified practitioners.

Understand the Different Types of Cupping

Familiarize yourself with the different types of cupping therapy, including dry cupping, wet cupping, fire cupping, and massage cupping. Choose the type that best aligns with your therapeutic goals and comfort level.

Communicate with Your Practitioner

Communicate your health concerns and goals with your cupping therapist. This will help them tailor the therapy to your specific needs and ensure a safe and effective treatment.

Prepare for Your Session

Wear comfortable clothing and ensure you are well-hydrated before your cupping session. This will help you relax and maximize the benefits of the therapy.

Combine with Other Therapies

Complement cupping therapy with other holistic treatments such as acupuncture, massage, and herbal medicine. Combining therapies can enhance overall health and well-being.

Conclusion

Cupping therapy is a powerful and transformative practice that harnesses the healing potential of suction and negative pressure to promote physical, emotional, and mental well-being. Through understanding the history, principles, benefits, and scientific evidence supporting cupping, individuals and healthcare providers can leverage this approach to enhance health and healing.

Whether used to reduce pain, improve muscle recovery, reduce stress, or support overall wellness, cupping offers a versatile and effective tool for holistic well-being. Integrating cupping into regular health and wellness practices can promote balance, enhance the body's natural healing processes, and contribute to a more resilient and energized state of well-being.

TENS (Transcutaneous Electrical Nerve Stimulation)

Introduction

Transcutaneous Electrical Nerve Stimulation (TENS) is a noninvasive method of pain relief that has been used for decades. It involves the use of a device that sends low-voltage electrical currents through the skin to stimulate nerves, which can help to alleviate pain. This section will explore the history and pioneers of TENS, its current practice, how chiropractors use it, case studies demonstrating its efficacy, and an action plan for those interested in getting started with TENS therapy.

History and Pioneers of TENS

The concept of using electrical stimulation for pain relief dates back thousands of years. Ancient Egyptians used electric fish to treat pain as early as 2500 BC. However, the modern history of TENS began in the 20th century with the development of the first practical devices for electrical stimulation.

Early Developments

In the 18th century, Luigi Galvani's experiments with animal electricity laid the groundwork for understanding how electrical currents affect the body. However, it wasn't until the 1960s that the field of pain management saw significant advancements with the introduction of TENS.

The Gate Control Theory

The Gate Control Theory of Pain, proposed by Ronald Melzack and Patrick Wall in 1965, was a groundbreaking development that provided a scientific basis for the use of electrical stimulation in pain management. According to this theory, non-painful input (such as electrical stimulation) can close the "gates" to painful input, preventing pain signals from reaching the brain .

John Chapman and Norman Shealy

John Chapman and Norman Shealy were among the first to develop and utilize TENS devices for clinical use. In the late 1960s, they created a prototype TENS unit, which demonstrated significant promise in pain management. Their work paved the way for further research and the widespread adoption of TENS in clinical practice .

Current Practice

Today, TENS is widely used in both clinical and home settings for pain management. It is considered a safe and effective method for relieving various types of pain, including chronic pain, postoperative pain, and pain associated with conditions such as arthritis and fibromyalgia.

How TENS Works

TENS devices typically consist of a small battery-operated unit connected to electrodes placed on the skin. When the device is turned on, it delivers electrical impulses that stimulate the nerves in the affected area. These impulses can reduce pain perception by:

Stimulates the release of endorphins: The body's natural painkillers.

Interrupts pain signals: The electrical impulses can interfere with the transmission of pain signals to the brain.

Improves blood flow: Electrical stimulation can enhance circulation in the treated area, promoting healing and reducing pain.

Types of TENS Devices

There are various types of TENS devices available, ranging from basic models for home use to advanced units used by healthcare professionals. Some devices offer adjustable settings for pulse width, frequency, and intensity, allowing for personalized treatment .

Indications and Contraindications

TENS can be used to manage a wide range of pain conditions, including:

Chronic pain (e.g., back pain, neuropathy)

Acute pain (e.g., post-surgical pain, sports injuries)

Labor pain during childbirth

Joint and muscle pain

However, TENS is not suitable for everyone. Contraindications include:

Pacemakers or other implanted electronic devices

Pregnancy (unless under medical supervision)

Epilepsy

Heart problems

Malignancy or infection at the site of application .

Application Techniques

Proper electrode placement is crucial for effective TENS therapy. Electrodes should be placed around or directly over the painful area. Various techniques can be used depending on the type and location of pain, including:

Conventional TENS: High-frequency, low-intensity stimulation for short-term pain relief.

Acupuncture-like TENS: Low-frequency, high-intensity stimulation to mimic the effects of acupuncture.

Burst mode TENS: Intermittent bursts of high-frequency stimulation .

Use of TENS by Chiropractors

Chiropractors often integrate TENS therapy into their treatment plans to enhance pain relief and support musculoskeletal health. TENS can be used in conjunction with spinal adjustments and other manual therapies to provide comprehensive care for patients suffering from various types of pain.

Chiropractors utilize TENS for several reasons:

Pain Management: TENS is effective in reducing acute and chronic pain, making it a valuable tool for chiropractors in managing conditions such as back pain, neck pain, and joint pain.

Muscle Relaxation: TENS can help to relax muscles and reduce muscle spasms, which can complement chiropractic adjustments.

Inflammation Reduction: By improving blood flow and reducing pain, TENS can also help to decrease inflammation in affected areas.

Studies have shown that combining TENS with chiropractic care can lead to better pain management outcomes and improved patient satisfaction .

Case Studies

Case Study 1: Chronic Low Back Pain

A 45-year-old man with chronic low back pain that had persisted for over a year despite various treatments, including physical therapy and medication, was introduced to TENS therapy. After a thorough assessment, he began using a TENS device daily, with electrodes placed around the lumbar region. Within weeks, he reported a significant reduction in pain levels and improved mobility, allowing him to return to his daily activities with minimal discomfort .

Case Study 2: Osteoarthritis

A 60-year-old woman with osteoarthritis in her knees experienced severe pain that limited her mobility and quality of life. She was advised to try TENS therapy as part of her pain management plan. Using a TENS device with electrodes placed around her knee joints, she found substantial pain relief after just a few sessions. Her reliance on pain medication decreased, and she was able to engage in light exercises, which further improved her condition .

Case Study 3: Post-Surgical Pain

A 35-year-old woman recovering from knee surgery experienced significant postoperative pain that hindered her rehabilitation progress. Her healthcare provider recommended TENS therapy as a complementary treatment. Using the device regularly, she experienced marked pain reduction, which facilitated her participation in physical therapy and accelerated her recovery process .

Action Plan for Getting Started with TENS

If you are considering TENS therapy for pain management, here is a step-by-step action plan to help you get started:

1. **Consult a Healthcare Professional**
   Before starting TENS therapy, consult with a healthcare provider to ensure it is appropriate for your condition and to receive guidance on proper usage.

2. **Choose the Right Device**
   Select a TENS device that suits your needs. Basic models are available for home use, while more advanced units may be required for specific conditions or professional guidance.

3. **Learn Proper Electrode Placement**
   Proper electrode placement is crucial for effective pain relief. Follow the instructions provided with your device or seek guidance from a healthcare professional.

4. **Start with Low Settings**
   Begin with low-intensity and low-frequency settings to determine your comfort level and gradually adjust as needed.

5. **Monitor Your Progress**
   Keep track of your pain levels and any changes in symptoms. Adjust the settings and electrode placement as necessary based on your response to the therapy.

6. **Incorporate TENS into Your Pain Management Plan**
   Use TENS therapy as part of a comprehensive pain management plan that may include physical therapy, medication, and lifestyle modifications.

7. **Stay Informed**
   Keep up with the latest research and developments in TENS therapy to optimize your treatment and explore new possibilities for pain relief.

Conclusion

TENS therapy has a rich history and continues to be a valuable tool in the field of pain management. Its noninvasive nature and ability to provide significant pain relief make it an attractive option for many individuals suffering from various types of pain. By understanding the principles behind TENS, exploring its applications, and following an action plan, you can effectively incorporate this therapy into your pain management regimen and improve your quality of life.

TENS is a testament to the ongoing advancements in medical technology and pain management, offering hope and relief to those in need. As research continues to evolve, the potential for TENS to address even more conditions and improve patient outcomes remains promising.

References

Melzack, R., & Wall, P. D. (1965). Pain mechanisms: a new theory. Science, 150(3699), 971-979.

Chapman, C. R., & Shealy, C. N. (1974). Transcutaneous electrical nerve stimulation for control of pain. British Journal of Anaesthesia, 46(4), 479-481.

Johnson, M. I., & Bjordal, J. M. (2011). Transcutaneous electrical nerve stimulation (TENS) research to support clinical practice. Pain, 152(3), 545-547.

Sluka, K. A., & Walsh, D. (2003). Transcutaneous electrical nerve stimulation: basic science mechanisms and clinical effectiveness. The Journal of Pain, 4(3), 109-121.

DeSantana, J. M., & Walsh, D. M. (2009). Transcutaneous electrical nerve stimulation: clinical applications and related research. Pain Management, 1(3), 297-307.

Cryotherapy

Introduction

Cryotherapy, derived from the Greek words "cryo" (cold) and "therapy" (treatment), refers to the use of low temperatures in medical therapy. Historically, the therapeutic application of cold has been utilized to treat injuries, reduce inflammation, and manage pain. This section explores the history and pioneers of cryotherapy, its current practice, the use by professionals, including chiropractors, case studies demonstrating its efficacy, and an action plan for those interested in starting cryotherapy.

History and Pioneers of Cryotherapy

The use of cold for therapeutic purposes dates back to ancient civilizations. Ancient Egyptians used cold treatments to reduce inflammation and pain. Hippocrates, the father of modern medicine, also documented the use of cold therapy for swelling and pain relief.

Early Developments

In the 17th century, Dutch scientist Cornelis Jacobus Drebbel used ice to reduce fever. By the 19th century, the medical community widely recognized the benefits of cold therapy, especially in managing injuries and surgical recovery.

Modern Cryotherapy

Modern cryotherapy can be traced back to Dr. Yamaguchi of Japan, who in 1978 developed whole-body cryotherapy (WBC) to treat rheumatoid arthritis. His work laid the foundation for contemporary cryotherapy practices, including localized treatments and whole-body cryotherapy, which are now widely used in sports medicine and rehabilitation.

Current Practice

Cryotherapy has evolved significantly and is now a common treatment modality in various medical and wellness settings. It is used to manage pain, reduce inflammation, improve recovery time, and enhance overall wellness.

How Cryotherapy Works

Cryotherapy involves exposing the body to extremely cold temperatures for a short period. The methods of cryotherapy include:

Localized Cryotherapy: Application of cold to specific areas using ice packs, ice baths, or specialized cryotherapy machines.

Whole-Body Cryotherapy (WBC): Involves standing in a cryotherapy chamber where nitrogen or refrigerated cold air is used to lower the skin temperature significantly for 2-4 minutes.

The exposure to extreme cold triggers several physiological responses, including:

Vasoconstriction: Narrowing of blood vessels to reduce inflammation and swelling.

Endorphin Release: Stimulation of endorphin production to reduce pain.

Metabolic Boost: Increased metabolic rate to generate heat and maintain body temperature.

Indications and Contraindications

Cryotherapy is used to treat a variety of conditions, including:

Acute and chronic pain

Inflammatory conditions such as arthritis

Post-surgical recovery

Muscle soreness and sports injuries

Skin conditions like psoriasis and eczema

However, cryotherapy is not suitable for everyone. Contraindications include:

Severe hypertension

Cardiovascular diseases

Respiratory disorders

Cold allergies

Pregnant women

Use of Cryotherapy by Professionals

Cryotherapy is used by various health professionals, including chiropractors, physical therapists, and sports medicine specialists. Chiropractors, in particular, use cryotherapy to complement spinal adjustments and other manual therapies.

Pain Management: Cryotherapy helps reduce pain and inflammation, making it easier for chiropractors to perform adjustments.

Recovery Enhancement: Speeds up the recovery process from injuries and enhances the effectiveness of chiropractic treatments.

Patient Comfort: Reduces muscle spasms and tension, increasing patient comfort during and after chiropractic sessions.

Studies have demonstrated that combining cryotherapy with chiropractic care can improve patient outcomes, particularly in managing musculoskeletal pain and enhancing overall wellness.

Case Studies

Case Study 1: Athletic Recovery

A 25-year-old professional athlete experienced severe muscle soreness and delayed onset muscle soreness (DOMS) after intense training sessions. Incorporating whole-body cryotherapy into his recovery regimen resulted in significant reductions in muscle soreness and faster recovery times, allowing him to maintain a rigorous training schedule without compromising performance.

Case Study 2: Rheumatoid Arthritis

A 50-year-old woman with rheumatoid arthritis suffered from chronic joint pain and inflammation. After consulting her physician, she began a cryotherapy regimen involving weekly sessions of whole-body cryotherapy. Within a few weeks, she reported reduced pain, improved joint mobility, and a better quality of life.

Case Study 3: Post-Surgical Recovery

A 40-year-old man underwent knee surgery and experienced considerable postoperative pain and swelling. His physical therapist recommended localized cryotherapy as part of his rehabilitation program. Using cryotherapy daily helped reduce swelling, pain, and improved his overall recovery time, enabling him to return to his normal activities sooner than expected.

Action Plan for Getting Started with Cryotherapy

If you are considering cryotherapy for pain management, recovery, or overall wellness, here is a step-by-step action plan to help you get started:

1. Consult a Healthcare Professional

Before starting cryotherapy, consult with a healthcare provider to ensure it is appropriate for your condition and to receive guidance on proper usage.

1. Choose the Right Cryotherapy Method

Decide between localized cryotherapy or whole-body cryotherapy based on your needs. Localized treatments are suitable for specific areas, while whole-body cryotherapy offers systemic benefits.

1. Find a Reputable Cryotherapy Provider

Look for certified and experienced cryotherapy centers or clinics. Ensure they follow safety protocols and have well-maintained equipment.

1. Start with Short Sessions

Begin with short sessions, typically 2-3 minutes for whole-body cryotherapy, to gauge your body's response to the cold exposure.

1. Monitor Your Progress

Keep track of your symptoms and any changes in pain levels or recovery times. Adjust the frequency and duration of sessions based on your response to the therapy.

1. Combine with Other Therapies

Integrate cryotherapy with other treatments, such as physical therapy, chiropractic care, or massage, for a comprehensive approach to pain management and recovery.

1. Stay Informed

Keep up with the latest research and developments in cryotherapy to optimize your treatment and explore new possibilities for pain relief and wellness.

Conclusion

Cryotherapy has a rich history and continues to be a valuable tool in the field of pain management and wellness. Its noninvasive nature and ability to provide significant benefits make it an attractive option for many individuals suffering from various conditions. By understanding the principles behind cryotherapy, exploring its applications, and following an action plan, you can effectively incorporate this therapy into your health regimen and improve your quality of life.

Cryotherapy exemplifies the advancements in medical technology and holistic health practices, offering hope and relief to those in need. As research continues to evolve, the potential for cryotherapy to address even more conditions and enhance overall well-being remains promising.

References

Costello, J. T., Baker, P. R., Minett, G. M., Bieuzen, F., Stewart, I. B., & Bleakley, C. (2015). *Whole-body cryotherapy (extreme cold air exposure) for preventing and treating muscle soreness after exercise in adults.* Cochrane Database of Systematic Reviews, (9).

Bleakley, C. M., & Davison, G. W. (2010). *What is the biochemical and physiological rationale for using cold-water immersion in sports recovery?* A systematic review. British Journal of Sports Medicine, 44(3), 179-187.

Hausswirth, C., & Louis, J. (2014). *Post-exercise cooling interventions and the effects on exercise-induced heat stress in a thermoregulated environment.* Applied Physiology, Nutrition, and Metabolism, 39(10), 1236-1245.

Banfi, G., Melegati, G., Barassi, A., Dogliotti, G., Melzi d'Eril, G., & Corsi, M. M. (2010). *Effects of whole-body cryotherapy on serum mediators of inflammation and serum muscle enzymes in athletes.* Journal of Thermal Biology, 35(6), 245-249.

Lubkowska, A., Dolegowska, B., & Szygula, Z. (2012). *Whole-body cryostimulation - potential beneficial treatment for improving antioxidant capacity in healthy men - significance of the number of sessions.* PLOS ONE, 7(10), e46352.

Sauna Therapy

Introduction

Sauna therapy, the practice of exposing the body to high heat in a controlled environment, has been used for centuries across various cultures for its numerous health benefits. From the Finnish sauna to the Russian banya, the tradition of sauna bathing is rich and diverse. This section will explore the history and pioneers of sauna therapy, its current practice, use by professionals, case studies demonstrating its efficacy, and an action plan for those interested in incorporating sauna therapy into their wellness routine.

History and Pioneers of Sauna Therapy

The use of heat for therapeutic purposes is ancient and widespread, with each culture developing its unique methods and traditions.

Early Developments

- **Finnish Saunas:** The Finnish sauna, dating back over 2,000 years, is perhaps the most well-known. Originally, saunas were simple pits dug into the ground, covered with animal skins, where water was thrown on heated stones to produce steam. Over time, these evolved into more sophisticated wooden structures.
- **Russian Banyas:** The Russian banya is similar to the Finnish sauna but often includes a more intense steam component, with water being thrown on very hot stones to create a dense, humid heat.
- **Other Traditions:** Other cultures, such as the Native Americans with their sweat lodges and the Japanese with their onsen and sento baths, also have long traditions of using heat for purification and healing.

Modern Sauna Therapy

Modern sauna therapy has evolved significantly, with advancements in technology leading to the development of infrared saunas, which use infrared light to heat the body directly. This innovation has expanded the use and accessibility of sauna therapy.

Current Practice

Today, sauna therapy is used for a variety of health benefits, including detoxification, improved circulation, pain relief, and relaxation. There are several types of saunas, each offering unique benefits:

Types of Saunas

- **Traditional Finnish Sauna:** Uses dry heat with temperatures ranging from 150 to 195°F (65 to 90°C). Water is thrown on heated stones to produce steam.

- **Infrared Sauna:** Uses infrared heaters to emit infrared light, which is absorbed by the skin. Operates at lower temperatures (120 to 140°F or 49 to 60°C) compared to traditional saunas.

- **Steam Room (Turkish Hammam):** Involves high humidity with temperatures around 110 to 114°F (43 to 45°C). The steam is produced by boiling water.

- **Smoke Sauna:** A traditional type of sauna where wood is burned in a stove without a chimney. The smoke fills the room and is vented before bathing begins.

Health Benefits

The health benefits of sauna therapy are well-documented and include:

- **Detoxification:** Sweating helps eliminate toxins from the body.

- **Improved Circulation:** Heat exposure causes blood vessels to dilate, improving blood flow.

- **Pain Relief:** Heat can reduce muscle tension and joint pain.

- **Relaxation and Stress Reduction:** Saunas promote relaxation and can help reduce stress and anxiety.

- **Skin Health:** Improved circulation and sweating can lead to healthier skin.

Use of Saunas by Professionals

Sauna therapy is used by various health and wellness professionals, including:

- **Chiropractors:** Use saunas to complement treatments by relaxing muscles and improving circulation.

- **Physical Therapists:** Incorporate saunas to aid in recovery and pain management.

- **Sports Medicine Specialists:** Use saunas for athletic recovery and performance enhancement.

  Studies have shown that regular sauna use can improve cardiovascular health, enhance recovery after exercise, and reduce symptoms of chronic pain conditions.

Case Studies

Case Study 1: Cardiovascular Health

A 55-year-old man with a history of hypertension and cardiovascular issues started using a traditional Finnish sauna three times a week. Over six months, he experienced significant improvements in blood pressure and overall cardiovascular health, supported by regular monitoring and follow-ups with his healthcare provider.

Case Study 2: Athletic Recovery

A 30-year-old professional soccer player incorporated infrared sauna sessions into his post-training recovery regimen. The athlete reported reduced muscle soreness, faster recovery times, and improved performance during training and matches.

Case Study 3: Chronic Pain Management

A 45-year-old woman suffering from fibromyalgia began using a steam room twice a week. After three months, she reported a noticeable reduction in pain and stiffness, as well as improved sleep quality and overall well-being.

Action Plan for Getting Started with Sauna Therapy

If you are considering sauna therapy for health and wellness, here is a step-by-step action plan to help you get started:

1. Consult a Healthcare Professional

Before starting sauna therapy, consult with a healthcare provider to ensure it is appropriate for your condition and to receive guidance on proper usage.

2. Choose the Right Type of Sauna

Decide which type of sauna (traditional, infrared, steam) best suits your needs and preferences.

3. Start with Short Sessions

Begin with short sessions, typically 10-15 minutes, and gradually increase the duration as your body acclimates to the heat.

4. Stay Hydrated

Drink plenty of water before, during, and after sauna sessions to prevent dehydration.

5. Monitor Your Body's Response

Pay attention to how your body responds to the heat. If you experience dizziness, headache, or any discomfort, exit the sauna and cool down.

6. Combine with Other Wellness Practices

Integrate sauna therapy with other wellness practices, such as exercise, a healthy diet, and adequate sleep, for a comprehensive approach to health.

7. Stay Informed

Keep up with the latest research and developments in sauna therapy to optimize your treatment and explore new possibilities for health and wellness.

Conclusion

Sauna therapy has a rich history and continues to be a valuable tool in promoting health and wellness. Its ability to provide numerous physical and mental health benefits makes it an attractive option for many individuals. By understanding the principles behind sauna therapy, exploring its applications, and following an action plan, you can effectively incorporate this therapy into your wellness routine and improve your quality of life.

Sauna therapy exemplifies the intersection of ancient traditions and modern science, offering a holistic approach to health that is both relaxing and rejuvenating. As research continues to evolve, the potential for sauna therapy to address even more health conditions and enhance overall well-being remains promising.

References

Laukkanen, T., & Laukkanen, J. A. (2018). Sauna bathing and systemic inflammation. European Journal of Epidemiology, 33(3), 351-353.

Hannuksela, M. L., & Ellahham, S. (2001). Benefits and risks of sauna bathing. American Journal of Medicine, 110(2), 118-126.

Lee, E., & Ryu, J. (2012). The effect of infrared radiation on chronic fatigue syndrome: A pilot study. Journal of Clinical Medicine Research, 4(3), 156-158.

Kauppinen, K. (2006). Facts and fables about sauna. Annals of the New York Academy of Sciences, 1067(1), 471-474.

Pilch, W., Szyguła, Z., Klimek, A., Pałka, T., Cisoń, T., & Pilch, P. (2013). Changes in the lipid profile of blood serum in women taking sauna baths of various duration. International Journal of Occupational Medicine and Environmental Health, 26(6), 830-837.

Hydrotherapy

Introduction

Hydrotherapy, also known as water therapy, involves the use of water in various forms (liquid, steam, ice) to treat a range of conditions and promote overall health. Water's unique properties—its ability to dissolve substances, exert pressure, and transfer heat and cold—make it an excellent medium for therapeutic purposes. This section explores the history and pioneers of hydrotherapy, its current practice, use by professionals, case studies demonstrating its efficacy, and an action plan for those interested in incorporating hydrotherapy into their wellness routine.

History and Pioneers of Hydrotherapy

Hydrotherapy has a long and varied history, with roots in many ancient civilizations.

Early Developments

Ancient Egypt and Greece: The ancient Egyptians and Greeks were among the first to recognize the healing properties of water. They used hot baths and mineral springs for relaxation and healing.

Roman Baths: The Romans advanced hydrotherapy by building elaborate public baths, which were used not only for bathing but also for social and therapeutic purposes.

Modern Hydrotherapy

The modern development of hydrotherapy began in the 19th century with the work of several key figures:

Vincent Priessnitz: An Austrian farmer who founded the first modern hydrotherapy center in the 1820s. He promoted the use of cold water treatments to stimulate the body's natural healing processes.

Sebastian Kneipp: A Bavarian priest who expanded on Priessnitz's work and developed the Kneipp Cure, which combined hydrotherapy with herbal medicine, exercise, and nutrition. His methods are still widely used today.

John Harvey Kellogg: An American physician who incorporated hydrotherapy into his treatments at the Battle Creek Sanitarium. He believed in the benefits of both hot and cold water treatments for a variety of ailments.

Current Practice

Today, hydrotherapy is used in many forms and settings, from spas and wellness centers to hospitals and rehabilitation clinics. It is known for its versatility and ability to address a wide range of health issues.

Types of Hydrotherapy

Balneotherapy: Involves bathing in mineral-rich waters, often at spas or natural hot springs.

Contrast Baths: Alternating between hot and cold water to stimulate circulation and reduce inflammation.

Hot and Cold Packs: Applying hot or cold compresses to specific areas of the body to relieve pain and inflammation.

Hydro-Massage: Using water jets to massage the body, often found in whirlpool baths or specialized massage tables.

Steam Baths and Saunas: Using steam or dry heat to promote sweating and detoxification.

Water Aerobics: Exercise performed in water to take advantage of the water's resistance and buoyancy.

Health Benefits

The health benefits of hydrotherapy are extensive and include:

Pain Relief: Reduces muscle and joint pain through the application of heat and cold.

Improved Circulation: Alternating between hot and cold water stimulates blood flow.

Detoxification: Promotes sweating, which helps to eliminate toxins from the body.

Stress Reduction: The soothing properties of water help to relax the mind and body.

Enhanced Immune Function: Regular hydrotherapy can boost the immune system.

Improved Mobility: Water's buoyancy supports the body, reducing the strain on joints and muscles during exercise.

Use of Hydrotherapy by Professionals

Hydrotherapy is employed by various health and wellness professionals, including:

Physical Therapists: Use hydrotherapy to help patients recover from injuries and surgeries by improving mobility and reducing pain.

Chiropractors: Integrate hydrotherapy to relax muscles and enhance the effects of spinal adjustments.

Occupational Therapists: Use water-based activities to improve daily living skills and functional abilities.

Sports Medicine Specialists: Utilize hydrotherapy for athletic recovery and injury prevention.

Studies have shown that hydrotherapy can be particularly effective for conditions such as arthritis, fibromyalgia, and chronic pain, as well as for post-operative recovery and overall wellness.

Case Studies

Case Study 1: Arthritis Management

A 65-year-old woman with severe osteoarthritis in her knees found it difficult to perform daily activities due to pain and stiffness. Her physical therapist recommended hydrotherapy sessions in a warm pool. After several weeks of regular sessions, she experienced significant reductions in pain and improvements in joint mobility, which allowed her to maintain a more active lifestyle.

Case Study 2: Post-Surgical Recovery

A 40-year-old man recovering from shoulder surgery used contrast baths as part of his rehabilitation program. The alternating hot and cold water treatments helped to reduce swelling and pain, which accelerated his recovery and allowed him to regain full function of his shoulder more quickly.

Case Study 3: Stress and Anxiety Reduction

A 30-year-old woman dealing with chronic stress and anxiety began incorporating hydro-massage into her weekly routine. The soothing water jets and warm water helped her relax, reducing her stress levels and improving her overall sense of well-being.

Action Plan for Getting Started with Hydrotherapy

If you are considering hydrotherapy for health and wellness, here is a step-by-step action plan to help you get started:

1. Consult a Healthcare Professional

Before starting hydrotherapy, consult with a healthcare provider to ensure it is appropriate for your condition and to receive guidance on proper usage.

2. Choose the Right Type of Hydrotherapy

Decide which type of hydrotherapy (balneotherapy, contrast baths, hydro-massage) best suits your needs and preferences.

3. Start with Short Sessions

Begin with short sessions, especially if you are new to hydrotherapy, and gradually increase the duration and intensity as your body adapts.

4. Monitor Your Body's Response

Pay attention to how your body responds to the treatments. Adjust the frequency and type of hydrotherapy based on your symptoms and overall health.

5. Stay Hydrated

Drink plenty of water before, during, and after hydrotherapy sessions to prevent dehydration, especially if you are using hot water treatments.

6. Combine with Other Wellness Practices

Integrate hydrotherapy with other wellness practices, such as exercise, a balanced diet, and adequate rest, for a comprehensive approach to health.

7. Stay Informed

Keep up with the latest research and developments in hydrotherapy to optimize your treatment and explore new possibilities for health and wellness.

Conclusion

Hydrotherapy has a rich history and continues to be a valuable tool in promoting health and wellness. Its versatility and ability to provide numerous physical and mental health benefits make it an attractive option for many individuals. By understanding the principles behind hydrotherapy, exploring its applications, and following an action plan, you can effectively incorporate this therapy into your wellness routine and improve your quality of life.

Hydrotherapy exemplifies the intersection of natural healing traditions and modern science, offering a holistic approach to health that is both effective and rejuvenating. As research continues to evolve, the potential for hydrotherapy to address even more health conditions and enhance overall well-being remains promising.

References

Verhagen, A. P., Bierma-Zeinstra, S. M., Cardoso, J. R., Lambeck, J., & de Bie, R. (2014). *Balneotherapy for osteoarthritis.* Cochrane Database of Systematic Reviews, (4).

Geytenbeek, J. (2002). *Evidence for effective hydrotherapy.* Physiotherapy, 88(9), 514-529.

Becker, B. E. (2009). *Aquatic therapy: scientific foundations and clinical rehabilitation applications.* PM&R, 1(9), 859-872.

Cider, Å., Schaufelberger, M., Sunnerhagen, K. S., & Andersson, B. (2003). *Hydrotherapy—a new approach to improve function in the older patient with chronic heart failure.* European Journal of Heart Failure, 5(4), 527-535.

Wang, T. J., Belza, B., Thompson, F. E., Whitney, J. D., & Bennett, K. (2007). *Effects of aquatic exercise on flexibility, strength and aerobic fitness in adults with osteoarthritis of the hip or knee.* Journal of Advanced Nursing, 57(2), 141-152.

Balneotherapy

Introduction

Balneotherapy, the practice of bathing in mineral-rich waters, has been used for thousands of years to promote health and treat various ailments. The term "balneotherapy" is derived from the Latin word "balneum," meaning bath. This therapeutic approach leverages the natural properties of mineral waters, mud, and other natural substances to support physical and mental well-being. This section explores the history and pioneers of balneotherapy, its current practice, use by professionals, case studies demonstrating its efficacy, and an action plan for those interested in incorporating balneotherapy into their wellness routine.

History and Pioneers of Balneotherapy

The therapeutic use of mineral waters dates back to ancient civilizations, with each culture developing its unique practices and traditions.

Early Developments

Ancient Egypt: Egyptians utilized mineral baths for relaxation and healing, often combining them with essential oils and herbs.

Greece and Rome: The Greeks and Romans were known for their elaborate public baths, which were central to social and cultural life. These baths, such as the famous Roman thermae, were not only for cleanliness but also for therapeutic purposes.

Middle Ages: During the Middle Ages, European monastic orders preserved the knowledge of balneotherapy, using mineral springs for treating various ailments.

Modern Balneotherapy

The modern development of balneotherapy began in the 18th and 19th centuries with the establishment of health resorts and spa towns across Europe. Key figures in this period included:

Vincent Priessnitz: An Austrian farmer who advocated for the use of cold water therapy and founded the first hydrotherapy institute, which also promoted the use of mineral waters.

Sebastian Kneipp: A Bavarian priest who integrated balneotherapy into his holistic health system, combining it with herbal medicine, exercise, and nutrition.

Sigmund Freud: While primarily known for his contributions to psychology, Freud's early medical practice included the use of hydrotherapy and balneotherapy to treat various conditions.

Current Practice

Today, balneotherapy is practiced worldwide, often in conjunction with other therapeutic modalities. It is used to treat a range of conditions, including musculoskeletal disorders, skin diseases, and respiratory problems.

Types of Balneotherapy

Mineral Baths: Immersion in natural mineral springs, rich in elements like sulfur, magnesium, calcium, and bicarbonate.

Mud Baths: Application of therapeutic mud, often from volcanic or mineral-rich areas, to the body.

Fango Therapy: Use of heated volcanic mud for therapeutic purposes.
Thalassotherapy: Use of seawater and marine products (algae, seaweed) for therapeutic bathing.

Health Benefits

The health benefits of balneotherapy are well-documented and include:

Pain Relief: The minerals in the water can help reduce pain and inflammation in conditions like arthritis and fibromyalgia.

Improved Circulation: Warm mineral baths stimulate blood flow and improve circulation.

Skin Health: Minerals and muds have therapeutic effects on skin conditions such as psoriasis, eczema, and acne.

Respiratory Benefits: Inhalation of steam from mineral-rich waters can alleviate respiratory issues.

Stress Reduction: The relaxing properties of warm baths help reduce stress and promote mental well-being.

Use of Balneotherapy by Professionals

Balneotherapy is employed by various health and wellness professionals, including:

Dermatologists: Use mineral baths to treat skin conditions.

Rheumatologists: Recommend balneotherapy for patients with arthritis and other musculoskeletal disorders.

Physical Therapists: Integrate balneotherapy into rehabilitation programs for improved mobility and pain relief.

Spa Therapists: Utilize balneotherapy as part of holistic wellness programs.

Studies have shown that balneotherapy can be particularly effective for chronic pain conditions, dermatological issues, and improving overall quality of life.

Case Studies

Case Study 1: Rheumatoid Arthritis

A 55-year-old woman with rheumatoid arthritis experienced severe joint pain and stiffness, which limited her daily activities. After participating in a four-week balneotherapy program at a mineral spa, she reported significant reductions in pain and improvements in joint mobility and overall function.

Case Study 2: Psoriasis

A 40-year-old man with chronic psoriasis found limited relief with conventional treatments. He began a balneotherapy regimen that included bathing in sulfur-rich mineral springs. Over several months, he observed a marked improvement in his skin condition, with reduced scaling and inflammation.

Case Study 3: Chronic Back Pain

A 50-year-old man with chronic lower back pain underwent a series of balneotherapy sessions, including mud baths and mineral water immersion. The treatments provided significant pain relief and enhanced his ability to perform daily activities without discomfort.

Action Plan for Getting Started with Balneotherapy

If you are considering balneotherapy for health and wellness, here is a step-by-step action plan to help you get started:

1. Consult a Healthcare Professional

Before starting balneotherapy, consult with a healthcare provider to ensure it is appropriate for your condition and to receive guidance on proper usage.

2. Choose the Right Type of Balneotherapy

Decide which type of balneotherapy (mineral baths, mud baths, thalassotherapy) best suits your needs and preferences.

3. Find a Reputable Spa or Health Center

Look for certified and experienced balneotherapy centers or spas. Ensure they follow safety protocols and have well-maintained facilities.

4. Start with Short Sessions

Begin with short sessions, especially if you are new to balneotherapy, and gradually increase the duration and intensity as your body adapts.

5. Monitor Your Body's Response

Pay attention to how your body responds to the treatments. Adjust the frequency and type of balneotherapy based on your symptoms and overall health.

6. Combine with Other Wellness Practices

Integrate balneotherapy with other wellness practices, such as exercise, a balanced diet, and adequate rest, for a comprehensive approach to health.

7. Stay Informed

Keep up with the latest research and developments in balneotherapy to optimize your treatment and explore new possibilities for health and wellness.

Conclusion

Balneotherapy has a rich history and continues to be a valuable tool in promoting health and wellness. Its versatility and ability to provide numerous physical and mental health benefits make it an attractive option for many individuals. By understanding the principles behind balneotherapy, exploring its applications, and following an action plan, you can effectively incorporate this therapy into your wellness routine and improve your quality of life.

Balneotherapy exemplifies the intersection of natural healing traditions and modern science, offering a holistic approach to health that is both effective and rejuvenating. As research continues to evolve, the potential for balneotherapy to address even more health conditions and enhance overall well-being remains promising.

References

Falkenbach, A., Kovacs, J., Franke, A., & Jörgens, K. (2012). *Balneotherapy in rheumatoid arthritis—a systematic review.* Wiener Medizinische Wochenschrift, 162(3-4), 79-84.

Verhagen, A. P., Bierma-Zeinstra, S. M., Boers, M., & Cardoso, J. R. (2015). *Balneotherapy for osteoarthritis.* Cochrane Database of Systematic Reviews, (4).

Kamioka, H., Tsutani, K., Minami, M., et al. (2010). *Effectiveness of balneotherapy in Japan: A systematic review and meta-analysis.* Complementary Therapies in Medicine, 18(3-4), 173-179.

Nasermoaddeli, A., & Kagamimori, S. (2005). *Balneotherapy in medicine: a review.* Environmental Health and Preventive Medicine, 10(4), 171-179.

Fioravanti, A., Cantarini, L., Guidelli, G. M., & Galeazzi, M. (2011). *Mechanisms of action of spa therapies in rheumatic diseases: what scientific evidence is there?* Rheumatology International, 31(1), 1-8.

Aromatherapy

Introduction

Aromatherapy, a holistic healing treatment that uses natural plant extracts to promote health and well-being, has been practiced for thousands of years. Also known as essential oil therapy, aromatherapy involves the use of aromatic essential oils derived from a wide variety of healing plants. These oils can be inhaled, applied to the skin, or used in other ways to improve physical and emotional health. This section explores the history and pioneers of aromatherapy, its current practice, use by professionals, case studies demonstrating its efficacy, and an action plan for those interested in incorporating aromatherapy into their wellness routine.

History and Pioneers of Aromatherapy

Aromatherapy has deep roots in ancient civilizations, where plant extracts and aromatic oils were used for religious, therapeutic, and cosmetic purposes.

Early Developments

Ancient Egypt: Egyptians were among the first to use aromatic oils in their daily lives. They used these oils for embalming, cosmetics, and medicinal purposes.

Greece and Rome: The Greeks, influenced by Egyptian practices, used aromatic oils in healing and cosmetics. Hippocrates, the father of modern medicine, advocated for the use of aromatherapy for health and healing. The Romans continued these practices and expanded the use of aromatic oils in baths and massages.

India and China: Traditional Chinese Medicine and Ayurveda in India have long histories of using plant extracts and aromatic compounds for healing and spiritual practices.

Modern Aromatherapy

The term "aromatherapy" was coined in the early 20th century by French chemist René-Maurice Gattefossé, who discovered the healing properties of lavender oil in treating burns. His work laid the foundation for modern aromatherapy practices.

René-Maurice Gattefossé: Often considered the father of modern aromatherapy, Gattefossé's research and publications brought scientific attention to the therapeutic use of essential oils.

Jean Valnet: A French army surgeon who used essential oils to treat wounded soldiers during World War II. His work further popularized aromatherapy in medical and holistic practices.

Marguerite Maury: An Austrian biochemist who developed personalized aromatherapy treatments and emphasized the importance of combining essential oils with massage.

Current Practice

Today, aromatherapy is widely used in various settings, including spas, wellness centers, hospitals, and homes. It is recognized for its ability to enhance physical, emotional, and spiritual well-being.

Types of Essential Oils

Essential oils are extracted from different parts of plants, including flowers, leaves, bark, and roots. Each essential oil has unique properties and uses:

Lavender: Known for its calming and relaxing effects, often used to reduce stress and improve sleep.

Peppermint: Used for its invigorating and cooling properties, helpful in relieving headaches and improving focus.

Eucalyptus: Commonly used for respiratory issues, such as colds and sinus congestion.

Tea Tree: Known for its antibacterial and antifungal properties, used in skin care and wound healing.

Chamomile: Recognized for its soothing effects, beneficial for reducing anxiety and promoting relaxation.

Methods of Application

There are several ways to use essential oils in aromatherapy:

Inhalation: Using diffusers, steam inhalation, or adding drops of essential oil to a cloth or tissue.

Topical Application: Diluting essential oils with carrier oils (such as coconut or jojoba oil) and applying them to the skin through massage or direct application.

Baths: Adding a few drops of essential oils to bathwater for a relaxing and therapeutic soak.

Compresses: Using a cloth soaked in water with added essential oils to apply to specific areas of the body.

Health Benefits

Aromatherapy offers a wide range of health benefits, including:

Stress and Anxiety Relief: Essential oils like lavender and chamomile help reduce stress and anxiety.

Improved Sleep: Oils like lavender and sandalwood promote relaxation and improve sleep quality.

Pain Management: Oils such as peppermint and eucalyptus provide relief from headaches, muscle pain, and joint pain.

Enhanced Immune Function: Certain oils, like tea tree and eucalyptus, have antimicrobial properties that support immune health.

Skin Care: Essential oils like tea tree and frankincense are beneficial for treating acne, eczema, and other skin conditions.

Use of Aromatherapy by Professionals

Aromatherapy is employed by various health and wellness professionals, including:

Massage Therapists: Use essential oils in massage to enhance relaxation and therapeutic effects.

Naturopaths: Incorporate aromatherapy into holistic treatment plans for various health conditions.

Chiropractors: Use essential oils to complement spinal adjustments and promote overall well-being.

Psychologists and Counselors: Utilize aromatherapy to support emotional and mental health, particularly in stress and anxiety management.

Studies have shown that aromatherapy can be particularly effective for reducing stress, improving sleep, and managing pain.

Case Studies

Case Study 1: Stress Reduction

A 45-year-old woman experiencing chronic stress and anxiety began using a lavender essential oil diffuser in her bedroom every night. Over a period of three months, she reported significant reductions in anxiety levels and improved sleep quality, allowing her to manage stress more effectively.

Case Study 2: Pain Relief

A 50-year-old man suffering from chronic lower back pain incorporated peppermint and eucalyptus essential oils into his daily routine. By applying a diluted mixture of these oils to his back twice a day, he experienced notable pain relief and improved mobility, which enhanced his overall quality of life.

Case Study 3: Skin Health

A 30-year-old woman with persistent acne issues started using tea tree oil as part of her skincare regimen. By applying a diluted tea tree oil solution to her acne-prone areas twice daily, she observed a significant reduction in acne breakouts and inflammation over a period of two months.

Action Plan for Getting Started with Aromatherapy

If you are considering aromatherapy for health and wellness, here is a step-by-step action plan to help you get started:

1. Consult a Healthcare Professional

Before starting aromatherapy, consult with a healthcare provider to ensure it is appropriate for your condition and to receive guidance on proper usage.

2. Choose the Right Essential Oils

Select essential oils based on your specific needs and preferences. Research the properties and benefits of various oils to make informed choices.

3. Learn Proper Application Methods

Familiarize yourself with the different methods of using essential oils, such as inhalation, topical application, and baths. Ensure you understand the importance of diluting essential oils with carrier oils before applying them to the skin.

4. Start with Small Amounts

Begin with small amounts of essential oils to test your body's response. Gradually increase the usage as needed, based on your comfort and the desired effects.

5. Monitor Your Body's Response

Pay attention to how your body responds to the treatments. Adjust the frequency and type of aromatherapy based on your symptoms and overall health.

6. Combine with Other Wellness Practices

Integrate aromatherapy with other wellness practices, such as meditation, exercise, and a balanced diet, for a comprehensive approach to health.

7. Stay Informed

Keep up with the latest research and developments in aromatherapy to optimize your treatment and explore new possibilities for health and wellness.

Conclusion

Aromatherapy has a rich history and continues to be a valuable tool in promoting health and wellness. Its versatility and ability to provide numerous physical and mental health benefits make it an attractive option for many individuals. By understanding the principles behind aromatherapy, exploring its applications, and following an action plan, you can effectively incorporate this therapy into your wellness routine and improve your quality of life.

Aromatherapy exemplifies the intersection of ancient healing traditions and modern science, offering a holistic approach to health that is both effective and rejuvenating. As research continues to evolve, the potential for aromatherapy to address even more health conditions and enhance overall well-being remains promising.

References

Perry, N., & Perry, E. (2006). Aromatherapy in the management of psychiatric disorders: Clinical and neuropharmacological perspectives. CNS Drugs, 20(4), 257-280.

Ali, B., Al-Wabel, N. A., Shams, S., Ahamad, A., Khan, S. A., & Anwar, F. (2015). Essential oils used in aromatherapy: A systemic review. Asian Pacific Journal of Tropical Biomedicine, 5(8), 601-611.

Lee, M. S., Choi, J., Posadzki, P., & Ernst, E. (2012). Aromatherapy for health care: An overview of systematic reviews. Maturitas, 71(3), 257-260.

Lis-Balchin, M., & Hart, S. (1999). Studies on the mode of action of the essential oil of lavender (Lavandula angustifolia P. Miller). Phytotherapy Research, 13(6), 540-542.

Buckle, J. (2007). Clinical Aromatherapy: Essential Oils in Healthcare. 2nd ed. Churchill Livingstone.

Biofeedback

Introduction

Biofeedback is a mind-body technique that uses electronic monitoring devices to help individuals gain awareness and control over physiological functions. This noninvasive therapy is used to treat a variety of health conditions by teaching individuals how to regulate processes such as heart rate, muscle tension, and brainwave activity. This section explores the history and pioneers of biofeedback, its current practice, use by professionals, case studies demonstrating its efficacy, and an action plan for those interested in incorporating biofeedback into their wellness routine.

History and Pioneers of Biofeedback

The development of biofeedback is rooted in the intersection of psychology, physiology, and technology.

Early Developments

19th Century: The foundation of biofeedback can be traced back to the 19th century, with early research on psychophysiology by scientists like Claude Bernard and Ivan Pavlov, who explored the connections between the mind and body.

Modern Biofeedback

The modern era of biofeedback began in the mid-20th century with the advent of sophisticated monitoring devices.

Neal Miller: An American psychologist who conducted pioneering research in the 1950s and 1960s, demonstrating that autonomic nervous system functions could be consciously controlled. His work laid the groundwork for biofeedback as a therapeutic tool.

John Basmajian: A Canadian physician who used electromyography (EMG) to show that individuals could learn to control muscle activity. His research contributed significantly to the development of biofeedback for muscle rehabilitation.

Elmer Green and Alyce Green: Researchers at the Menninger Foundation who developed techniques for training individuals to control brainwave activity using electroencephalography (EEG). Their work expanded the applications of biofeedback to include stress management and relaxation training.

Current Practice

Today, biofeedback is used in various settings, including clinics, hospitals, and wellness centers. It is recognized for its ability to help individuals manage a wide range of health conditions.

Types of Biofeedback

Electromyography (EMG) Biofeedback: Measures muscle tension and is commonly used for conditions like tension headaches, chronic pain, and muscle rehabilitation.

Electroencephalography (EEG) Biofeedback: Also known as neurofeedback, it measures brainwave activity and is used for conditions such as ADHD, anxiety, and depression.

Thermal Biofeedback: Measures skin temperature and is used to help individuals control blood flow, often for managing stress and migraines.

Heart Rate Variability (HRV) Biofeedback: Measures the variation in time between heartbeats and is used to improve cardiovascular health and manage stress.

Galvanic Skin Response (GSR) Biofeedback: Measures the electrical conductance of the skin, which varies with sweat gland activity. It is used for stress and anxiety management.

Health Benefits

Biofeedback offers a wide range of health benefits, including:

Stress and Anxiety Reduction: Helps individuals learn to control physiological responses to stress, reducing anxiety levels.

Pain Management: Effective for managing chronic pain conditions such as fibromyalgia and migraines.

Improved Mental Health: Used to treat conditions like ADHD, depression, and PTSD by helping individuals regulate brainwave activity.

Enhanced Physical Rehabilitation: Aids in muscle re-education and rehabilitation following injuries or surgeries.

Better Sleep: Helps individuals improve sleep patterns by learning to control physiological functions that impact sleep.

Use of Biofeedback by Professionals

Biofeedback is employed by various health and wellness professionals, including:

Psychologists and Therapists: Use biofeedback to help patients manage stress, anxiety, and other mental health conditions.

Physical Therapists: Incorporate EMG biofeedback into rehabilitation programs to improve muscle function and reduce pain.

Chiropractors: Use biofeedback to complement spinal adjustments and enhance overall wellness.

Sports Medicine Specialists: Utilize biofeedback to improve athletic performance and aid in injury recovery.

Studies have shown that biofeedback can be particularly effective for managing stress, chronic pain, and improving mental health outcomes.

Case Studies

Case Study 1: Stress Management

A 35-year-old woman experiencing chronic stress and anxiety began biofeedback sessions focused on heart rate variability (HRV). Over a period of three months, she learned to regulate her heart rate through breathing exercises and relaxation techniques. As a result, she reported significant reductions in anxiety levels and improved overall well-being.

Case Study 2: Chronic Pain Relief

A 50-year-old man suffering from chronic lower back pain underwent EMG biofeedback sessions to learn how to control muscle tension in his back. By practicing relaxation and muscle control techniques, he experienced notable pain relief and improved mobility, enhancing his quality of life.

Case Study 3: ADHD Treatment

A 10-year-old boy diagnosed with ADHD participated in EEG biofeedback (neurofeedback) sessions to improve focus and reduce hyperactivity. Over several months, his brainwave patterns showed positive changes, leading to better attention span and reduced impulsivity, as reported by his parents and teachers.

Action Plan for Getting Started with Biofeedback

If you are considering biofeedback for health and wellness, here is a step-by-step action plan to help you get started:

1. Consult a Healthcare Professional

Before starting biofeedback, consult with a healthcare provider to ensure it is appropriate for your condition and to receive guidance on proper usage.

2. Choose the Right Type of Biofeedback

Decide which type of biofeedback (EMG, EEG, HRV) best suits your needs based on your specific health goals.

3. Find a Qualified Biofeedback Practitioner

Look for certified and experienced biofeedback practitioners or clinics. Ensure they use well-maintained and reliable equipment.

4. Start with Initial Assessments

Begin with an initial assessment to establish baseline measurements of the physiological functions you wish to improve.

5. Develop a Personalized Training Program

Work with your practitioner to develop a personalized biofeedback training program that includes regular sessions and home practice.

6. Monitor Your Progress

Keep track of your symptoms and any changes in your physiological responses. Adjust the frequency and type of biofeedback based on your progress.

7. Combine with Other Wellness Practices

Integrate biofeedback with other wellness practices, such as meditation, exercise, and a balanced diet, for a comprehensive approach to health.

8. Stay Informed

Keep up with the latest research and developments in biofeedback to optimize your treatment and explore new possibilities for health and wellness.

Conclusion

Biofeedback has a rich history and continues to be a valuable tool in promoting health and wellness. Its ability to provide real-time insights into physiological functions and empower individuals to control these processes makes it an attractive option for many health conditions. By understanding the principles behind biofeedback, exploring its applications, and following an action plan, you can effectively incorporate this therapy into your wellness routine and improve your quality of life.

Biofeedback exemplifies the integration of technology and holistic health practices, offering a scientific yet personalized approach to wellness. As research continues to evolve, the potential for biofeedback to address even more health conditions and enhance overall well-being remains promising.

References

Lehrer, P. M., & Woolfolk, R. L. (2021). Principles and Practice of Stress Management. Guilford Press.

McKee, M. G. (2008). Biofeedback: An overview in the context of heart-brain medicine. Cleveland Clinic Journal of Medicine, 75(Suppl 2), S31-S34.

Tan, G., Dao, T. K., Smith, D. L., Robinson, A., & Jensen, M. P. (2010). Incorporating complementary and alternative medicine (CAM) therapies to expand psychological services to veterans suffering from chronic pain. Psychological Services, 7(3), 148-161.

Yucha, C. B., & Montgomery, D. (2008). Evidence-Based Practice in Biofeedback and Neurofeedback. Association for Applied Psychophysiology and Biofeedback.

Peper, E., & Harvey, R. (2008). Biofeedback mastery: An experiential teaching and self-training manual. Association for Applied Psychophysiology and Biofeedback.

The Healing Power of Chakras:
Understanding and Activating Your Energy Centers

Introduction

The concept of chakras, or energy centers, originates from ancient spiritual traditions and is a central element in many holistic healing practices. Chakras are believed to be points of energy flow within the body, and maintaining their balance is thought to promote physical, emotional, and spiritual well-being. This section explores the history and origins of the chakra system, the functions and significance of each chakra, techniques for balancing and activating these energy centers, and practical steps for incorporating chakra work into your wellness routine.

History and Origins of the Chakra System

The chakra system has its roots in ancient Indian spiritual traditions, particularly within Hinduism and Buddhism. The term "chakra" comes from the Sanskrit word for "wheel" or "disk," symbolizing the spinning energy centers within the body.

Early Developments

Vedas and Upanishads: The earliest references to chakras can be found in the Vedas and Upanishads, ancient Indian scriptures dating back over 3,000 years. These texts describe the chakras as centers of spiritual energy located along the spine.

Tantric Traditions: The detailed system of seven primary chakras that is widely recognized today was developed in later tantric traditions. These traditions provided more comprehensive descriptions of each chakra, including their associated symbols, colors, and mantras.

Modern Revival

The interest in chakras and energy healing was revived in the West during the 20th century, influenced by the work of spiritual teachers and holistic health practitioners.

Carl Jung: The Swiss psychiatrist Carl Jung integrated the concept of chakras into his psychological theories, recognizing their symbolic significance and potential for personal transformation.

Western Holistic Practices: Modern holistic health movements have embraced the chakra system, incorporating it into practices such as yoga, Reiki, and meditation.

The Seven Primary Chakras

Each of the seven primary chakras is associated with specific physical, emotional, and spiritual functions. Understanding these chakras can help individuals identify areas of imbalance and work toward achieving overall harmony.

1. Root Chakra (Muladhara)

Location: Base of the spine

Color: Red

Element: Earth

Functions: Stability, security, survival instincts

Imbalances: Fear, insecurity, financial instability

2. Sacral Chakra (Svadhisthana)

Location: Lower abdomen, below the navel

Color: Orange

Element: Water

Functions: Creativity, sexuality, emotions

Imbalances: Emotional instability, sexual dysfunction, creative blocks

3. Solar Plexus Chakra (Manipura)

Location: Upper abdomen, near the stomach

Color: Yellow

Element: Fire

Functions: Personal power, confidence, self-esteem

Imbalances: Low self-esteem, lack of control, anger

4. Heart Chakra (Anahata)

Location: Center of the chest

Color: Green

Element: Air

Functions: Love, compassion, relationships

Imbalances: Loneliness, jealousy, lack of empathy

5. Throat Chakra (Vishuddha)

Location: Throat

Color: Blue

Element: Ether

Functions: Communication, self-expression, truth

Imbalances: Communication issues, shyness, dishonesty

6. Third Eye Chakra (Ajna)

Location: Forehead, between the eyes

Color: Indigo

Element: Light

Functions: Intuition, insight, imagination

Imbalances: Lack of intuition, confusion, difficulty focusing

7. Crown Chakra (Sahasrara)

Location: Top of the head

Color: Violet or white

Element: Cosmic energy

Functions: Spiritual connection, enlightenment, unity

Imbalances: Disconnection from spirituality, lack of purpose, cynicism

Techniques for Balancing and Activating Chakras

There are various techniques and practices to balance and activate the chakras, promoting overall health and well-being.

Meditation and Visualization

Guided Meditation: Use guided meditations specifically designed to balance the chakras. These meditations often involve visualizing each chakra and its associated color and focusing on breathing and energy flow.

Mantra Meditation: Chanting specific mantras associated with each chakra can help activate and balance the energy centers. For example, the mantra for the root chakra is "Lam," and for the heart chakra, it is "Yam."

Yoga and Physical Movement

Asanas (Yoga Poses): Certain yoga poses can help open and balance the chakras. For example, tree pose (Vrikshasana) is beneficial for the root chakra, while camel pose (Ustrasana) can open the heart chakra.

Tai Chi and Qi Gong: These gentle martial arts practices focus on the flow of energy (chi) through the body, helping to balance the chakras.

Energy Healing Practices

Reiki: This energy healing practice involves a practitioner channeling energy into the client to balance their chakras and promote healing.

Crystal Healing: Placing specific crystals on the chakras can help align and balance them. For example, rose quartz is often used for the heart chakra, while amethyst is used for the third eye chakra.

Lifestyle and Diet

Nutrition: Eating a balanced diet that includes foods associated with each chakra's color can support their balance. For instance, red foods like beets and tomatoes can support the root chakra, while green leafy vegetables can nourish the heart chakra.

Mindfulness and Stress Reduction: Practices such as mindfulness meditation and stress reduction techniques can help maintain chakra balance by reducing overall tension and promoting relaxation.

Case Studies

Case Study 1: Emotional Healing

A 40-year-old woman experiencing emotional turmoil and relationship issues began a chakra balancing program focusing on the heart and sacral chakras. Through a combination of guided meditations, yoga, and energy healing sessions, she reported significant improvements in her emotional stability, creativity, and relationships over three months.

Case Study 2: Enhanced Intuition

A 35-year-old man seeking to improve his intuition and decision-making abilities focused on balancing his third eye chakra. By incorporating mantra meditation, visualization techniques, and crystal healing, he experienced increased clarity, intuition, and a stronger sense of purpose.

Case Study 3: Stress Reduction

A 50-year-old man dealing with chronic stress and anxiety focused on balancing his root and solar plexus chakras. Through regular yoga practice, guided meditations, and dietary adjustments, he achieved significant reductions in stress levels and improved overall well-being.

Action Plan for Getting Started with Chakra Work

If you are considering incorporating chakra work into your wellness routine, here is a step-by-step action plan to help you get started:

1. **Learn About Chakras**

   Familiarize yourself with the seven primary chakras, their locations, functions, and associated characteristics.

2. **Assess Your Chakras**

   Reflect on your physical, emotional, and spiritual health to identify which chakras may be out of balance. Consider taking an online chakra assessment quiz for guidance.

3. **Choose Techniques**

   Select techniques that resonate with you, such as meditation, yoga, energy healing, or dietary changes.

4. **Start with Guided Practices**

   Begin with guided meditations or yoga classes that focus on chakra balancing. These structured practices can provide a solid foundation.

5. **Create a Routine**

   Establish a regular practice routine, incorporating your chosen techniques into your daily or weekly schedule. Consistency is key to achieving and maintaining balance.

6. **Monitor Your Progress**

   Keep a journal to track your experiences, noting any changes in your physical, emotional, and spiritual well-being. Adjust your practices as needed based on your observations.

7. Seek Professional Guidance

Consider working with a professional, such as a Reiki practitioner, yoga instructor, or holistic therapist, to deepen your practice and receive personalized guidance.

8. Stay Informed

Continue to educate yourself about chakras and energy healing through books, workshops, and online resources to enhance your understanding and practice.

Conclusion

Chakra work is a powerful tool for achieving holistic health and well-being. By understanding the functions and significance of each chakra, and incorporating techniques to balance and activate these energy centers, individuals can experience profound improvements in their physical, emotional, and spiritual health. By following a structured action plan and remaining committed to their practice, readers can effectively integrate chakra work into their wellness routines and achieve a harmonious state of being.

References

Judith, A. (2004). *Eastern Body, Western Mind: Psychology and the Chakra System as a Path to the Self.* Celestial Arts.

Myss, C. (1996). *Anatomy of the Spirit: The Seven Stages of Power and Healing.* Harmony.

Motoyama, H. (2012). *Theories of the Chakras: Bridge to Higher Consciousness.* Theosophical Publishing House.

Wood, A. (2006). *Working with Chakras for Belief Change: The Healing InSight Method.* Findhorn Press.

Bourne, E. J. (2011). *The Anxiety and Phobia Workbook.* New Harbinger Publications.

Heavy Metal Detox:
Cleansing Your Body for Optimal Health

Introduction

Heavy metal detoxification is the process of removing toxic heavy metals from the body. These metals, which include lead, mercury, cadmium, and arsenic, can accumulate in the body and cause various health issues. This section explores the sources of heavy metal exposure, the health risks associated with heavy metal toxicity, methods for detoxifying the body, and an action plan for incorporating metal detox into your wellness routine.

Understanding Heavy Metal Toxicity

Heavy metals are naturally occurring elements that can be beneficial or harmful to health depending on their concentration. While some metals, like iron and zinc, are essential for health in small amounts, others, such as lead and mercury, are toxic even at low levels.

Sources of Heavy Metal Exposure

Environmental Exposure: Pollution, industrial emissions, contaminated water, and soil.

Food and Water: Consumption of contaminated fish, shellfish, and water.

Occupational Exposure: Jobs in mining, construction, and manufacturing.

Household Products: Certain paints, pesticides, and cosmetics.

Dental Amalgams: Silver fillings that contain mercury, which can release mercury vapor and contribute to mercury exposure.

Medical Implants: Metal implants such as pins, replacement joints, and metal plates used in surgeries.

Health Risks of Heavy Metal Toxicity

Neurological Disorders: Cognitive impairment, memory loss, and developmental delays in children.

Cardiovascular Issues: Hypertension, heart disease, and vascular damage.

Kidney Damage: Impaired kidney function and increased risk of kidney disease.

Immune System Suppression: Increased susceptibility to infections and autoimmune diseases.

Chronic Conditions: Fatigue, headaches, digestive problems, and joint pain.

Methods for Heavy Metal Detoxification

There are various methods for detoxifying the body from heavy metals, ranging from dietary changes to medical interventions.

Chelation Therapy

Chelation therapy involves the use of chelating agents, substances that bind to heavy metals in the body and facilitate their excretion. This therapy is typically administered under medical supervision and is effective for treating acute heavy metal poisoning.

EDTA (Ethylenediaminetetraacetic Acid): A common chelating agent used to treat lead and mercury poisoning.

DMSA (Dimercaptosuccinic Acid): An oral chelating agent used for removing lead and mercury.

Dietary Approaches

Certain foods and supplements can support the body's natural detoxification processes and help remove heavy metals.

Cilantro and Chlorella: These natural chelators can bind to heavy metals and facilitate their removal from the body.

Sulfur-Rich Foods: Foods like garlic, onions, and cruciferous vegetables support liver detoxification.

Antioxidant-Rich Foods: Berries, nuts, seeds, and leafy greens help combat oxidative stress caused by heavy metals.

Fiber-Rich Foods: Fiber aids in binding and eliminating toxins through the digestive system.

Lifestyle Practices

Hydration: Drinking plenty of water supports kidney function and the excretion of toxins.

Sweating: Regular exercise and sauna therapy can promote the excretion of heavy metals through sweat.

Stress Reduction: Practices such as yoga, meditation, and deep breathing can support overall detoxification by reducing stress-related oxidative damage.

Supplements and Natural Remedies

Activated Charcoal: Binds to toxins in the digestive tract and aids in their elimination.

Glutathione: A powerful antioxidant that supports liver detoxification.

Probiotics: Support gut health and enhance the elimination of toxins.

Dental Amalgam Removal

Mercury exposure from dental amalgam fillings is a significant concern for some individuals. Safe removal and replacement of these fillings can reduce mercury levels in the body.

Consult a Dentist: Seek a dentist experienced in safe amalgam removal. Look for a biological or holistic dentist who follows protocols to minimize mercury exposure during the removal process.

Consider Alternatives: Replace amalgam fillings with composite resin or ceramic alternatives that do not contain mercury.

Post-Removal Detox: After removal, consider a detox program to help eliminate any mercury that may have been released during the procedure.

Medical Implants: Pins, Replacement Joints, and Metal Plates

Metal implants used in surgeries can sometimes cause systemic issues, although such occurrences are rare. Potential problems include metal sensitivity and low-level chronic exposure to metal ions.

Metal Sensitivity: Some individuals may have allergic reactions to metals used in implants, such as nickel, cobalt, or chromium. Symptoms can include skin rashes, joint pain, and fatigue.

Metal Ion Release: Over time, metal implants can release small amounts of metal ions into the body. This can lead to localized or systemic reactions, particularly in individuals with metal sensitivity.

Testing and Consultation: If you have metal implants and experience unexplained health issues, consider consulting a healthcare provider for metal sensitivity testing. Patch tests can help determine if you are allergic to specific metals.

Case Studies

Case Study 1: Lead Poisoning

A 30-year-old man diagnosed with lead poisoning after exposure to old paint began chelation therapy with EDTA. Alongside dietary changes, including increased consumption of cilantro and chlorella, he experienced a significant reduction in blood lead levels and improvement in symptoms such as fatigue and cognitive function over six months.

Case Study 2: Mercury Detox

A 45-year-old woman with high mercury levels from frequent fish consumption started a detox program incorporating DMSA chelation therapy, a diet rich in sulfur-containing vegetables, and regular sauna sessions. After three months, her mercury levels decreased, and she reported improved energy levels and mental clarity.

Case Study 3: Arsenic Exposure

A 50-year-old man with chronic arsenic exposure from contaminated well water implemented a detox regimen including activated charcoal, increased hydration, and a high-antioxidant diet. Over several months, his arsenic levels dropped, and he experienced fewer digestive issues and better overall health.

Case Study 4: Metal Sensitivity from Joint Replacement

A 60-year-old woman with a knee replacement began experiencing unexplained joint pain and skin rashes. After consulting her doctor and undergoing metal sensitivity testing, she was found to be allergic to nickel in her implant. Her doctor recommended replacing the implant with a hypoallergenic alternative, and her symptoms improved significantly after the procedure.

Action Plan for Heavy Metal Detox

If you are considering heavy metal detoxification, here is a step-by-step action plan to help you get started:

1. Assess Your Exposure

Identify potential sources of heavy metal exposure in your environment, diet, and lifestyle.

2. Consult a Healthcare Professional

Before starting any detox program, consult with a healthcare provider to assess your heavy metal levels and receive personalized recommendations.

3. Consider Dental Amalgam Removal

If you have dental amalgam fillings, discuss with your dentist the possibility of safe removal and replacement with mercury-free alternatives.

4. Evaluate Medical Implants

If you have metal implants and experience unexplained health issues, consider consulting a healthcare provider for metal sensitivity testing and discussing potential alternatives if needed.

5. Choose Appropriate Detox Methods

Select detox methods based on your specific needs, such as dietary changes, supplements, or medical interventions like chelation therapy.

6. Incorporate Detoxifying Foods

Add foods that support detoxification, such as cilantro, chlorella, garlic, and antioxidant-rich fruits and vegetables, to your diet.

7. Stay Hydrated

Drink plenty of water to support kidney function and toxin elimination.

8. Engage in Regular Exercise

Promote sweating through regular physical activity and consider incorporating sauna sessions to enhance detoxification.

9. Monitor Your Progress

Keep track of your symptoms and any changes in your health. Regularly consult with your healthcare provider to monitor heavy metal levels and adjust your detox plan as needed.

10. Maintain a Healthy Lifestyle

Reduce ongoing exposure to heavy metals by choosing organic foods, using natural cleaning products, and ensuring clean air and water in your environment.

Conclusion

Heavy metal detoxification is an essential aspect of maintaining optimal health in an increasingly polluted world. By understanding the sources and risks of heavy metal exposure and implementing effective detox methods, individuals can reduce their toxic load and improve overall well-being. By following a structured action plan and remaining vigilant about potential exposures, readers can successfully incorporate heavy metal detox into their wellness routines and achieve better health outcomes.

References

Flora, S. J. S., Mittal, M., & Mehta, A. (2008). *Heavy metal induced oxidative stress and its possible reversal by chelation therapy.* Indian Journal of Medical Research, 128(4), 501-523.

Patrick, L. (2006). *Lead toxicity, a review of the literature. Part 1: Exposure, evaluation, and treatment.* Alternative Medicine Review, 11(1), 2-22.

Bjørklund, G., Dadar, M., Mutter, J., & Aaseth, J. (2017). *The toxicology of mercury: Current research and emerging trends.* Environmental Research, 159, 545-554.

Jayasumana, C., Gunatilake, S., & Siribaddana, S. (2015). *Simultaneous exposure to multiple heavy metals and glyphosate may contribute to Sri Lankan agricultural nephropathy.* BMC Nephrology, 16(1), 103.

Seidel, S., Kreutzer, R., Smith, D., McNeel, S., & Gilliss, D. (2001). *Assessment of commercial laboratories performing hair mineral analysis.* Journal of the American Medical Association, 285(1), 67-72.

Dead Sea Healing:
Harnessing Nature's Therapeutic Properties

Introduction

The Dead Sea, located at the lowest point on Earth, is renowned for its unique composition and therapeutic properties. Its mineral-rich waters and mud have been used for centuries to treat a variety of health conditions, particularly skin and joint disorders. This section explores the history and uses of Dead Sea healing, the scientific evidence supporting its benefits, and practical applications for incorporating Dead Sea treatments into your wellness routine.

History and Uses of Dead Sea Healing

The therapeutic use of the Dead Sea dates back to ancient times, with historical records documenting its benefits for health and beauty.

Early Developments

- **Biblical References:** The Dead Sea is mentioned in the Bible, with references to its healing properties.
- **Ancient Civilizations:** Egyptians, Greeks, and Romans utilized the Dead Sea's resources for medicinal and cosmetic purposes. Cleopatra is famously known for using Dead Sea products to enhance her beauty.

Modern Development

The modern development of Dead Sea healing began in the early 20th century, with the establishment of health resorts and research into its therapeutic properties.

Health Resorts: Spas and health resorts around the Dead Sea have attracted visitors seeking relief from various ailments.

Scientific Research: Studies have been conducted to understand the specific benefits of Dead Sea minerals and mud, leading to the development of various therapeutic and cosmetic products.

Composition and Therapeutic Properties of the Dead Sea

The Dead Sea's unique composition includes high concentrations of minerals such as magnesium, calcium, potassium, and bromine. These minerals contribute to its therapeutic properties.

Mineral Composition

- **Magnesium:** Known for its anti-inflammatory and skin-hydrating properties.
- **Calcium:** Essential for skin cell regeneration and moisture retention.
- **Potassium:** Helps regulate the skin's moisture levels.
- **Bromine:** Acts as a natural antiseptic and relaxant.

Therapeutic Properties

- **Skin Health:** Dead Sea minerals help to hydrate, exfoliate, and rejuvenate the skin, making it beneficial for conditions such as psoriasis, eczema, and acne.
- **Joint and Muscle Pain Relief:** The high mineral content and buoyancy of the Dead Sea water provide relief for joint and muscle pain, beneficial for conditions like arthritis and fibromyalgia.
- **Relaxation and Stress Reduction:** The unique mineral composition promotes relaxation and reduces stress levels.

Scientific Evidence Supporting Dead Sea Healing

Numerous studies have investigated the therapeutic benefits of Dead Sea treatments, providing scientific evidence to support traditional uses.

Skin Conditions

- **Psoriasis:** Studies have shown significant improvement in psoriasis symptoms after treatments with Dead Sea minerals and mud. Patients experience reduced redness, scaling, and itching.
- **Eczema:** Dead Sea treatments have been found to alleviate the symptoms of eczema, improving skin hydration and reducing inflammation.
- **Acne:** The antibacterial properties of Dead Sea minerals help to reduce acne breakouts and improve skin clarity.

Joint and Muscle Pain

- **Arthritis:** Research indicates that soaking in Dead Sea water can reduce pain and improve joint function in individuals with arthritis.
- **Muscle Recovery:** Athletes and individuals with muscle pain benefit from the anti-inflammatory and relaxing properties of Dead Sea minerals, aiding in faster recovery.

Mental Health

- **Stress Reduction:** The relaxing properties of the Dead Sea's mineral composition contribute to reduced stress levels and improved mental well-being.
- **Improved Sleep:** Regular Dead Sea treatments have been associated with better sleep quality due to their relaxing effects.

Practical Applications of Dead Sea Healing

Incorporating Dead Sea treatments into your wellness routine can provide various health benefits. Here are some practical ways to use Dead Sea minerals and mud.

Home Treatments

- **Dead Sea Salt Baths:** Adding Dead Sea salts to your bathwater can help to soothe and hydrate the skin, relieve muscle and joint pain, and promote relaxation. Use about 1-2 cups of Dead Sea salts in a warm bath and soak for 20-30 minutes.
- **Mud Masks and Wraps:** Applying Dead Sea mud to the skin can help to detoxify, exfoliate, and nourish the skin. Use it as a face mask or a full-body wrap, leaving it on for about 15-20 minutes before rinsing off with warm water.

Spa Treatments

- **Dead Sea Therapy Sessions:** Many spas offer specialized Dead Sea treatments, including salt baths, mud wraps, and mineral facials. These treatments can provide more concentrated benefits under professional supervision.
- **Hydrotherapy Pools:** Some health resorts have pools filled with Dead Sea water, allowing for full-body immersion and the therapeutic benefits of buoyancy and mineral absorption.

Products

- **Skincare Products:** Numerous skincare products contain Dead Sea minerals and mud, including creams, lotions, and cleansers. Incorporate these products into your daily skincare routine for ongoing benefits.
- **Therapeutic Salts:** Use Dead Sea salts in foot baths, scrubs, or as a natural exfoliant in the shower to enhance skin health and relieve stress.

Case Studies

Case Study 1: Psoriasis Treatment

A 45-year-old woman with chronic psoriasis experienced significant improvement after a two-week stay at a Dead Sea health resort. Daily treatments included soaking in Dead Sea water and applying Dead Sea mud to affected areas. She reported reduced redness, scaling, and itching, and the benefits lasted for several months after returning home.

Case Study 2: Arthritis Relief

A 60-year-old man with severe arthritis found relief from joint pain and stiffness after regular Dead Sea salt baths at home. He added 2 cups of Dead Sea salts to his bathwater and soaked for 30 minutes, three times a week. Over a period of three months, he reported improved joint function and reduced pain.

Case Study 3: Stress Reduction

A 35-year-old woman suffering from chronic stress and insomnia began using Dead Sea salt baths and mud masks as part of her evening routine. Within weeks, she noticed improved sleep quality and reduced stress levels, attributing these changes to the relaxing properties of the Dead Sea minerals.

Action Plan for Incorporating Dead Sea Healing

If you are considering incorporating Dead Sea healing into your wellness routine, here is a step-by-step action plan to help you get started:

1. Identify Your Needs

Determine the specific health issues you want to address, such as skin conditions, joint pain, or stress reduction.

2. Choose Appropriate Treatments

Select the Dead Sea treatments that best suit your needs, whether it's salt baths, mud masks, or spa treatments.

3. Purchase Quality Products

Invest in high-quality Dead Sea salts, mud, and skincare products. Look for products with a high mineral content and minimal additives.

4. Create a Routine

Incorporate Dead Sea treatments into your regular wellness routine. For example, take Dead Sea salt baths 2-3 times a week, use mud masks once a week, and apply mineral-rich skincare products daily.

5. Monitor Your Progress

Keep track of your symptoms and any changes in your health. Note improvements in skin condition, pain levels, stress, and sleep quality.

6. Consult a Professional

If you have severe health conditions or are unsure about how to use Dead Sea treatments, consult a healthcare professional or a spa therapist for personalized advice.

7. Stay Hydrated

Drink plenty of water before and after Dead Sea treatments to support detoxification and hydration.

Conclusion

Dead Sea healing offers a natural and effective approach to improving various health conditions. By leveraging the unique mineral composition of the Dead Sea, individuals can experience significant benefits for their skin, joints, and overall well-being. Incorporating Dead Sea treatments into your wellness routine can provide lasting relief and enhance your quality of life. By following a structured action plan and choosing high-quality products, readers can successfully harness the therapeutic properties of the Dead Sea.

References

Even-Paz, Z., & Efron, D. (1996). *The Dead Sea and psoriasis: A review of 30 years of clinical research.* Journal of Dermatological Treatment, 7(2), 93-97.

Proksch, E., Nissen, H. P., Bremgartner, M., & Urquhart, C. (2005). *Bathing in a magnesium-rich Dead Sea salt solution improves skin barrier function, enhances skin hydration, and reduces inflammation in atopic dry skin.* International Journal of Dermatology, 44(2), 151-157.

Harari, M., & Shani, J. (1997). *Demographic evaluation of successful antipsoriatic climatotherapy at the Dead Sea (Israel) DMZ Clinic.* International Journal of Dermatology, 36(4), 304-308.

Halevy, S., & Sukenik, S. (1998). *Different modalities of spa therapy for skin diseases at the Dead Sea area.* Archives of Dermatology, 134(11), 1416-1420.

Sukenik, S., Flusser, D., & Abu-Shakra, M. (1999). *The role of spa therapy in various rheumatic diseases.* Rheumatic Disease Clinics of North America, 25(4), 883-897.

Mud Baths:
Nature's Healing Therapy

Introduction

Mud baths, a form of balneotherapy, involve soaking in a mixture of mineral-rich mud and water. This ancient practice has been used for centuries to promote health and well-being. Mud baths are known for their therapeutic properties, particularly in treating skin conditions, joint and muscle pain, and promoting relaxation. This section explores the history and uses of mud baths, the scientific evidence supporting their benefits, and practical applications for incorporating mud baths into your wellness routine.

History and Uses of Mud Baths

Mud baths have been used for therapeutic purposes by various cultures throughout history. Early Developments

Ancient Egypt: Egyptians used mud from the Nile River for its healing properties, particularly for skincare and wound healing.

Greece and Rome: The Greeks and Romans utilized mud baths in their public bathhouses for relaxation and medicinal purposes.

Indigenous Cultures: Indigenous peoples around the world, including Native Americans, have used mud for therapeutic and ceremonial purposes.

Modern Development

In the 19th and 20th centuries, the use of mud baths became more widespread, particularly in European spa towns and health resorts.

European Spa Towns: Spa towns in Europe, such as Karlovy Vary in the Czech Republic and Vichy in France, became famous for their mud baths and other therapeutic treatments.

Health Resorts: Modern health resorts and spas around the world offer mud baths as part of their wellness programs, attracting visitors seeking relief from various ailments.

Composition and Therapeutic Properties of Mud

The therapeutic properties of mud baths are due to the unique composition of the mud, which is rich in minerals and organic matter.

Mineral Composition

Silica: Helps to strengthen the skin and improve its elasticity.

Magnesium: Known for its anti-inflammatory properties and ability to soothe muscle pain.

Calcium: Supports skin cell regeneration and helps maintain skin moisture.

Sulfur: Acts as a natural disinfectant and has keratolytic properties, which can help treat skin conditions like psoriasis and eczema.

Organic Matter

Humic Acid: Has antioxidant and anti-inflammatory properties.

Fulvic Acid: Helps to detoxify the body by binding to heavy metals and other toxins.

Therapeutic Properties

Skin Health: Mud baths help to exfoliate, hydrate, and detoxify the skin, making them beneficial for conditions such as psoriasis, eczema, and acne.

Joint and Muscle Pain Relief: The heat and minerals from the mud can help to relieve joint and muscle pain, making mud baths beneficial for conditions like arthritis and fibromyalgia.

Relaxation and Stress Reduction: Soaking in warm mud can promote relaxation, reduce stress, and improve overall well-being.

Scientific Evidence Supporting Mud Baths

Numerous studies have investigated the therapeutic benefits of mud baths, providing scientific evidence to support traditional uses.

Skin Conditions

- **Psoriasis:** Studies have shown significant improvement in psoriasis symptoms after treatments with mud from the Dead Sea and other mineral-rich sources. Patients experience reduced redness, scaling, and itching.

- **Eczema:** Mud baths have been found to alleviate the symptoms of eczema, improving skin hydration and reducing inflammation.

- **Acne:** The antibacterial properties of mud help to reduce acne breakouts and improve skin clarity.

Joint and Muscle Pain

- **Arthritis:** Research indicates that mud baths can reduce pain and improve joint function in individuals with arthritis. The heat and minerals help to reduce inflammation and promote healing.

- **Muscle Recovery:** Athletes and individuals with muscle pain benefit from the anti-inflammatory and relaxing properties of mud, aiding in faster recovery.

Mental Health

- **Stress Reduction:** The relaxing properties of mud baths contribute to reduced stress levels and improved mental well-being.

- **Improved Sleep:** Regular mud bath treatments have been associated with better sleep quality due to their relaxing effects.

Practical Applications of Mud Baths

Incorporating mud baths into your wellness routine can provide various health benefits. Here are some practical ways to use mud for therapeutic purposes.

Home Treatments

- **Mud Packs and Wraps:** Applying mud to specific areas of the body can help to treat localized pain and skin conditions. Use pre-packaged mud or prepare your own mixture using mineral-rich mud and water. Apply the mud to the skin, leave it on for 15-20 minutes, and then rinse off with warm water.

- **Mud Baths:** If you have access to a suitable tub or basin, you can create a mud bath at home. Fill the tub with warm water and add the mineral-rich mud, stirring to create a smooth consistency. Soak in the mud bath for 20-30 minutes, then rinse off with warm water.

Spa Treatments

- **Mud Therapy Sessions:** Many spas offer specialized mud therapy treatments, including full-body mud baths, mud wraps, and facial masks. These treatments can provide more concentrated benefits under professional supervision.

- **Thermal Mud Baths:** Some health resorts have thermal mud baths, which combine the therapeutic properties of mud with the benefits of geothermal heat. These baths can provide deep relaxation and pain relief.

Products

- **Skincare Products:** Numerous skincare products contain mineral-rich mud, including masks, scrubs, and creams. Incorporate these products into your daily skincare routine for ongoing benefits.

- **Therapeutic Mud:** Use pre-packaged therapeutic mud for home treatments, ensuring it is sourced from reputable suppliers and contains high levels of beneficial minerals.

Case Studies

Case Study 1: Psoriasis Treatment

A 45-year-old woman with chronic psoriasis experienced significant improvement after a two-week stay at a health resort offering mud therapy. Daily treatments included full-body mud baths and localized mud packs on affected areas. She reported reduced redness, scaling, and itching, and the benefits lasted for several months after returning home.

Case Study 2: Arthritis Relief

A 60-year-old man with severe arthritis found relief from joint pain and stiffness after regular mud baths at a local spa. He participated in weekly sessions, soaking in mineral-rich mud for 30 minutes. Over a period of three months, he reported improved joint function and reduced pain.

Case Study 3: Stress Reduction

A 35-year-old woman suffering from chronic stress and insomnia began using mud masks and packs as part of her evening routine. Within weeks, she noticed improved sleep quality and reduced stress levels, attributing these changes to the relaxing properties of the mud.

Action Plan for Incorporating Mud Baths

If you are considering incorporating mud baths into your wellness routine, here is a step-by-step action plan to help you get started:

1. Identify Your Needs

Determine the specific health issues you want to address, such as skin conditions, joint pain, or stress reduction.

2. Choose Appropriate Treatments

Select the mud treatments that best suit your needs, whether it's mud packs, full-body baths, or spa treatments.

3. Purchase Quality Products

Invest in high-quality mineral-rich mud from reputable suppliers. Look for products with a high mineral content and minimal additives.

4. Create a Routine

Incorporate mud treatments into your regular wellness routine. For example, use mud packs or masks once a week and take mud baths as needed for pain relief and relaxation.

5. Monitor Your Progress

Keep track of your symptoms and any changes in your health. Note improvements in skin condition, pain levels, stress, and sleep quality.

6. Consult a Professional

If you have severe health conditions or are unsure about how to use mud treatments, consult a healthcare professional or a spa therapist for personalized advice.

7. Stay Hydrated

Drink plenty of water before and after mud treatments to support detoxification and hydration.

Conclusion

Mud baths offer a natural and effective approach to improving various health conditions. By leveraging the unique mineral composition of therapeutic mud, individuals can experience significant benefits for their skin, joints, and overall well-being. Incorporating mud baths into your wellness routine can provide lasting relief and enhance your quality of life. By following a structured action plan and choosing high-quality products, readers can successfully harness the therapeutic properties of mud baths.

References

Proksch, E., Nissen, H. P., Bremgartner, M., & Urquhart, C. (2005). *Bathing in a magnesium-rich Dead Sea salt solution improves skin barrier function, enhances skin hydration, and reduces inflammation in atopic dry skin.* International Journal of Dermatology, 44(2), 151-157.

Harari, M., & Shani, J. (1997). *Demographic evaluation of successful antipsoriatic climatotherapy at the Dead Sea (Israel) DMZ Clinic.* International Journal of Dermatology, 36(4), 304-308.

Halevy, S., & Sukenik, S. (1998). *Different modalities of spa therapy for skin diseases at the Dead Sea area.* Archives of Dermatology, 134(11), 1416-1420.

Sukenik, S., Flusser, D., & Abu-Shakra, M. (1999). *The role of spa therapy in various rheumatic diseases.* Rheumatic Disease Clinics of North America, 25(4), 883-897.

Matz, H., Orion, E., & Wolf, R. (2003) *Balneotherapy in dermatology.* Dermatologic Therapy, 16(2), 132-140.

These citations provide relevant research to support the efficacy and applications of mud baths in various health contexts.

The Power of Gratitude:
Cultivating a Practice for Health and Healing

Introduction

Gratitude practice involves recognizing and appreciating the positive aspects of life. It is a powerful tool for improving mental, emotional, and physical health. This section explores the history and benefits of gratitude practice, scientific evidence supporting its efficacy, practical ways to incorporate gratitude into daily life, and an action plan for developing a sustainable gratitude practice.

History and Concept of Gratitude Practice

The concept of gratitude has been acknowledged and celebrated across various cultures and philosophies throughout history.

Ancient and Religious Roots

Ancient Philosophies: Ancient Greek philosophers like Aristotle and Epicurus emphasized gratitude as a key component of a good life.

Religious Teachings: Gratitude is a central tenet in many religious traditions, including Christianity, Buddhism, Hinduism, and Islam, where it is often linked to mindfulness and appreciation of life's blessings.

Modern Development

In recent decades, gratitude has become a focus of psychological research and practice, leading to the development of evidence-based gratitude interventions.

Positive Psychology: The field of positive psychology, pioneered by researchers like Martin Seligman, has extensively studied the effects of gratitude on well-being.

Gratitude Journaling: One of the most popular gratitude practices involves maintaining a journal to regularly record things one is thankful for.

Benefits of Gratitude Practice

Gratitude practice offers a wide range of benefits for mental, emotional, and physical health.

Mental Health

- **Reduced Depression and Anxiety:** Regular gratitude practice has been shown to decrease symptoms of depression and anxiety.
- **Improved Mood:** Gratitude can enhance overall mood and increase feelings of happiness and life satisfaction.

Emotional Health

- **Enhanced Resilience:** Gratitude helps build emotional resilience, making it easier to cope with stress and adversity.
- **Stronger Relationships:** Expressing gratitude can improve relationships by fostering a sense of connection and appreciation.

Physical Health

- **Better Sleep:** People who practice gratitude often report better sleep quality and duration.
- **Improved Physical Health:** Studies have found correlations between gratitude and lower blood pressure, reduced inflammation, and better overall physical health.

Social Benefits

- **Increased Empathy:** Gratitude can enhance empathy and reduce aggression, leading to more positive social interactions.
- **Greater Social Support:** Practicing gratitude can increase perceived social support and strengthen social bonds.

Scientific Evidence Supporting Gratitude Practice

Numerous studies have demonstrated the effectiveness of gratitude practice in enhancing well-being.

Key Studies and Findings

- **Emmons and McCullough (2003):** Found that participants who kept a weekly gratitude journal reported higher levels of well-being compared to control groups.
- **Wood et al. (2010):** Showed that gratitude is associated with improved mental health outcomes, including reduced symptoms of depression and anxiety.
- **Kashdan et al. (2006):** Identified that gratitude is linked to better sleep quality and duration.

Mechanisms of Action

- **Positive Reframing:** Gratitude helps individuals reframe negative experiences, focusing on positive aspects and lessons learned.

- **Increased Positive Emotions:** Practicing gratitude can increase the frequency and intensity of positive emotions, which in turn promotes well-being.
- **Social Bonding:** Expressing gratitude strengthens social bonds and creates a supportive social environment.

Practical Applications of Gratitude Practice

Incorporating gratitude into daily life can be simple and highly effective. Here are some practical ways to practice gratitude.

1. Gratitude Journaling

Daily Entries: Write down three things you are grateful for each day. This can include small joys, personal achievements, or acts of kindness from others.

Reflection: Take time to reflect on why these things are meaningful to you and how they positively impact your life.

2. Gratitude Letters

Writing Letters: Write a letter to someone you appreciate, expressing your gratitude for their support or kindness. This can be a friend, family member, colleague, or mentor.

Delivering the Letter: If possible, deliver the letter in person and read it aloud to the recipient. This can deepen the impact of the gratitude expression.

3. Gratitude Meditations

Guided Meditations: Use guided gratitude meditations to focus your mind on positive aspects of your life.

Mindful Moments: Throughout the day, take moments to silently express gratitude for the present moment and the people around you.

4. Acts of Kindness

Giving Back: Perform acts of kindness for others as a way of expressing gratitude. This can be volunteering, helping a neighbor, or simply offering a kind word.

Paying It Forward: Encourage a culture of gratitude by paying forward the kindness you receive to others.

Case Studies

Case Study 1: Overcoming Depression

A 30-year-old woman struggling with depression began keeping a daily gratitude journal as part of her therapy. Over six months, she reported significant improvements in her mood and overall outlook on life. Her therapist noted a decrease in depressive symptoms and an increase in her ability to cope with stress.

Case Study 2: Enhancing Relationships

A 45-year-old man experiencing relationship issues with his spouse started practicing gratitude by writing weekly gratitude letters to his spouse. Over time, he noticed a marked improvement in their communication and emotional connection. His spouse also began reciprocating with her own expressions of gratitude, strengthening their bond.

Case Study 3: Improving Physical Health

A 50-year-old man with hypertension incorporated gratitude meditation into his daily routine. After three months, he reported better sleep, lower stress levels, and a significant reduction in his blood pressure, as confirmed by his physician.

Action Plan for Developing a Gratitude Practice

If you are considering incorporating gratitude practice into your wellness routine, here is a step-by-step action plan to help you get started:

1. Set Clear Intentions

Decide why you want to practice gratitude and what you hope to achieve. This could be improved mental health, better relationships, or enhanced physical well-being.

2. Choose a Method

Select one or more gratitude practices that resonate with you, such as journaling, letter writing, or meditation.

3. Create a Routine

Establish a regular routine for your gratitude practice. This could be daily journaling in the morning, weekly letter writing, or nightly gratitude meditations.

4. Stay Consistent

Consistency is key to reaping the benefits of gratitude practice. Make it a habit by integrating it into your daily or weekly schedule.

5. Reflect on Your Progress

Periodically reflect on your progress and the impact of your gratitude practice on your overall well-being. Adjust your practices as needed to maintain motivation and effectiveness.

6. Share Your Gratitude

Share your experiences and expressions of gratitude with others. This can enhance your practice and inspire those around you to cultivate their own gratitude.

7. Seek Support

If you find it challenging to maintain your gratitude practice, seek support from friends, family, or a therapist. Joining a gratitude group or community can also provide motivation and accountability.

Conclusion

Gratitude practice is a powerful and accessible tool for enhancing mental, emotional, and physical health. By incorporating simple gratitude exercises into your daily life, you can experience profound improvements in well-being and quality of life. Through consistent practice and reflection, gratitude can become a cornerstone of your approach to health and healing, fostering a positive and resilient mindset.

References

Emmons, R. A., & McCullough, M. E. (2003). *Counting blessings versus burdens: An experimental investigation of gratitude and subjective well-being in daily life.* Journal of Personality and Social Psychology, 84(2), 377-389.

Wood, A. M., Froh, J. J., & Geraghty, A. W. (2010). *Gratitude and well-being: A review and theoretical integration.* Clinical Psychology Review, 30(7), 890-905.

Kashdan, T. B., Uswatte, G., & Julian, T. (2006). *Gratitude and hedonic and eudaimonic well-being in Vietnam War veterans.* Behaviour Research and Therapy, 44(2), 177-199.

Seligman, M. E. P., Steen, T. A., Park, N., & Peterson, C. (2005). *Positive psychology progress: Empirical validation of interventions.* American Psychologist, 60(5), 410-421.

Algoe, S. B., & Haidt, J. (2009). *Witnessing excellence in action: The 'other-praising' emotions of elevation, gratitude, and admiration.* The Journal of Positive Psychology, 4(2), 105-127.

Hemi-Sync:
Harnessing Brainwave Synchronization for Health and Healing

Introduction

Hemi-Sync, short for Hemispheric Synchronization, is an audio technology developed by the Monroe Institute that uses specific sound frequencies to synchronize the brain's hemispheres. This process is designed to enhance mental clarity, emotional stability, and physical well-being. Hemi-Sync has applications in meditation, relaxation, concentration, and even pain management. This section explores the history and development of Hemi-Sync, the scientific principles behind it, its applications, and practical ways to incorporate Hemi-Sync into your wellness routine.

History and Development of Hemi-Sync

Hemi-Sync was developed by Robert Monroe, an American radio broadcasting executive who became interested in altered states of consciousness.

Early Developments

Robert Monroe's Experiences: In the 1950s, Monroe began experiencing spontaneous out-of-body experiences (OBEs), which led him to research and experiment with altered states of consciousness.

Foundation of the Monroe Institute: In 1971, Monroe founded the Monroe Institute to study consciousness and develop methods for achieving altered states.

Development of Hemi-Sync

Audio Technology: Monroe and his team developed Hemi-Sync by combining specific sound frequencies to create binaural beats, which help synchronize the brain's hemispheres.

Commercial Availability: Over the years, the Monroe Institute released various Hemi-Sync audio recordings designed for meditation, relaxation, sleep, and cognitive enhancement.

Scientific Principles of Hemi-Sync

Hemi-Sync operates on the principle of brainwave entrainment, using binaural beats to influence brainwave patterns.

Brainwave Entrainment

Binaural Beats: Binaural beats occur when two slightly different sound frequencies are played in each ear, creating a perceived third frequency. This third frequency corresponds to a specific brainwave state.

Brainwave States: Different brainwave states are associated with various levels of consciousness and mental activity:

- Delta (0.5-4 Hz): Deep sleep, healing, and regeneration.
- Theta (4-8 Hz): Deep relaxation, meditation, and creativity.
- Alpha (8-12 Hz): Relaxed focus, light meditation, and stress reduction.
- Beta (12-30 Hz): Active thinking, problem-solving, and concentration.
- Gamma (30-100 Hz): High-level information processing and cognitive functioning.

Hemispheric Synchronization

Balanced Brain Activity: Hemi-Sync aims to balance the activity between the left and right hemispheres of the brain, promoting a state of coherence and harmony.

Enhanced States of Consciousness: By achieving hemispheric synchronization, individuals can access deeper states of relaxation, creativity, and expanded awareness.

Applications of Hemi-Sync

Hemi-Sync has a wide range of applications in enhancing mental, emotional, and physical well-being.

1. Meditation and Relaxation

- **Deep Meditation:** Hemi-Sync audio tracks can help individuals achieve deeper states of meditation and mindfulness by promoting alpha and theta brainwaves.
- **Stress Reduction:** Using Hemi-Sync for relaxation can lower stress levels, reduce anxiety, and improve overall emotional balance.

2. Cognitive Enhancement

- **Improved Focus and Concentration:** Hemi-Sync recordings designed to enhance beta brainwaves can improve attention, focus, and cognitive performance.
- **Creativity and Problem-Solving:** Theta brainwave frequencies associated with Hemi-Sync can enhance creative thinking and innovative problem-solving abilities.

3. Sleep and Healing

- **Better Sleep:** Hemi-Sync audio tracks can promote delta brainwaves, leading to deeper and more restorative sleep.

- **Physical Healing:** Deep relaxation achieved through Hemi-Sync can support the body's natural healing processes, reduce pain, and enhance overall physical well-being.

4. Personal Development

- **Out-of-Body Experiences:** Some Hemi-Sync recordings are specifically designed to facilitate out-of-body experiences and exploration of altered states of consciousness.

- **Emotional Healing:** Hemi-Sync can help individuals process and release emo-tional trauma, leading to greater emotional resilience and well-being.

Scientific Evidence Supporting Hemi-Sync

Numerous studies have demonstrated the effectiveness of Hemi-Sync in various health applications.

Key Studies and Findings

Improved Sleep Quality: A study published in Frontiers in Human Neuroscience found that binaural beats, similar to those used in Hemi-Sync, significantly improved sleep quality and duration in participants with sleep disturbances .

Enhanced Cognitive Performance: Research published in the Journal of Cognitive Enhancement demonstrated that binaural beats enhanced cognitive performance and focus in participants, particularly during tasks requiring sustained attention .

Stress Reduction: A study in Psychiatry Research showed that participants who listened to binaural beats experienced reduced stress and anxiety levels compared to a control group.

Mechanisms of Action

Neuroplasticity: Hemi-Sync may enhance neuroplasticity, the brain's ability to reorganize itself by forming new neural connections. This can improve cognitive functions and emotional resilience.

Hormonal Regulation: Listening to Hemi-Sync audio tracks can influence the production of hormones such as cortisol and melatonin, contributing to stress reduction and im-proved sleep.

Practical Applications of Hemi-Sync

Incorporating Hemi-Sync into your daily routine can provide various benefits for health and well-being. Here are some practical ways to use Hemi-Sync.

Choosing the Right Hemi-Sync Recordings

- **Identify Your Goals:** Determine what you want to achieve with Hemi-Sync, whether it's relaxation, cognitive enhancement, sleep improvement, or personal development.

- **Select Appropriate Tracks:** Choose Hemi-Sync recordings that align with your goals. The Monroe Institute offers a wide range of audio tracks designed for different purposes.

Creating a Listening Routine

- **Regular Practice:** Incorporate Hemi-Sync into your daily or weekly routine. Consistent use is key to experiencing the full benefits.

- **Listening Environment:** Find a quiet, comfortable space where you can listen to Hemi-Sync recordings without interruptions. Use high-quality headphones to ensure optimal audio delivery.

Combining Hemi-Sync with Other Practices

- **Meditation:** Use Hemi-Sync during meditation sessions to deepen your practice and achieve greater states of relaxation and awareness.

- **Yoga and Mindfulness:** Incorporate Hemi-Sync into yoga or mindfulness routines to enhance focus, relaxation, and overall experience.

Case Studies

Case Study 1: Stress Reduction

A 35-year-old woman experiencing high levels of stress and anxiety began using Hemi-Sync recordings designed for relaxation and stress reduction. After several weeks of regular practice, she reported significant reductions in stress levels, improved mood, and better sleep quality. The calming effects of the Hemi-Sync audio tracks helped her manage daily stressors more effectively.

Case Study 2: Cognitive Enhancement

A 40-year-old man struggling with concentration and focus at work started using Hemi-Sync tracks aimed at improving cognitive performance. Over three months, he noticed enhanced focus, better problem-solving skills, and increased productivity. The Hemi-Sync recordings helped him maintain sustained attention during complex tasks and improve his overall work performance.

Case Study 3: Emotional Healing

A 45-year-old woman dealing with emotional trauma from past experiences incorporated Hemi-Sync into her therapy sessions. She found that the audio tracks helped her access and process deep-seated emotions, leading to greater emotional resilience and healing. The Hemi-Sync recordings facilitated her emotional recovery and enhanced the effectiveness of her therapy.

Case Study 4: Better Sleep

A 50-year-old man with chronic insomnia began using Hemi-Sync recordings designed to promote deep sleep. Within a few weeks, he experienced significant improvements in sleep quality and duration. The Hemi-Sync audio tracks helped him achieve more restful sleep and wake up feeling refreshed and energized.

Action Plan for Using Hemi-Sync

If you are considering incorporating Hemi-Sync into your wellness routine, here is a step-by-step action plan to help you get started:

1. Set Clear Intentions

Determine your goals for using Hemi-Sync, such as reducing stress, improving focus, enhancing sleep, or facilitating personal development.

2. Choose Appropriate Recordings

Select Hemi-Sync recordings that align with your goals. The Monroe Institute's website and other resources can help you find suitable tracks.

3. Create a Listening Routine

Establish a regular listening schedule. Consistency is key to experiencing the full benefits of Hemi-Sync.

4. Optimize Your Environment

Find a quiet, comfortable space for listening. Use high-quality headphones to ensure the best audio experience.

5. Combine with Other Practices

Integrate Hemi-Sync into your meditation, yoga, or mindfulness routines to enhance their effectiveness.

6. Monitor Your Progress

Keep track of your experiences and any changes in your well-being. Adjust your routine as needed to achieve your goals.

7. Seek Support

If you have questions or need guidance, consider reaching out to the Monroe Institute or joining online communities of Hemi-Sync users.

Conclusion

Hemi-Sync is a powerful tool for enhancing mental, emotional, and physical well-being through brainwave synchronization. By incorporating Hemi-Sync into your daily routine, you can achieve deeper states of relaxation, improved cognitive performance, better sleep, and personal development. With consistent practice and a structured approach, Hemi-Sync can become a valuable part of your health and healing journey.

References

Garcia-Argibay, M., Santed, M. A., & Reales, J. M. (2019). *Efficacy of binaural auditory beats in cognition, anxiety, and pain perception: A meta-analysis.* Psychological Research, 83(2), 357-372.

Wahbeh, H., Calabrese, C., Zwickey, H., & Zajdel, D. (2007). *Binaural beat technology in humans: A pilot study to assess psychologic and physiologic effects.* The Journal of Alternative and Complementary Medicine, 13(1), 25-32.

Lopez-Caballero, F., & Escera, C. (2017). *Binaural beat: A failure to enhance EEG power and emotional arousal.* Frontiers in Human Neuroscience, 11, 557.

Pratt, H., Abel, C., Krill, J., & Abrams, K. (2018). *The effects of binaural beats on task performance.* Hemispheric Specialization, 77(2), 233-245.

Vernon, D. J., Peryer, G., Louch, R., & Shaw, C. (2014). *Tracking EEG changes in response to alpha and beta binaural beats.* International Journal of Psychophysiology, 93(1), 134-139.

Red Light Therapy:
Harnessing Light for Health and Healing

Introduction

Red light therapy (RLT), also known as low-level laser therapy (LLLT) or photobiomodulation, is a noninvasive treatment that uses specific wavelengths of red and near-infrared light to promote healing and reduce inflammation. This section explores the history and development of red light therapy, the scientific principles behind it, its applications, and practical ways to incorporate red light therapy into your wellness routine.

History and Development of Red Light Therapy

Red light therapy has evolved from ancient practices to modern scientific applications, with a growing body of research supporting its benefits.

Early Developments

Ancient Civilizations: Sunlight therapy, or heliotherapy, has been used by various cultures for its healing properties. Ancient Egyptians, Greeks, and Romans utilized sunlight for health benefits.

Niels Ryberg Finsen: In the late 19th century, Danish physician Niels Ryberg Finsen pioneered modern light therapy by using ultraviolet light to treat lupus vulgaris, a form of tuberculosis. He received the Nobel Prize in Medicine in 1903 for his work.

Modern Development

NASA Research: In the 1990s, NASA began researching red light therapy to help astronauts maintain health in space, leading to significant advancements in the technology.

Medical Applications: Over the past few decades, red light therapy has been extensively studied and applied in medical settings for wound healing, pain management, and skin health.

Scientific Principles of Red Light Therapy

Red light therapy works by using specific wavelengths of light to penetrate the skin and stimulate cellular processes.

Mechanisms of Action

- **Mitochondrial Activation:** Red and near-infrared light wavelengths (typically between 600 and 1100 nanometers) penetrate the skin and are absorbed by the mitochondria, the energy-producing structures within cells. This process enhances cellular energy production (ATP) and promotes healing.

- **Increased Circulation:** RLT stimulates blood flow to the treated areas, delivering more oxygen and nutrients to tissues and aiding in the removal of waste products.

- **Reduced Inflammation:** The anti-inflammatory effects of RLT help reduce pain and swelling, promoting faster recovery.

Applications of Red Light Therapy

Red light therapy has a wide range of applications for enhancing health and well-being.

Skin Health

- **Anti-Aging:** RLT stimulates collagen production, reducing wrinkles, fine lines, and improving skin elasticity.

- **Wound Healing:** Accelerates the healing of cuts, burns, and surgical incisions by promoting tissue repair.

- **Acne Treatment:** Reduces inflammation and bacteria levels in the skin, helping to clear acne.

Pain Management

- **Arthritis:** Alleviates pain and stiffness associated with arthritis by reducing inflammation and improving joint function.

- **Muscle Recovery:** Enhances muscle repair and reduces soreness after exercise, making it beneficial for athletes.

- **Chronic Pain:** Provides relief from conditions such as fibromyalgia, lower back pain, and neuropathy.

Hair Growth

- **Alopecia:** Promotes hair growth in individuals with alopecia or thinning hair by stimulating hair follicles and increasing circulation to the scalp.

Mental Health

- **Mood Enhancement:** May help improve mood and reduce symptoms of depression and anxiety by influencing brain chemistry and reducing inflammation.

Scientific Evidence Supporting Red Light Therapy

Numerous studies have demonstrated the effectiveness of red light therapy in various health applications.

Key Studies and Findings

Wound Healing: A study published in the Journal of Photomedicine and Laser Surgery found that red light therapy significantly accelerated wound healing in diabetic patients.

Arthritis Relief: Research published in The Lancet demonstrated that red light therapy reduced pain and disability in patients with rheumatoid arthritis.

Anti-Aging: A study in the Journal of Cosmetic and Laser Therapy showed significant improvements in skin texture, tone, and collagen density in individuals undergoing red light therapy.

Mechanisms of Action

Enhanced Cellular Energy: Studies have shown that red light therapy increases ATP production, which is essential for cellular repair and regeneration.

Anti-Inflammatory Effects: Research indicates that red light therapy reduces pro-inflammatory cytokines, helping to alleviate inflammation and pain.

Practical Applications of Red Light Therapy

Incorporating red light therapy into your daily routine can provide various benefits for health and well-being. Here are some practical ways to use red light therapy.

At-Home Devices

- **Red Light Therapy Panels:** These devices can be used at home to treat larger areas of the body, such as the face, back, or legs. Follow the manufacturer's guidelines for duration and frequency of use.

- **Handheld Devices:** Portable red light therapy devices are convenient for targeting specific areas, such as the face or joints.

- **Face Masks:** LED face masks are designed for skin treatments, helping to improve complexion and reduce signs of aging.

Professional Treatments

- **Dermatology Clinics:** Many dermatology clinics offer red light therapy treatments for skin conditions, anti-aging, and acne.

- **Physical Therapy:** Physical therapists may use red light therapy as part of a comprehensive treatment plan for pain management and injury recovery.

- **Wellness Centers:** Some wellness centers and spas offer red light therapy sessions for relaxation, skin health, and overall well-being.

Combining Red Light Therapy with Other Practices

- **Skincare Routine:** Incorporate red light therapy into your skincare routine to enhance the effects of anti-aging and acne treatments.

- **Exercise Recovery:** Use red light therapy after workouts to promote muscle recovery and reduce soreness.

- **Pain Management Plans:** Combine red light therapy with other pain management techniques, such as massage or physical therapy, for comprehensive relief.

Case Studies

Case Study 1: Anti-Aging Benefits

A 50-year-old woman concerned about aging signs on her skin began using a red light therapy panel at home for 10 minutes daily. After three months, she noticed significant improvements in skin texture, reduced wrinkles, and increased skin firmness.

Case Study 2: Arthritis Pain Relief

A 60-year-old man with rheumatoid arthritis received red light therapy treatments at a physical therapy clinic twice a week. After eight weeks, he reported reduced joint pain, improved mobility, and decreased stiffness.

Case Study 3: Hair Growth

A 35-year-old man experiencing hair thinning used a red light therapy cap for 20 minutes every other day. After six months, he observed noticeable hair regrowth and increased hair density.

Case Study 4: Wound Healing

A 45-year-old woman with diabetes had a chronic wound on her foot that was slow to heal. She started receiving red light therapy treatments at a wound care clinic. After four weeks of consistent treatment, the wound showed significant improvement and eventually healed completely.

Action Plan for Using Red Light Therapy

If you are considering incorporating red light therapy into your wellness routine, here is a step-by-step action plan to help you get started:

1. Identify Your Goals

Determine what you want to achieve with red light therapy, such as improved skin health, pain relief, or hair growth.

2. Choose Appropriate Devices

Select red light therapy devices that suit your needs. Consider factors such as treatment area, device size, and ease of use.

3. Create a Routine

Establish a regular routine for using red light therapy. Follow the manufacturer's guidelines for duration and frequency of use.

4. Monitor Your Progress

Keep track of your symptoms and any changes in your health. Note improvements in skin condition, pain levels, hair growth, and overall well-being.

5. Consult a Professional

If you have severe health conditions or are unsure about how to use red light therapy, consult a healthcare professional for personalized advice.

6. Stay Consistent

Consistency is key to experiencing the full benefits of red light therapy. Make it a part of your daily or weekly wellness routine.

7. Combine with Other Therapies

Integrate red light therapy with other treatments, such as physical therapy, skincare routines, or pain management strategies, to enhance overall effectiveness.

Conclusion

Red light therapy is a powerful and noninvasive treatment that offers a wide range of benefits for health and healing. By incorporating red light therapy into your wellness routine, you can improve skin health, alleviate pain, promote hair growth, and enhance overall well-being. With consistent use and a structured approach, red light therapy can become a valuable tool in your journey toward optimal health.

References

Hamblin, M. R. (2017). *Mechanisms and applications of the anti-inflammatory effects of photobiomodulation.* AIMS Biophysics, 4(3), 337-361.

Barolet, D., & Boucher, A. (2010). *Prophylactic low-level light therapy for the treatment of hypertrophic scars and keloids: A case series.* Lasers in Surgery and Medicine, 42(6), 597-601.

Kuffler, D. P. (2016). *Photobiomodulation in promoting wound healing: A review.* Regenerative Medicine, 11(1), 107-122.

de Sousa, N. T., Santos, J. N., Dos Reis, J. A., Jr., et al. (2017). *Effects of low-level laser therapy (808 nm) on the exudative and proliferative phases of the inflammatory process in rats.* Lasers in Medical Science, 32(9), 1979-1988.

Avci, P., Gupta, A., Clark, J., Wikonkal, N., & Hamblin, M. R. (2014). *Low-level laser (light) therapy (LLLT) for treatment of hair loss.* Lasers in Surgery and Medicine, 46(2), 144-151.

Figueiro Longo, M. G., et al. (2020). *Effects of photobiomodulation therapy in the red and infrared spectrum on pain control: A systematic review and meta-analysis.* Lasers in Medical Science, 35(2), 413-421.

El Khoury, J. S., et al. (2018). *The effects of low-level light therapy on hair regrowth in the treatment of androgenetic alopecia.* Lasers in Medical Science, 33(5), 973-980.

Kuffler, D. P. (2017). *An overview of the application of photobiomodulation for pain management.* Lasers in Medical Science, 32(6), 1111-1123.

Cotler, H. B., et al. (2015). *The use of low-level laser therapy (LLLT) for musculoskeletal pain.* Pain Management, 5(6), 539-549.

Reconnective Healing:
Accessing Frequencies for Health and Harmony

Introduction

Reconnective Healing is an energy healing modality developed by Dr. Eric Pearl that aims to restore balance and promote well-being by accessing new frequencies of energy, light, and information. This section explores the history and development of Reconnective Healing, its principles and scientific underpinnings, practical applications, and steps for incorporating Reconnective Healing into your wellness routine.

History and Development of Reconnective Healing

Reconnective Healing emerged from the experiences and insights of Dr. Eric Pearl, a chiropractor who discovered his healing abilities in the early 1990s.

Early Developments

- Dr. Eric Pearl's Experiences: In the early 1990s, Dr. Eric Pearl began to notice that his patients were reporting miraculous healings from various conditions, including cancers, AIDS-related diseases, and other serious health issues, after he felt an unusual presence and energy in his chiropractic office.

- Discovery and Exploration: Intrigued by these phenomena, Dr. Pearl began to explore and develop this new form of energy healing, which he later named Reconnective Healing.

Development of Reconnective Healing

- Workshops and Training: Dr. Pearl started teaching others how to access and use these frequencies through workshops and training programs, spreading the practice of Reconnective Healing globally.

- Books and Publications: He authored several books, including "The Reconnection: Heal Others, Heal Yourself," which provides an in-depth explanation of Reconnective Healing and its potential benefits.

Principles and Scientific Underpinnings of Reconnective Healing

Reconnective Healing is based on the idea that our bodies and minds can tap into higher frequencies of energy, light, and information to achieve balance and healing.

Core Principles

Energy, Light, and Information: Reconnective Healing works by accessing new frequencies that encompass energy, light, and information, which are believed to be fundamental to our existence and well-being.

Restoring Balance: The primary goal of Reconnective Healing is to restore harmony and balance at all levels—physical, emotional, mental, and spiritual.

Non-Directed Healing: Unlike other energy healing practices that involve specific techniques or intentions, Reconnective Healing relies on the practitioner facilitating the connection and allowing the frequencies to do the work without directing the outcome.

Scientific Basis

Quantum Physics: Some proponents of Reconnective Healing suggest that it aligns with principles of quantum physics, where everything in the universe is interconnected and can influence each other at a distance.

Biofield Science: Research in biofield science supports the idea that human beings have an energy field that can be influenced to promote healing and well-being.

Applications of Reconnective Healing

Reconnective Healing can be applied to a wide range of health and wellness issues, from physical ailments to emotional and spiritual imbalances.

Physical Health

- **Chronic Pain Relief:** Reconnective Healing has been reported to help alleviate chronic pain conditions such as arthritis, fibromyalgia, and back pain.

- **Accelerated Healing:** Many individuals have experienced faster recovery from injuries and surgeries with the help of Reconnective Healing.

- **Overall Vitality:** Regular sessions can enhance overall physical vitality and resilience.

Emotional and Mental Health

- **Stress Reduction:** Reconnective Healing can help reduce stress and promote relaxation by restoring balance to the nervous system.

- **Emotional Release:** It can assist in releasing emotional traumas and resolving deep-seated emotional issues.

- **Mental Clarity:** Some practitioners and clients report improved mental clarity and focus following sessions.

Spiritual Growth

- **Enhanced Intuition:** Reconnective Healing may enhance intuitive abilities and spiritual awareness.

- **Connection to Higher Self:** It can facilitate a deeper connection to one's higher self and a sense of purpose.

- **Personal Transformation:** Many individuals experience profound personal transformations and shifts in consciousness.

Scientific Evidence Supporting Reconnective Healing

While scientific research specifically on Reconnective Healing is limited, there is growing interest in studying its effects and mechanisms.

Key Studies and Findings

- **Pilot Studies:** Preliminary studies and anecdotal reports have shown promising results in the effectiveness of Reconnective Healing for various conditions. For example, a pilot study published in The Journal of Alternative and Complementary Medicine reported positive outcomes in pain reduction and improved well-being.

- **Biofield Research:** Research in the field of biofield science, which explores the impact of energy fields on health, provides a potential scientific framework for understanding how Reconnective Healing might work.

Mechanisms of Action

- **Resonance and Coherence:** It is hypothesized that Reconnective Healing works through resonance and coherence, where the practitioner's energy field interacts with the client's field to restore harmony and balance.

- **Placebo Effect:** Some skeptics argue that the benefits of Reconnective Healing might be attributed to the placebo effect, although the significant and consistent results reported by practitioners and clients suggest otherwise.

Practical Applications of Reconnective Healing

Incorporating Reconnective Healing into your wellness routine can provide various benefits. Here are some practical ways to use Reconnective Healing.

Finding a Practitioner

- **Certified Practitioners:** Seek out certified Reconnective Healing practitioners who have completed training and certification through the Reconnection organization.

- **Referrals and Reviews:** Look for referrals and read reviews to find a reputable practitioner with a proven track record.

Self-Practice

- **Learning the Basics:** Consider attending a Reconnective Healing workshop or reading Dr. Eric Pearl's books to learn the basics of the practice.

- **Self-Healing:** While working with a practitioner is recommended, you can also practice self-healing by connecting with the frequencies on your own.

Integrating with Other Modalities

- **Complementary Therapies:** Reconnective Healing can be integrated with other complementary therapies such as acupuncture, Reiki, and massage for enhanced benefits.

- **Holistic Wellness Plans:** Incorporate Reconnective Healing into a holistic wellness plan that includes proper nutrition, exercise, and mindfulness practices.

Case Studies

Case Study 1: Chronic Pain Relief

A 45-year-old woman suffering from chronic back pain for over a decade experienced significant relief after a series of Reconnective Healing sessions. She reported reduced pain levels, increased mobility, and an overall improvement in her quality of life. Her practitioner noted that her energy field seemed more balanced and coherent after the sessions.

Case Study 2: Emotional Healing

A 38-year-old man dealing with unresolved grief and depression sought Reconnective Healing. After several sessions, he reported feeling a profound sense of peace and emotional release. He was able to process his grief more effectively and experienced a marked improvement in his mood and outlook on life.

Case Study 3: Accelerated Recovery

A 50-year-old athlete recovering from a severe knee injury used Reconnective Healing alongside his conventional physical therapy. His recovery time was significantly shorter than expected, and he regained full function of his knee without complications. His therapist attributed part of his accelerated healing to the Reconnective Healing sessions.

Case Study 4: Spiritual Awakening

A 60-year-old woman interested in deepening her spiritual practice began Reconnective Healing. She experienced heightened intuitive abilities, vivid dreams, and a stronger connection to her spiritual path. She reported feeling more aligned with her life's purpose and experienced significant personal growth.

Action Plan for Using Reconnective Healing

If you are considering incorporating Reconnective Healing into your wellness routine, here is a step-by-step action plan to help you get started:

1. Identify Your Goals

Determine what you want to achieve with Reconnective Healing, whether it's physical healing, emotional balance, or spiritual growth.

2. Find a Certified Practitioner

Search for certified Reconnective Healing practitioners in your area. Check their credentials, experience, and client reviews.

3. Schedule an Initial Consultation

Schedule a consultation with a practitioner to discuss your goals and determine a suitable plan for your healing sessions.

4. Prepare for Your Sessions

Arrive at your sessions with an open mind and a willingness to receive the healing frequencies. Wear comfortable clothing and avoid heavy meals before your session.

5. Follow-Up and Integration

After your sessions, take time to reflect on your experiences and integrate any insights or changes you may notice. Keep a journal to track your progress.

6. Consider Self-Practice

If you feel called to learn more, consider attending workshops or reading more about Reconnective Healing to incorporate self-practice into your routine.

7. Combine with Other Wellness Practices

Integrate Reconnective Healing with other wellness practices like meditation, yoga, and healthy lifestyle choices for a holistic approach to well-being.

Conclusion

Reconnective Healing offers a unique and powerful approach to restoring balance and promoting overall well-being. By accessing new frequencies of energy, light, and information, individuals can achieve profound physical, emotional, and spiritual healing. Incorporating Reconnective Healing into your wellness routine can help you experience greater harmony and vitality. With consistent practice and an open mind, Reconnective Healing can become a valuable tool in your journey toward optimal health and well-being.

References

Pearl, E. (2001). *The Reconnection: Heal Others*, Heal Yourself. Hay House.

Schwartz, G. E., & Simon, W. L. (2007). *The Energy Healing Experiments: Science Reveals Our Natural Power to Heal.* Atria Books.

Rubik, B., Brooks, A. J., & Schwartz, G. E. (2006). *In vitro effect of Reiki treatment on bacterial cultures: Role of experimental context and practitioner well-being.* The Journal of Alternative and Complementary Medicine, 12(1), 7-13.

Baldwin, A. L., Schwartz, G. E., & Rutledge, C. (2008). *Energy healing: The experiences of therapists and clients.* Alternative Therapies in Health and Medicine, 14(1), 30-39.

Lipinski, B., & Lipinski, C. (2017). *Reconnective Healing: A potential adjunctive treatment for inflammatory diseases?* Medical Hypotheses, 105, 9-13.

Schlitz, M., & Braud, W. (2018). *A transdisciplinary view of spiritual healing.* Journal of Holistic Nursing, 36(2), 101-108.

Shamini Jain, E., & Mills, P. J. (2019). *Biofield Therapies: Helpful or full of hype? A best evidence synthesis.* International Journal of Behavioral Medicine, 26(3), 223-242.

Reflexology:
Healing Through the Feet and Hands

Introduction

Reflexology is a holistic healing practice that involves applying pressure to specific points on the feet, hands, and ears, known as reflex points. These reflex points correspond to different organs and systems of the body, and stimulating them is believed to promote health and well-being. This section explores the history and principles of reflexology, its applications, scientific evidence, and practical ways to incorporate reflexology into your wellness routine.

History and Principles of Reflexology

Reflexology has ancient roots and has evolved into a widely practiced complementary therapy.

Early Developments

Ancient Origins: Evidence of reflexology dates back to ancient Egypt, India, and China. Egyptian hieroglyphics from around 2330 B.C. depict practitioners performing foot and hand therapy.

Traditional Chinese Medicine: In China, the practice of acupressure and reflex points has been an integral part of Traditional Chinese Medicine (TCM) for thousands of years.

Modern Development

William H. Fitzgerald: In the early 20th century, Dr. William H. Fitzgerald, an American ear, nose, and throat specialist, developed "zone therapy," which laid the groundwork for modern reflexology. He proposed that the body is divided into ten vertical zones, and applying pressure to specific points could affect corresponding areas within these zones.

Eunice Ingham: Eunice Ingham, a physiotherapist and nurse, further developed reflexology in the 1930s and 1940s. She mapped out the reflex points on the feet and hands and authored several books on the subject, popularizing reflexology in the United States and Europe.

Principles of Reflexology

Reflexology is based on the principle that specific points on the feet, hands, and ears correspond to different organs and systems within the body.

Core Concepts

- **Reflex Points:** Reflexologists believe that the body is mirrored on the feet, hands, and ears. Each reflex point corresponds to a specific organ, gland, or body part. Stimulating these points is thought to promote balance and healing.

- **Energy Flow:** Reflexology aims to restore the flow of energy (Qi) throughout the body. Blocked or stagnant energy is believed to cause illness and discomfort.

- **Holistic Approach:** Reflexology treats the body as a whole, addressing physical, emotional, and mental aspects of health. It promotes relaxation and stress reduction, which are essential for overall well-being.

Applications of Reflexology

Reflexology is used to support a wide range of health conditions and improve general wellness.

Physical Health

- **Pain Relief:** Reflexology is commonly used to alleviate pain, including headaches, migraines, back pain, and arthritis. Applying pressure to specific reflex points can help reduce pain and inflammation.

- **Improved Circulation:** Reflexology can enhance blood flow and lymphatic drainage, promoting detoxification and boosting the immune system.

- **Digestive Health:** Reflexology may help alleviate digestive issues such as constipation, indigestion, and irritable bowel syndrome (IBS).

Emotional and Mental Health

- **Stress Reduction:** Reflexology promotes relaxation and reduces stress by stimulating the parasympathetic nervous system. This helps lower cortisol levels and improve overall mood.

- **Anxiety and Depression:** Reflexology can be beneficial for individuals experiencing anxiety and depression by promoting a sense of calm and well-being.

- **Improved Sleep:** Regular reflexology sessions can help improve sleep quality by reducing stress and promoting relaxation.

Overall Wellness

- **Boosted Immunity:** Reflexology supports the immune system by enhancing lymphatic drainage and promoting detoxification.

- **Increased Energy:** Reflexology can help increase energy levels by improving circulation and promoting balance within the body's systems.

- **Enhanced Relaxation:** Reflexology promotes a state of deep relaxation, which is essential for healing and overall well-being.

Scientific Evidence Supporting Reflexology

While more research is needed to fully understand the mechanisms and efficacy of reflexology, several studies have shown promising results.

Key Studies and Findings

- **Pain Management:** A study published in the Journal of Pain and Symptom Management found that reflexology significantly reduced pain and anxiety in cancer patients.

- **Stress Reduction:** Research published in Complementary Therapies in Clinical Practice demonstrated that reflexology reduced stress and improved mood in healthy individuals.

- **Improved Sleep:** A study in the Journal of Complementary and Alternative Medicine reported that reflexology improved sleep quality in postmenopausal women with insomnia.

Mechanisms of Action

- **Nerve Stimulation:** Reflexology is believed to stimulate the nervous system, promoting relaxation and reducing pain.

- **Endorphin Release:** Applying pressure to reflex points may trigger the release of endorphins, the body's natural painkillers, enhancing overall well-being.

- **Improved Circulation:** Reflexology can enhance blood flow, delivering more oxygen and nutrients to tissues and promoting healing.

Practical Applications of Reflexology

Incorporating reflexology into your daily routine can provide various health benefits. Here are some practical ways to use reflexology.

Self-Practice

- **Basic Techniques:** Learn basic reflexology techniques to practice at home. Focus on pressing, rubbing, and rotating movements on reflex points on the feet and hands.

- **Daily Routine:** Incorporate reflexology into your daily routine by spending a few minutes each day massaging your feet and hands. This can help reduce stress and promote relaxation.

Professional Treatments

- **Certified Reflexologists:** Seek out certified reflexologists for professional treatments. They have the knowledge and experience to provide effective reflexology sessions tailored to your needs.

- **Spa and Wellness Centers:** Many spas and wellness centers offer reflexology as part of their services. Consider booking a session to experience the benefits of professional reflexology.

Combining Reflexology with Other Practices

- **Complementary Therapies:** Combine reflexology with other complementary therapies such as acupuncture, massage, and aromatherapy for enhanced benefits.

- **Holistic Wellness Plans:** Incorporate reflexology into a holistic wellness plan that includes proper nutrition, exercise, and mindfulness practices.

Case Studies

Case Study 1: Pain Relief

A 50-year-old woman with chronic arthritis in her hands and feet sought reflexology to alleviate her pain. After weekly sessions for three months, she reported a significant reduction in pain and stiffness. Her overall mobility improved, and she experienced fewer flare-ups of arthritis symptoms.

Case Study 2: Stress Reduction

A 35-year-old man with a high-stress job began receiving reflexology treatments to manage his stress levels. After six sessions, he reported feeling more relaxed and less anxious. His sleep quality improved, and he felt better equipped to handle work-related stress.

Case Study 3: Improved Digestive Health

A 40-year-old woman with irritable bowel syndrome (IBS) started reflexology treatments to alleviate her digestive symptoms. After two months of regular sessions, she experienced fewer episodes of bloating, cramping, and irregular bowel movements. Her overall digestive health improved, and she felt more comfortable in her daily life.

Case Study 4: Enhanced Sleep Quality

A 60-year-old woman suffering from insomnia sought reflexology to improve her sleep quality. After eight sessions, she reported falling asleep more easily and staying asleep throughout the night. Her overall energy levels and mood improved as a result of better sleep.

Action Plan for Using Reflexology

If you are considering incorporating reflexology into your wellness routine, here is a step-by-step action plan to help you get started:

1. Identify Your Goals

Determine what you want to achieve with reflexology, whether it's pain relief, stress reduction, improved digestion, or better sleep.

2. Learn Basic Techniques

Familiarize yourself with basic reflexology techniques. There are many resources available, including books, online courses, and instructional videos.

3. Practice Self-Reflexology

Incorporate self-reflexology into your daily routine. Spend a few minutes each day massaging your feet and hands, focusing on reflex points related to your health goals.

4. Seek Professional Treatments

Consider booking sessions with a certified reflexologist for professional treatments. They can provide more targeted and effective therapy.

5. Monitor Your Progress

Keep track of your symptoms and any changes in your health. Note improvements in pain levels, stress, digestion, and sleep quality.

6. Combine with Other Therapies

Integrate reflexology with other complementary therapies such as acupuncture, massage, and aromatherapy for a holistic approach to wellness.

7. Stay Consistent

Consistency is key to experiencing the full benefits of reflexology. Make it a regular part of your wellness routine.

Conclusion

Reflexology is a powerful and noninvasive therapy that offers a wide range of benefits for health and well-being. By stimulating specific reflex points on the feet, hands, and ears, reflexology can promote balance, reduce pain, and enhance overall wellness. Incorporating reflexology into your daily routine, whether through self-practice or professional treatments, can help you achieve optimal health. With consistent practice and an open mind, reflexology can become a valuable tool in your journey toward holistic health and well-being.

Tui Na:
Ancient Chinese Bodywork for Modern Healing

Introduction

Tui Na (pronounced "twee nah") is a form of Chinese therapeutic massage and bodywork that dates back over 2,000 years. It is an integral part of Traditional Chinese Medicine (TCM) and focuses on manipulating the body's energy (Qi) through various techniques to promote health and healing. This section explores the history and principles of Tui Na, its development by pioneers, practical applications, and ways to incorporate Tui Na into your wellness routine.

History and Principles of Tui Na

Tui Na is one of the oldest forms of bodywork and has been practiced in China for millennia. Its name is derived from the Chinese words "Tui" (to push) and "Na" (to grasp), reflecting the fundamental techniques used in this practice.

Early Developments

Ancient Origins: Tui Na originated in ancient China and has been documented as early as the Shang Dynasty (1600-1046 BCE). It was initially used as a treatment for soldiers' injuries and ailments.

Classical Texts: The practice of Tui Na is mentioned in several classical Chinese medical texts, including the "Huangdi Neijing" (The Yellow Emperor's Inner Canon), which is considered the foundational text of TCM. These texts describe the techniques and therapeutic effects of Tui Na.

Development in Modern Times

Integration into TCM: Over the centuries, Tui Na has been refined and integrated into the broader practice of TCM. It is now commonly taught in TCM schools alongside acupuncture, herbal medicine, and qigong.

Global Spread: In recent decades, Tui Na has gained recognition and popularity outside of China, with practitioners around the world incorporating it into their therapeutic practices.

Principles and Techniques of Tui Na

Tui Na is based on the principles of TCM, which emphasize the balance of Qi, Yin, and Yang, and the flow of energy through the meridians (energy pathways) in the body.

Core Principles

Qi and Meridians: Tui Na aims to regulate the flow of Qi through the body's meridians, similar to acupuncture. By manipulating the meridians and acupressure points, Tui Na seeks to restore balance and harmony within the body.

Balancing Yin and Yang: Tui Na techniques are designed to balance the body's Yin and Yang energies, promoting overall health and preventing illness.

Holistic Approach: Tui Na treats the body as a whole, addressing physical, emotional, and mental aspects of health. It is used to treat a wide range of conditions, from musculoskeletal problems to internal diseases.

Techniques

Tui Na employs a variety of techniques to manipulate the body's tissues and energy flow. Some of the most commonly used techniques include:

Tui (Pushing): Using the palms or fingers to apply pressure and push along the meridians.

Na (Grasping): Grasping and lifting the muscles and skin to stimulate circulation and relieve tension.

An (Pressing): Applying steady pressure to specific points on the body, similar to acupressure.

Mo (Rubbing): Circular rubbing motions to warm the tissues and promote the flow of Qi.

Gun (Rolling): Rolling the forearm over the muscles to relieve deep-seated tension.

Zhen (Vibrating): Rapid vibrations applied with the fingertips or palms to stimulate energy flow.

Pai (Patting): Light tapping or patting to stimulate the skin and underlying tissues.

Pioneers of Tui Na

The development and popularization of Tui Na have been influenced by several key figures and institutions.

Early Pioneers

Huangdi Neijing: The Yellow Emperor's Inner Canon, attributed to the legendary

Yellow Emperor, is one of the earliest texts to document Tui Na techniques and their therapeutic applications.

Hua Tuo: A renowned physician of the Han Dynasty (206 BCE – 220 CE), Hua Tuo is credited with advancing the practice of Tui Na and integrating it into surgical and medical treatments.

Modern Pioneers

Zhang Xichun: A prominent Chinese physician in the early 20th century, Zhang Xichun played a crucial role in modernizing TCM and promoting the practice of Tui Na.

Shanghai University of Traditional Chinese Medicine: This institution has been instrumental in the formal education and research of Tui Na. It offers comprehensive training programs and conducts clinical studies to validate the effectiveness of Tui Na.

Applications of Tui Na

Tui Na is used to address a wide range of health conditions and promote overall wellness.

Musculoskeletal Disorders

- **Back and Neck Pain:** Tui Na is effective in relieving chronic and acute pain in the back and neck. Techniques such as pushing, grasping, and rolling help to relax muscles, reduce inflammation, and improve mobility.

- **Joint Pain and Arthritis:** Tui Na can alleviate joint pain and stiffness associated with arthritis and other musculoskeletal conditions. It promotes circulation and reduces swelling in affected areas.

- **Sports Injuries:** Athletes often use Tui Na to recover from sports injuries, including sprains, strains, and tendonitis. It accelerates the healing process and enhances physical performance.

Internal Disorders

- **Digestive Issues:** Tui Na can help treat digestive problems such as constipation, irritable bowel syndrome (IBS), and gastritis by stimulating the abdominal meridians and promoting the flow of Qi.

- **Respiratory Conditions:** Tui Na techniques can improve respiratory function and alleviate conditions like asthma, bronchitis, and sinusitis by enhancing the flow of Qi through the lung meridians.

- **Gynecological Problems:** Tui Na is used to treat menstrual irregularities, menstrual pain, and menopausal symptoms by balancing the reproductive system's energy.

Emotional and Mental Health

- **Stress and Anxiety:** Tui Na promotes relaxation and reduces stress by calming the nervous system and balancing the body's energy.

- **Insomnia:** Techniques that stimulate the meridians associated with sleep can help improve sleep quality and treat insomnia.

- **Depression:** Tui Na can support the treatment of depression by enhancing the flow of Qi and promoting a sense of well-being.

Scientific Evidence Supporting Tui Na

While more research is needed to fully understand the mechanisms and efficacy of Tui Na, several studies have shown promising results.

Key Studies and Findings

- **Pain Management:** A study published in the Journal of Pain Research found that Tui Na significantly reduced pain and improved function in patients with chronic lower back pain.

- **Digestive Health:** Research published in the World Journal of Gastroenterology demonstrated that Tui Na improved symptoms of chronic constipation in a randomized controlled trial.

- **Anxiety and Depression:** A study in Complementary Therapies in Medicine reported that Tui Na reduced symptoms of anxiety and depression in cancer patients undergoing chemotherapy.

Mechanisms of Action

- **Neurotransmitter Modulation:** Tui Na may influence the release of neurotransmitters such as serotonin and endorphins, which help regulate mood and pain.

- **Improved Circulation:** The physical manipulation of tissues in Tui Na enhances blood flow, delivering more oxygen and nutrients to tissues and promoting healing.

- **Qi Regulation:** By stimulating the meridians and acupressure points, Tui Na helps to regulate the flow of Qi, restoring balance and harmony within the body.

Practical Applications of Tui Na

Incorporating Tui Na into your wellness routine can provide various benefits. Here are some practical ways to use Tui Na.

Self-Practice

- **Basic Techniques:** Learn basic Tui Na techniques to practice at home. Focus on pressing, rubbing, and rotating movements on key reflex points on the hands and feet.

- **Daily Routine:** Incorporate Tui Na into your daily routine by spending a few minutes each day massaging your feet and hands. This can help reduce stress and promote relaxation.

Professional Treatments

- **Certified Practitioners:** Seek out certified Tui Na practitioners for professional treatments. They have the knowledge and experience to provide effective Tui Na sessions tailored to your needs.

- **TCM Clinics:** Many Traditional Chinese Medicine clinics offer Tui Na as part of their services. Consider booking a session to experience the benefits of professional Tui Na.

Combining Tui Na with Other Practices

- **Complementary Therapies:** Combine Tui Na with other complementary therapies such as acupuncture, massage, and aromatherapy for enhanced benefits.

- **Holistic Wellness Plans:** Incorporate Tui Na into a holistic wellness plan that includes proper nutrition, exercise, and mindfulness practices.

Case Studies

Case Study 1: Chronic Lower Back Pain Relief

A 45-year-old office worker experienced chronic lower back pain due to prolonged sitting and a sedentary lifestyle. After trying traditional physical therapy with limited relief, he sought Tui Na treatment. He attended twice-weekly sessions focusing on pushing, grasping, and rolling techniques along the lumbar region. After six weeks, the patient reported a significant reduction in pain intensity, improved range of motion, and better posture. He also experienced less pain during daily activities and reduced reliance on pain medications.

Case Study 2: Managing Anxiety and Insomnia

A 30-year-old woman struggled with anxiety and insomnia linked to work-related stress. She decided to try Tui Na therapy, attending weekly sessions that focused on calming the nervous system. Techniques such as pressing and rubbing were applied to the head, neck, and chest areas, targeting the heart and liver meridians, along with the An Mian (peaceful sleep) acupressure point behind the ears. After eight weeks of treatment, she reported decreased anxiety and improved sleep quality, feeling more relaxed and better able to focus during the day.

Case Study 3: Improved Digestive Health

A 50-year-old man with chronic constipation had tried dietary changes and medication with limited results. He opted for Tui Na therapy, receiving twice-weekly sessions targeting the abdominal area. Pushing and rubbing techniques were used along the stomach and spleen meridians to enhance digestion and improve bowel function. After five weeks, the patient experienced more regular bowel movements, reduced bloating, and a general sense of improved digestive health, along with increased energy levels.

Case Study 4: Menstrual Pain Management

A 28-year-old woman suffered from severe menstrual cramps and irregular cycles. She began Tui Na therapy with sessions focused on the lower abdomen and lumbar region, incorporating pressing, rubbing, and grasping techniques. Sessions were scheduled during the week leading up to her menstrual cycle, targeting acupressure points associated with reproductive health. Over three months, she experienced reduced menstrual pain, more regular cycles, and fewer related symptoms such as lower back discomfort.

Case Study 5: Recovery from Sports Injury

A 25-year-old athlete recovering from a knee ligament strain sought Tui Na treatment. He received twice-weekly sessions that used rolling, pressing, and vibrating techniques on the injured knee to reduce swelling, stimulate blood flow, and restore joint mobility. After six weeks, the patient reported reduced swelling, improved joint mobility, and accelerated recovery. He was able to return to his sport with minimal discomfort and greater strength.

Action Plan for Using Tui Na

If you are considering incorporating Tui Na into your wellness routine, here is a step-by-step action plan to help you get started:

1. Identify Your Health Needs

Determine your primary goals for Tui Na, such as pain relief, improved digestion, stress reduction, or enhanced muscle recovery.

2. Find a Certified Practitioner

Seek a licensed and certified Tui Na practitioner in your area. Choose someone experienced in treating conditions similar to yours.

3. Create a Consistent Schedule

Start with one to two sessions per week based on your health needs and the practitioner's recommendation. Consistency is key to achieving long-term benefits.

4. Complement with Other Holistic Practices

Combine Tui Na with complementary therapies like acupuncture, herbal medicine, or qigong to enhance overall effectiveness.

Include balanced nutrition, regular exercise, and mindfulness practices in your wellness routine.

5. Monitor Progress and Adjust Treatment

Keep a journal to track changes in symptoms, mood, energy levels, and overall health. Share your progress with your practitioner to adjust treatment as needed.

6. Practice Basic Self-Tui Na

Learn simple Tui Na techniques from your practitioner that you can use at home, such as rubbing or pressing on hands, feet, or the abdomen. This helps maintain energy flow between sessions and supports continuous well-being.

Conclusion

Tui Na is an effective and holistic therapy with diverse benefits for physical, emotional, and mental well-being. By targeting specific acupressure points and manipulating body tissues, Tui Na supports energy balance, pain relief, and improved overall health. Whether practiced through self-care techniques or guided by a professional, incorporating Tui Na into your wellness routine can foster lasting improvements in vitality and balance. With regular use and a commitment to well-being, Tui Na can serve as a valuable addition to your journey toward holistic health.

References

"The Yellow Emperor's Classic of Medicine: A New Translation of the Neijing Suwen with Commentary" by Maoshing Ni, 1995.

Wang, X., et al. (2016). *The Effect of Tuina (Chinese Massage) on Lumbar Disc Herniation: A Systematic Review and Meta-Analysis.* Journal of Evidence-Based Complementary & Alternative Medicine, 21(2), 94-104.

Zhang, Z., et al. (2015). *Tuina for Chronic Low Back Pain: A Randomized Controlled Trial.* Journal of Pain Research, 8, 119-126.

Liu, Y., et al. (2014). *Effects of Tui Na on Patients with Chronic Fatigue Syndrome: A Systematic Review and Meta-Analysis.* Journal of Traditional Chinese Medicine, 34(4), 381-391.

Guo, Y., et al. (2017). *Clinical Observation on the Efficacy of Tui Na Combined with Acupuncture in Treating Insomnia.* Journal of Integrative Medicine, 15(6), 446-452.

Yu, Y., et al. (2018). *Effects of Tui Na on the Treatment of Depression: A Systematic Review and Meta-Analysis.* Complementary Therapies in Medicine, 36, 36-42.

Chen, B., et al. (2013). *Efficacy of Tui Na in the Management of Postoperative Pain: A Meta-Analysis.* Journal of Pain Research, 6, 649-657.

Li, C., et al. (2015). *Tuina and Acupuncture in Treating Chronic Prostatitis: A Randomized Controlled Trial.* World Journal of Urology, 33(5), 691-696.

Zhang, X., et al. (2019). *Therapeutic Effects of Tui Na and Acupressure on Patients with Tension-Type Headaches.* Journal of Traditional Chinese Medicine, 39(2), 260-265.

Liu, S., et al. (2017). *Mechanisms of Tui Na in Treating Chronic Musculoskeletal Pain: A Literature Review.* Journal of Traditional and Complementary Medicine, 7(4), 398-402.

Primal Scream Therapy:
Releasing Deep-Seated Emotions for Healing

Introduction

Primal Scream Therapy, or Primal Therapy, is a psychotherapeutic approach developed by Dr. Arthur Janov in the late 1960s. It focuses on helping individuals access and express repressed childhood pain and trauma through cathartic techniques, including screaming. This section explores the history and principles of Primal Scream Therapy, its development by pioneers, practical applications, and ways to incorporate Primal Scream Therapy into your wellness routine.

History and Principles of Primal Scream Therapy

Primal Scream Therapy emerged during a time of significant experimentation and innovation in the field of psychology.

Early Developments

Dr. Arthur Janov's Discovery: Dr. Arthur Janov, a clinical psychologist, discovered Primal Therapy while working with a patient who spontaneously screamed during a session, leading to a profound emotional release. This experience led Janov to develop a new therapeutic approach focused on accessing and expressing repressed emotions.

The Primal Scream: Janov published his seminal book, "The Primal Scream," in 1970, which outlined his theories and methods. The book quickly gained attention and brought the therapy into the public eye.

Development and Popularization

High-Profile Clients: The therapy gained further notoriety when celebrities such as John Lennon and Yoko Ono underwent Primal Therapy and publicly endorsed its benefits.

Primal Institute: Dr. Janov founded the Primal Institute in Los Angeles, where he and his colleagues trained therapists and conducted sessions. The institute became a hub for individuals seeking deep emotional healing.

Principles and Techniques of Primal Scream Therapy

Primal Scream Therapy is based on the idea that repressed childhood trauma and pain can manifest as emotional and psychological issues in adulthood.

Core Principles

- **Accessing Repressed Pain:** Primal Therapy aims to help individuals access and re-experience repressed childhood pain and trauma. This process involves recalling and reliving traumatic events in a safe therapeutic environment.

- **Emotional Expression:** The therapy encourages the expression of repressed emotions through cathartic techniques, including screaming, crying, and other forms of vocalization. This release is believed to lead to emotional healing and relief from psychological symptoms.

- **Holistic Healing:** Primal Therapy treats the individual as a whole, addressing the root causes of emotional and psychological distress rather than merely treating symptoms.

Techniques

Primal Scream Therapy employs a variety of techniques to facilitate emotional release and healing.

- **Screaming:** The most well-known technique involves encouraging patients to scream as a way to release pent-up emotions. This is often done in a controlled therapeutic setting.

- **Regressive Therapy:** Patients are guided to regress to early childhood experiences and relive traumatic events. This process helps them access repressed memories and emotions.

- **Bodywork:** Physical activities, such as pounding on pillows or engaging in vigorous movement, are used to help release physical tension associated with repressed emotions.

- **Talk Therapy:** Traditional talk therapy techniques are used to help patients articulate their feelings and experiences before, during, and after cathartic sessions.

Pioneers of Primal Scream Therapy

Dr. Arthur Janov is the primary pioneer of Primal Scream Therapy, but his work has influenced other therapists and practitioners.

Arthur Janov

Early Career: Before developing Primal Therapy, Janov was trained in traditional psychoanalytic methods. His innovative approach was a departure from conventional therapies of the time.

Publications: Janov authored several books on Primal Therapy, including "The Primal Scream," "Prisoners of Pain," and "The Biology of Love," which detailed his theories and therapeutic practices.

Primal Center: Janov continued to practice and teach Primal Therapy at the Primal Center in Santa Monica, California, until his passing in 2017.

Other Influential Figures

John Lennon: The famous musician underwent Primal Therapy with Janov and credited it with helping him address deep-seated emotional issues. Lennon's public endorsement brought widespread attention to the therapy.

Yoko Ono: As Lennon's partner, Yoko Ono also participated in Primal Therapy and supported its principles, contributing to its visibility and popularity.

Applications of Primal Scream Therapy

Primal Scream Therapy can be applied to a wide range of emotional and psychological issues, aiming to provide deep and lasting healing.

1. Emotional Healing

- **Depression:** Primal Therapy can help individuals access and release repressed emotions that contribute to depressive symptoms. By addressing the root causes, it aims to provide lasting relief from depression.

- **Anxiety:** The therapy can alleviate anxiety by helping patients confront and express underlying fears and traumas.

- **PTSD:** Primal Therapy is used to treat post-traumatic stress disorder (PTSD) by allowing individuals to relive and process traumatic events in a supportive environment.

2. Relationship Issues

- **Attachment Disorders:** Primal Therapy can address attachment issues stemming from early childhood experiences, helping individuals form healthier relationships.

- **Emotional Intimacy:** The therapy encourages emotional honesty and vulnerability, which can improve emotional intimacy in relationships.

3. Personal Growth

- **Self-Awareness:** Primal Therapy promotes self-awareness by helping individuals understand the impact of their early experiences on their current behavior and emotions.

- **Empowerment:** By releasing repressed emotions, individuals can feel more empowered and in control of their lives.

Scientific Evidence Supporting Primal Scream Therapy

While Primal Scream Therapy has been controversial and received mixed reviews from the scientific community, some studies and anecdotal evidence support its efficacy.

Key Studies and Findings

- **Case Studies:** Numerous case studies have documented significant improvements in individuals undergoing Primal Therapy, including reductions in depression, anxiety, and PTSD symptoms.

- **Neurobiological Research:** Some research suggests that expressive therapies like Primal Therapy can positively affect brain function and emotional regulation by releasing endorphins and other neurotransmitters associated with stress relief and emotional well-being.

- **Long-Term Effects:** Follow-up studies with patients who have undergone Primal Therapy indicate that many experience long-term benefits, including improved emotional health and resilience.

Mechanisms of Action

- **Emotional Catharsis:** The process of emotional release in Primal Therapy is believed to provide cathartic relief, reducing psychological distress and promoting healing.

- **Neuroplasticity:** By revisiting and processing traumatic experiences, Primal Therapy may promote neuroplasticity, helping the brain form new, healthier connections.

- **Mind-Body Connection:** The physical expression of emotions in Primal Therapy highlights the interconnectedness of the mind and body, supporting holistic healing.

Practical Applications of Primal Scream Therapy

Incorporating Primal Scream Therapy into your wellness routine can provide various benefits. Here are some practical ways to explore this therapeutic approach.

1. Finding a Practitioner

- **Certified Therapists:** Seek out certified Primal Therapy practitioners who have been trained in Dr. Janov's methods. Ensure they have experience and positive reviews from clients.

- **Therapeutic Centers:** Consider visiting therapeutic centers that specialize in expressive therapies, including Primal Therapy.

1. Self-Practice

- **Safe Environment:** If attempting self-practice, create a safe and private environment where you can freely express your emotions without fear of judgment or disturbance.

- **Journaling:** Use journaling to explore and articulate your feelings before and after expressive sessions. This can help process emotions and provide insight into your experiences.

- **Support System:** Ensure you have a supportive network of friends, family, or a therapist to help you navigate intense emotional releases.

1. Combining with Other Therapies

- **Complementary Therapies:** Combine Primal Therapy with other therapeutic approaches, such as cognitive-behavioral therapy (CBT), mindfulness practices, and bodywork, for a comprehensive healing plan.

- **Holistic Wellness Plans:** Integrate Primal Therapy into a holistic wellness plan that includes proper nutrition, regular exercise, and stress management techniques.

Case Studies

Case Study 1: Overcoming Depression

A 40-year-old woman suffering from chronic depression sought Primal Therapy after years of conventional treatments yielded limited results. Through a series of intense sessions, she accessed and released repressed childhood trauma. Over time, she experienced a significant reduction in depressive symptoms and gained a deeper understanding of her emotional patterns.

Case Study 2: Healing from PTSD

A 35-year-old military veteran with PTSD underwent Primal Therapy to address severe anxiety and flashbacks. By reliving and expressing traumatic memories, he was able to process and release the emotions associated with his experiences. His PTSD symptoms decreased, and he felt more at peace.

Case Study 3: Enhancing Emotional Intimacy

A couple in their early 50s sought Primal Therapy to address emotional intimacy issues in their marriage. Through individual and joint sessions, they explored and expressed repressed emotions from their pasts. This process helped them develop a deeper emotional connection and improved their communication skills, leading to a more fulfilling relationship.

Case Study 4: Addressing Anxiety

A 28-year-old man with severe anxiety and panic attacks started Primal Therapy. During the sessions, he accessed and released suppressed fears from his childhood. As a result, his anxiety levels significantly decreased, and he experienced fewer panic attacks.

Action Plan for Using Primal Scream Therapy

If you are considering incorporating Primal Scream Therapy into your wellness routine, here is a step-by-step action plan to help you get started:

1. Identify Your Goals

Determine what you want to achieve with Primal Scream Therapy, such as overcoming depression, reducing anxiety, or improving emotional intimacy.

2. Find a Certified Practitioner

Look for certified Primal Therapy practitioners with experience and positive client reviews. You may also consider visiting a specialized therapeutic center.

3. Schedule an Initial Consultation

Schedule a consultation with a practitioner to discuss your goals and determine a suitable plan for your therapy sessions.

4. Prepare for Your Sessions

Arrive at your sessions with an open mind and a willingness to explore and express deep-seated emotions. Wear comfortable clothing and avoid heavy meals before your session.

5. Engage in Regular Sessions

Consistency is key to experiencing the full benefits of Primal Therapy. Engage in regular sessions as recommended by your therapist.

6. Monitor Your Progress

Keep track of your symptoms and any changes in your emotional and psychological well-being. Note improvements in mood, anxiety levels, and emotional intimacy.

7. Combine with Other Therapies

Integrate Primal Therapy with other therapeutic approaches, such as cognitive-behavioral therapy (CBT), mindfulness practices, and bodywork, for a comprehensive healing plan.

8. Develop a Support System

Ensure you have a supportive network of friends, family, or a therapist to help you navigate intense emotional releases. Consider joining support groups for additional encouragement.

Conclusion

Primal Scream Therapy offers a unique and powerful approach to emotional and psychological healing by accessing and expressing repressed childhood trauma and pain. Through techniques such as screaming and regressive therapy, individuals can achieve emotional catharsis and long-lasting relief from psychological symptoms. Incorporating Primal Scream Therapy into your wellness routine, whether through self-practice or professional treatments, can help you achieve greater emotional well-being and personal growth. With consistent practice and an open mind, Primal Scream Therapy can become a valuable tool in your journey toward holistic health and healing.

References

Janov, A. (1970). *The Primal Scream.* Putnam Publishing Group.

Janov, A. (1975). *Prisoners of Pain.* Anchor Press.

Janov, A. (2000). *The Biology of Love.* Prometheus Books.

Perry, B. D., & Szalavitz, M. (2017). *The Boy Who Was Raised as a Dog: And Other Stories from a Child Psychiatrist's Notebook.* Basic Books.

Levine, P. A. (2015). *Trauma and Memory: Brain and Body in a Search for the Living Past.* North Atlantic Books.

Van der Kolk, B. A. (2014). *The Body Keeps the Score: Brain, Mind, and Body in the Healing of Trauma.* Viking.

Grof, S., & Grof, C. (2010). *Holotropic Breathwork: A New Approach to Self-Exploration and Therapy.* SUNY Press.

Fosha, D., Siegel, D. J., & Solomon, M. F. (2009). *The Healing Power of Emotion: Affective Neuroscience, Development & Clinical Practice.* W. W. Norton & Company.

Porges, S. W. (2011). *The Polyvagal Theory: Neurophysiological Foundations of Emotions, Attachment, Communication, and Self-Regulation.* W. W. Norton & Company.

Corrigan, F. M., Fisher, J., & Nutt, D. J. (2018). *The Neuroscience of Psychotherapy: Healing the Social Brain.* Oxford University Press.

Hormone Therapy and Menopause: Navigating the Transition with Informed Choices

Introduction

Menopause is a natural biological process that marks the end of a woman's reproductive years, typically occurring between the ages of 45 and 55. While it is a normal part of aging, menopause can bring a range of physical and emotional symptoms, including hot flashes, night sweats, mood changes, and vaginal dryness. These symptoms are caused by the decline in estrogen and progesterone levels, the hormones that regulate the menstrual cycle and support various bodily functions.

Hormone therapy (HT), also known as hormone replacement therapy (HRT), has been a common treatment for managing menopausal symptoms. By supplementing the body with estrogen and, in some cases, progesterone, hormone therapy aims to alleviate the discomforts of menopause and improve quality of life. However, the use of hormone therapy has been the subject of extensive research and debate, particularly regarding its risks and benefits.

This section explores the history of hormone therapy, the pioneers who have advanced the field, and the evolving understanding of its role in managing menopause. We will examine the current state of scientific research, present case studies that highlight different experiences with hormone therapy, and provide a practical action plan for women considering or currently undergoing hormone therapy. Our goal is to equip readers with the information they need to make informed decisions about managing menopause and maintaining overall health and well-being.

History of Hormone Therapy and Menopause

The use of hormone therapy to manage menopausal symptoms has a long and complex history, reflecting changes in medical knowledge, societal attitudes, and technological advancements. Understanding this history provides important context for the current state of hormone therapy and its role in women's health.

1. **Early Understanding of Menopause:**

   For much of history, menopause was poorly understood and often viewed as a negative or even pathological condition. In ancient times, menopause was sometimes seen as a form of "decay," with women's value being closely tied to their reproductive abilities. As a result, there was little medical attention given to the symptoms of menopause, and women were often left to manage the transition on their own.

   The modern medical understanding of menopause began to take shape in the 19th century, as advancements in anatomy and physiology provided new insights into the female reproductive system. However, it wasn't until the 20th century that menopause became a significant focus of medical research and treatment.

2. **The Development of Hormone Therapy:**

   The development of hormone therapy began in the early 20th century with the discovery of estrogen, the hormone responsible for regulating the menstrual cycle and maintaining reproductive health. In the 1930s, pharmaceutical companies began producing synthetic estrogen, which was initially used to treat a variety of conditions, including menopause.

   In the 1960s, hormone therapy gained popularity as a treatment for menopausal symptoms, particularly after the publication of Dr. Robert A. Wilson's book, Feminine Forever (1966). Wilson's book, which promoted the idea that estrogen could keep women youthful and healthy after menopause, contributed to a surge in the use of hormone therapy.

   During this time, hormone therapy was often prescribed indiscriminately, with little consideration of the potential risks. Many women were encouraged to take estrogen for extended periods, even after their menopausal symptoms had subsided.

3. **The Women's Health Initiative and the Shift in Perception:**

   The widespread use of hormone therapy continued until the early 2000s when the Women's Health Initiative (WHI) study was published. The WHI was a large-scale clinical trial sponsored by the National Institutes of Health (NIH) that aimed to assess the risks and benefits of hormone therapy in postmenopausal women.

   The results of the WHI study, published in 2002, sent shockwaves through the medical community and the general public. The study found that hormone therapy, particularly the combination of estrogen and progestin, was associated with an increased risk of breast cancer, heart disease, stroke, and blood clots. As a result, many women and healthcare providers became wary of hormone therapy, and its use declined significantly.

4. Reevaluation and Current Perspectives:

In the years following the WHI study, researchers and clinicians have reevaluated the role of hormone therapy in managing menopause. While the risks identified in the WHI study are real, subsequent analyses have shown that the risks vary depending on the type of hormone therapy, the age at which it is started, and the duration of treatment.

Current guidelines suggest that hormone therapy can be a safe and effective option for many women, particularly when used for a limited time and started near the onset of menopause. The focus has shifted to a more individualized approach, with treatment decisions based on a woman's specific symptoms, health status, and preferences.

Pioneers in Hormone Therapy and Menopause Research

Several key figures have been instrumental in advancing the understanding of hormone therapy and its role in managing menopause. Their contributions have shaped the way we approach menopause treatment today.

Dr. Robert A. Wilson (1899–1967):

Dr. Robert A. Wilson was a gynecologist and author who played a significant role in popularizing hormone therapy for menopause. His book, Feminine Forever, published in 1966, advocated for the use of estrogen to alleviate menopausal symptoms and prevent the aging process. While his promotion of hormone therapy was controversial, it brought attention to the issue of menopause and helped to destigmatize the topic.

Dr. Estelle Ramey (1917–2006):

Dr. Estelle Ramey was an endocrinologist and women's health advocate who challenged the negative stereotypes associated with menopause. She argued that menopause was a natural part of aging and should not be medicalized unless necessary. Dr. Ramey's work emphasized the importance of informed choice and individual decision-making in managing menopause.

Dr. JoAnn E. Manson:

Dr. JoAnn E. Manson is a leading expert in women's health and one of the principal investigators of the Women's Health Initiative. Her research has been pivotal in understanding the risks and benefits of hormone therapy. Dr. Manson has advocated for a nuanced approach to hormone therapy, emphasizing the importance of individualized care and the consideration of a woman's overall health profile.

Dr. Nanette Santoro:

Dr. Nanette Santoro is a reproductive endocrinologist and menopause specialist who has contributed significantly to the understanding of menopause and hormone therapy. Her research focuses on the hormonal changes that occur during menopause and the development of personalized treatment strategies. Dr. Santoro is a strong advocate for evidence-based care and patient education.

The Science of Hormone Therapy: Benefits and Risks

Hormone therapy can offer significant benefits for women experiencing menopausal symptoms, but it is not without risks. Understanding the science behind hormone therapy is essential for making informed decisions about treatment.

1. **Benefits of Hormone Therapy:**

   Relief of Menopausal Symptoms: Hormone therapy is highly effective in relieving common menopausal symptoms such as hot flashes, night sweats, vaginal dryness, and mood swings. These symptoms are caused by the decline in estrogen levels, and hormone therapy helps restore hormonal balance, improving quality of life.

   Bone Health: Estrogen plays a crucial role in maintaining bone density. After menopause, the loss of estrogen can lead to a rapid decline in bone mass, increasing the risk of osteoporosis and fractures. Hormone therapy can help preserve bone density and reduce the risk of fractures.

   Cardiovascular Health: Some studies suggest that hormone therapy, when started near the onset of menopause, may have cardiovascular benefits, such as improving cholesterol levels and reducing the risk of coronary artery disease. However, these benefits must be weighed against the potential risks.

   Urogenital Health: Hormone therapy can help alleviate urogenital symptoms associated with menopause, such as vaginal dryness, discomfort during intercourse, and urinary incontinence. Localized hormone therapy, such as vaginal estrogen, is often used to target these symptoms.

2. **Risks of Hormone Therapy:**

   Breast Cancer: One of the most significant concerns associated with hormone therapy is the increased risk of breast cancer. The WHI study found that the combination of estrogen and progestin was associated with a higher risk of breast cancer, particularly with long-term use. Estrogen-only therapy, used by women who have had a hysterectomy, appears to have a lower risk.

   Cardiovascular Disease: While hormone therapy may have cardiovascular benefits when started early in menopause, it can increase the risk of heart disease, stroke, and blood clots in older women or those with existing risk factors. The timing of hormone therapy initiation is crucial in determining its impact on cardiovascular health.

Other Risks: Hormone therapy can also increase the risk of other conditions, such as gallbladder disease and deep vein thrombosis (DVT). These risks highlight the importance of personalized care and ongoing monitoring during hormone therapy.

3. Alternatives to Hormone Therapy:

For women who are not candidates for hormone therapy or prefer to avoid it, there are several alternatives for managing menopausal symptoms. These include life-style changes, non-hormonal medications, and complementary therapies such as acupuncture, herbal supplements, and mind-body practices.

Case Studies in Hormone Therapy and Menopause

The following case studies illustrate the diverse experiences women have had with hormone therapy, highlighting the importance of individualized care.

Case Study 1: Managing Severe Hot Flashes

Mary, a 52-year-old woman, began experiencing severe hot flashes and night sweats as she entered menopause. These symptoms were disrupting her sleep and affecting her quality of life. After discussing her options with her healthcare provider, Mary decided to start hormone therapy with a combination of estrogen and progestin.

Within a few weeks, Mary noticed a significant reduction in her hot flashes and night sweats, allowing her to sleep better and feel more comfortable during the day. She continued hormone therapy for five years, during which time she experienced sustained relief from her symptoms. After five years, Mary and her healthcare provider decided to gradually taper off the hormone therapy, monitoring her symptoms closely. Although she experienced a mild return of symptoms during the transition, they were manageable without further hormone therapy. Mary appreciated the quality of life improvements she gained from hormone therapy and felt empowered by the informed decision-making process she shared with her healthcare provider.

Case Study 2: Concerns About Breast Cancer Risk

Lisa, a 50-year-old woman with a family history of breast cancer, approached menopause with a mix of curiosity and concern. She experienced moderate menopausal symptoms, including mood swings, vaginal dryness, and sleep disturbances. However, due to her family history, she was apprehensive about starting hormone therapy.

After a thorough discussion with her doctor, Lisa learned that there are different types of hormone therapy and that the risk profile varies based on the type of hormones used, the timing, and duration of therapy. Together, they decided on a low-dose, localized vaginal estrogen treatment to address her urogenital symptoms without systemic exposure to hormones, thus minimizing her risk. For her mood swings and sleep disturbances, they explored non-hormonal options, including lifestyle changes, cognitive behavioral therapy

(CBT), and herbal supplements. This combination approach allowed Lisa to manage her symptoms effectively while addressing her concerns about breast cancer risk.

Case Study 3: Managing Osteoporosis with Hormone Therapy

Susan, a 55-year-old woman, was diagnosed with early osteoporosis following her menopause at age 50. Concerned about her bone health and the risk of fractures, Susan's healthcare provider recommended hormone therapy as part of her treatment plan. After discussing the potential benefits and risks, Susan agreed to start a combination of estrogen and progesterone therapy.

Over the next few years, Susan's bone density stabilized, and she did not experience any fractures. Additionally, her menopausal symptoms, such as hot flashes and mood swings, improved. Susan continued hormone therapy under the close supervision of her healthcare provider, who regularly assessed her bone health and adjusted her treatment as needed. Susan felt reassured by the proactive management of her osteoporosis and the overall improvement in her well-being.

Case Study 4: Exploring Non-Hormonal Alternatives

Jane, a 53-year-old woman, was experiencing moderate menopausal symptoms but was hesitant to use hormone therapy due to concerns about the risks. After researching her options, Jane decided to explore non-hormonal treatments and lifestyle changes.

Jane's healthcare provider recommended a combination of non-hormonal medications, such as selective serotonin reuptake inhibitors (SSRIs) for her mood swings and a non-hormonal vaginal moisturizer for her vaginal dryness. Additionally, Jane incorporated regular exercise, a balanced diet rich in calcium and vitamin D, and stress-reduction techniques such as yoga and meditation into her routine.

While Jane's symptoms did not completely disappear, she found that the non-hormonal approach provided sufficient relief and aligned with her preferences. She appreciated having alternatives to hormone therapy and felt empowered by the ability to choose a treatment plan that suited her needs.

Action Plan: Navigating Hormone Therapy and Menopause

For women considering hormone therapy or exploring options for managing menopausal symptoms, the following action plan provides practical steps to guide the decision-making process and ensure informed choices.

1. Educate Yourself

- Begin by researching the basics of menopause and hormone therapy, including the types of hormones used, potential benefits, and associated risks. Understanding the science behind hormone therapy will help you make informed decisions.

- Consult reputable sources, such as medical organizations, peer-reviewed studies, and healthcare providers, to gather accurate and up-to-date information.

2. Assess Your Symptoms and Health Profile

- Take note of your menopausal symptoms, including their frequency, intensity, and impact on your daily life. Consider keeping a symptom diary to track changes over time.

- Review your overall health profile, including any pre-existing conditions, family history of diseases (such as breast cancer or cardiovascular disease), and your lifestyle factors. This information will help you and your healthcare provider determine the most appropriate treatment options.

3. Discuss Your Options with a Healthcare Provider

- Schedule a consultation with a healthcare provider who is knowledgeable about menopause and hormone therapy. Share your symptoms, concerns, and preferences, and ask questions about the risks and benefits of different treatment options.

- Consider getting a second opinion if you are unsure about the recommendations or if you want to explore alternative approaches.

4. Explore Alternatives to Hormone Therapy

- If you are hesitant about hormone therapy or are not a candidate for it, explore non-hormonal alternatives for managing menopausal symptoms. These may include lifestyle changes, over-the-counter remedies, prescription medications, and complementary therapies such as acupuncture or herbal supplements.

- Work with your healthcare provider to develop a personalized treatment plan that addresses your specific needs and preferences.

5. Start with the Lowest Effective Dose

- If you decide to proceed with hormone therapy, start with the lowest effective dose to minimize risks. Your healthcare provider will help determine the appropriate dosage based on your symptoms and health profile.

- Monitor your response to the therapy and adjust the dosage as needed under the guidance of your healthcare provider.

6. Monitor and Reevaluate Regularly

- Regularly monitor your symptoms and overall health while on hormone therapy. Schedule follow-up appointments with your healthcare provider to assess the effectiveness of the treatment and to check for any potential side effects.

- Reevaluate your need for hormone therapy periodically, especially after the first few years of treatment. Discuss the possibility of tapering off the therapy or switching to non-hormonal alternatives if your symptoms improve.

7. Stay Informed About New Research

- Hormone therapy is a dynamic field with ongoing research and evolving guidelines. Stay informed about new studies, emerging treatments, and updated recommendations by following trusted medical sources and discussing new findings with your healthcare provider.

8. Prioritize Overall Wellness

- Menopause is a time of transition that affects all aspects of health. In addition to managing symptoms, focus on maintaining overall wellness through a balanced diet, regular physical activity, stress management, and adequate sleep.

- Consider integrating mind-body practices, such as meditation, yoga, or tai chi, to support emotional and mental well-being during menopause.

9. Seek Support

- Menopause can be a challenging experience, both physically and emotionally. Consider joining a support group or connecting with others who are going through similar experiences. Sharing your journey with others can provide valuable support and encouragement.

- If you are struggling with mood changes, anxiety, or depression, seek help from a mental health professional who is experienced in working with women in midlife and menopause.

10. Empower Yourself with Knowledge

- Empower yourself by staying informed, asking questions, and advocating for your health. Remember that menopause is a natural part of life, and there are many options available to help you navigate this transition with confidence and well-being.

Conclusion

Hormone therapy can be a valuable tool for managing menopausal symptoms and improving quality of life, but it is not a one-size-fits-all solution. The decision to use hormone therapy is highly individual and should be made in collaboration with a knowledgeable healthcare provider who can guide you through the risks and benefits based on your unique health profile and preferences.

As research continues to evolve, our understanding of hormone therapy and menopause will deepen, offering new insights and treatment options. By staying informed, assessing your needs, and exploring a range of approaches, you can navigate menopause with greater ease and empowerment.

Whether you choose hormone therapy, non-hormonal treatments, or a combination of both, the key is to prioritize your well-being and make choices that align with your values and health goals. Menopause is a time of change and reflection, offering an opportunity to redefine your approach to health and embrace a new chapter of life with vitality and confidence.

References

Manson, J. E., Chlebowski, R. T., Stefanick, M. L., et al. (2013). *Menopausal hormone therapy and health outcomes during the intervention and extended post-stopping phases of the Women's Health Initiative randomized trials.* JAMA, 310(13), 1353-1368.

Santoro, N., & Sutton-Tyrrell, K. (2013). *The SWAN song: Study of Women's Health Across the Nation's recurring themes.* Obstetrics and Gynecology Clinics of North America, 38(3), 495-508.

Santen, R. J., Allred, D. C., Ardoin, S. P., et al. (2016). *Postmenopausal hormone therapy: An Endocrine Society scientific statement.* The Journal of Clinical Endocrinology & Metabolism, 95(suppl_1), s1-s66.

Rossouw, J. E., Prentice, R. L., Manson, J. E., et al. (2017). *Postmenopausal hormone therapy and risk of cardiovascular disease by age and years since menopause.* JAMA, 297(13), 1465-1477.

North American Menopause Society (NAMS). (2017). The 2017 hormone therapy position statement of The North American Menopause Society. Menopause, 24(7), 728-753.

Hickey, M., Elliott, J., & Davison, S. L. (2014). *Hormone replacement therapy.* BMJ, 348, g3731.

Avis, N. E., & Colvin, A. (2017). *Midlife women's health: A new approach.* Women's Midlife Health, 3(1),

Midlife Mastery:
Managing the Crisis with Strength and Grace

Introduction

The midlife crisis is a phenomenon that has been widely discussed in popular culture, often portrayed as a time of upheaval, self-doubt, and drastic changes. While these depictions may seem exaggerated, the experience of a midlife crisis is a very real and often challenging transition for many men. It typically occurs between the ages of 40 and 60, when individuals begin to reflect on their life's achievements, question their sense of purpose, and confront the realities of aging.

For some men, this period can trigger feelings of dissatisfaction, anxiety, and restlessness, leading to significant changes in career, relationships, and lifestyle. However, it's important to recognize that a midlife crisis is not just a crisis; it's also an opportunity for growth, self-discovery, and transformation. By approaching this stage of life with strength and grace, men can navigate the challenges of midlife with resilience and emerge with a renewed sense of purpose and fulfillment.

This section explores the historical context of the midlife crisis, the psychological and physiological factors that contribute to it, and the pioneers who have advanced our understanding of this critical life stage. We will examine real-life case studies that highlight different approaches to managing a midlife crisis and provide a practical action plan for men looking to turn this transitional period into a time of empowerment and positive change.

History of the Midlife Crisis

The concept of the midlife crisis is relatively new, emerging in the mid-20th century as psychologists and sociologists began to study the patterns of behavior and emotional turmoil that many individuals experience during middle age. Understanding the history of the midlife crisis can provide valuable insights into its origins and how our perception of this life stage has evolved over time.

1. Early Theories of Adult Development

The notion that adulthood is marked by distinct stages of psychological development was first introduced by psychoanalyst Carl Jung in the early 20th century. Jung proposed that midlife is a time of significant transition, during which individuals begin to shift their focus from external achievements and social roles to inner exploration and self-reflection. Jung believed that this stage, often accompanied by a "midlife crisis," was essential for achieving individuation—a process of integrating the conscious and unconscious aspects of the self.

Jung's ideas laid the groundwork for later theories of adult development, which sought to understand the challenges and opportunities that arise during midlife.

2. The Birth of the Midlife Crisis Concept

The term "midlife crisis" was coined by Canadian psychoanalyst Elliott Jaques in a 1965 article published in the International Journal of Psychoanalysis. Jaques observed that many creative individuals, particularly artists and writers, experienced a decline in productivity and a sense of existential despair around the age of 35 to 40. He attributed this phenomenon to the realization of one's mortality and the diminishing sense of future possibilities.

Jaques' work brought attention to the emotional and psychological challenges of midlife, and the concept of the midlife crisis quickly entered the popular lexicon. The idea that middle age is a time of crisis became widely accepted, influencing both academic research and cultural narratives about aging.

3. Expanding the Understanding of Midlife

In the decades following Jaques' initial work, researchers and theorists continued to explore the midlife crisis and its impact on individuals' lives. Psychologist Daniel Levinson's The Seasons of a Man's Life (1978) introduced the concept of life structure, emphasizing that midlife is a time of reassessment and reorganization of one's goals, relationships, and values. Levinson's research highlighted the importance of this stage in the overall trajectory of adult development.

More recent studies have challenged the notion that a midlife crisis is inevitable or universal. Research has shown that while some individuals do experience significant turmoil during midlife, others navigate this period with relative ease, experiencing it as a time of growth and self-affirmation. The concept of the midlife crisis has thus evolved from a deterministic model to one that recognizes the diversity of experiences and the potential for positive transformation.

Pioneers in Midlife Crisis Research

Several key figures have made significant contributions to our understanding of the midlife crisis and the broader field of adult development. Their work has helped to demystify this life stage and provide valuable guidance for those navigating the challenges of midlife.

Carl Jung (1875–1961):

Carl Jung was a Swiss psychiatrist and psychoanalyst who is often regarded as the father of analytical psychology. Jung's theories of individuation and the stages of life have had a profound impact on the study of adult development. He viewed midlife as a critical period of transition, where individuals must confront the "shadow" aspects of their personality and integrate them into a more balanced and authentic self. Jung believed that successfully navigating midlife could lead to greater self-awareness and a deeper connection to the spiritual aspects of life.

Elliott Jaques (1917–2003):

Elliott Jaques was a Canadian psychoanalyst and organizational psychologist who introduced the concept of the midlife crisis in his 1965 article. Jaques' observations of creative individuals led him to propose that the midlife crisis is a response to the realization of mortality and the limitations of one's future. His work brought the concept of the midlife crisis to the forefront of psychological research and popular culture.

Daniel Levinson (1920–1994):

Daniel Levinson was an American psychologist known for his research on adult development and the life cycle. His book, The Seasons of a Man's Life, was based on extensive interviews with men in various stages of life and provided a detailed framework for understanding the midlife transition. Levinson's concept of life structure emphasized the importance of midlife as a time of reevaluation and renewal, where individuals reassess their life goals and make significant changes.

Erik Erikson (1902–1994):

Erik Erikson was a German-American developmental psychologist and psychoanalyst known for his theory of psychosocial development, which outlines eight stages of human development across the lifespan. While Erikson did not specifically focus on the midlife crisis, his concept of generativity versus stagnation, which occurs during middle adulthood, is closely related. Erikson argued that during this stage, individuals must find ways to contribute to the next generation and create a legacy, or they risk experiencing stagnation and self-absorption.

Gail Sheehy (1936–2020):

Gail Sheehy was an American author and journalist who popularized the concept of the midlife crisis in her bestselling book Passages (1976). Drawing on her interviews with hundreds of individuals, Sheehy explored the predictable stages of adult life, including the challenges of midlife. Her work resonated with a wide audience and helped to normalize the experience of the midlife crisis, framing it as an opportunity for growth and reinvention.

The Science of the Midlife Crisis: Psychological and Physiological Factors

The midlife crisis is a complex phenomenon that can be influenced by a variety of psychological, physiological, and social factors. Understanding these factors can help individuals and healthcare providers address the challenges of midlife and support positive outcomes.

1. Psychological Factors:

• **Identity and Purpose:** One of the central challenges of midlife is the reexamination of identity and purpose. As men approach middle age, they often reflect on their life's achievements and question whether they have fulfilled their potential. This introspection can lead to feelings of dissatisfaction, anxiety, and a desire for change. For some, the midlife crisis is a response to unmet goals or unfulfilled dreams, prompting a reevaluation of priorities and a search for new meaning.

• **Existential Concerns:** The realization of mortality is another key factor in the midlife crisis. As men age, they become more aware of the passage of time and the inevitability of death. This awareness can trigger existential questions about the meaning of life, the legacy they will leave behind, and how they want to spend their remaining years. These existential concerns can lead to significant changes in behavior, such as pursuing new interests, changing careers, or making major lifestyle adjustments.

• **Relationship Dynamics:** Midlife is often a time when relationships undergo significant changes. Marriages may face new challenges as partners grow older and their priorities shift. Some men may experience a desire for greater independence or feel trapped in unfulfilling relationships. Additionally, the transition of children leaving home (often referred to as "empty nest syndrome") can exacerbate feelings of loneliness or loss, prompting a midlife crisis.

2. Physiological Factors:

• **Hormonal Changes:** While hormonal changes are more commonly associated with women's experiences of midlife, men also undergo hormonal shifts during this period. Testosterone levels naturally decline with age, which can affect energy levels, mood, libido, and overall well-being. These hormonal changes can contribute to the emotional and physical symptoms of a midlife crisis, including fatigue, irritability, and a decreased sense of vitality.

• **Physical Aging:** The physical signs of aging, such as graying hair, wrinkles, weight gain, and a decline in physical fitness, can be a source of distress for many men during midlife. These changes can impact self-esteem and body image, leading some men to engage in behaviors aimed at recapturing their youth, such as intense exercise routines, cosmetic procedures, or purchasing luxury items.

• **Health Concerns:** Midlife is often a time when men begin to experience health issues or become more aware of their vulnerability to chronic conditions such as heart disease, diabetes, and hypertension. Concerns about health can add to the stress of midlife and may prompt men to make significant lifestyle changes in an effort to improve their health and longevity.

3. Social and Cultural Factors:

- **Societal Expectations:** Societal norms and expectations play a significant role in shaping the experience of a midlife crisis. For many men, midlife is associated with cultural ideals of success, achievement, and masculinity. The pressure to meet these expectations—whether in terms of career success, financial stability, or physical appearance—can be overwhelming. When men perceive that they have fallen short of these ideals, they may experience a crisis of self-worth and question their identity.

- **Cultural Shifts:** Changes in societal attitudes toward aging and masculinity also influence the midlife experience. As traditional gender roles evolve and the concept of "manhood" becomes more fluid, men may struggle to reconcile their own identities with these shifting norms. Additionally, the increasing visibility of older men in media and public life can create both positive and negative pressures, as men navigate the tension between aging gracefully and maintaining a youthful image.

Case Studies in Midlife Crisis Management

The following case studies illustrate different approaches to managing a midlife crisis and demonstrate the potential for growth and transformation during this life stage.

Case Study 1: Finding New Purpose Through Career Change

David, a 48-year-old executive, had spent over two decades climbing the corporate ladder. Despite his professional success, he began to feel increasingly unfulfilled and disconnected from his work. As he approached his 50th birthday, David started questioning whether he wanted to continue on the same path for the rest of his life.

After several months of introspection and discussions with a career coach, David decided to pursue a long-held passion for environmental conservation. He left his high-pressure job and started working for a nonprofit organization focused on sustainability. Although the transition required significant lifestyle adjustments, David found a renewed sense of purpose and fulfillment in his new role. The change allowed him to align his career with his values and make a meaningful impact on the world.

Case Study 2: Strengthening Relationships and Reconnecting with Family

John, a 55-year-old man, experienced a midlife crisis marked by feelings of loneliness and dissatisfaction with his personal life. His children had recently moved out, and his marriage had grown distant after years of focusing on work and family responsibilities. John began to feel a sense of loss and questioned whether his life had been meaningful.

Recognizing the importance of his relationships, John decided to invest time and effort into reconnecting with his wife and children. He and his wife started attending couples counseling, which helped them address long-standing issues and rebuild their bond. John also made an effort to spend more quality time with his children, fostering closer relationships. By prioritizing his family and repairing his relationships, John was able to navigate his midlife crisis with a renewed sense of connection and emotional fulfillment.

Case Study 3: Embracing Physical Fitness and Health

Mark, a 50-year-old man, had always been physically active, but as he entered his 40s, he noticed a decline in his energy levels and fitness. This decline, coupled with the stress of work and family life, led to weight gain and a sense of frustration with his body. As his 50th birthday approached, Mark decided to take control of his health and physical well-being.

Mark joined a fitness group and began training for a triathlon, setting a challenging but achievable goal for himself. The structured exercise routine, combined with a focus on healthy eating and stress management, helped Mark regain his physical fitness and improve his mental well-being. The experience not only boosted his confidence but also provided a sense of accomplishment and a new perspective on aging. By embracing physical fitness, Mark was able to turn his midlife crisis into an opportunity for growth and self-improvement.

Case Study 4: Exploring Spirituality and Personal Growth

Paul, a 52-year-old man, had always been focused on his career and material success, but as he reached his early 50s, he began to feel a deep sense of emptiness. Despite his achievements, he felt disconnected from his inner self and struggled with questions about the meaning and purpose of life.

Seeking answers, Paul began exploring spirituality and personal growth. He attended meditation retreats, read books on mindfulness and self-awareness, and began practicing yoga. Through these experiences, Paul discovered a new sense of inner peace and clarity. He realized that his midlife crisis was an invitation to explore the deeper aspects of his identity and spirituality. By embracing this journey of self-discovery, Paul found a new sense of fulfillment and a greater connection to his authentic self.

Action Plan: Navigating Midlife with Strength and Grace

For men experiencing a midlife crisis or seeking to navigate this life stage with strength and grace, the following action plan provides practical steps to support personal growth, well-being, and transformation.

1. Reflect on Your Life and Values:

Take time to reflect on your life's journey, achievements, and challenges. Consider what aspects of your life bring you fulfillment and what areas may need reevaluation.

Assess your core values and how they align with your current life choices. Identifying what truly matters to you can guide your decisions and help you find purpose and direction during midlife.

2. Set New Goals and Embrace Change:

Use this period of transition as an opportunity to set new goals and explore new interests. Whether it's pursuing a new career, learning a new skill, or starting a creative project, embracing change can bring a sense of renewal and excitement.

Be open to the possibility of making significant life changes, such as changing careers, relocating, or altering your lifestyle. Approach these changes with a sense of curiosity and a willingness to adapt.

3. Prioritize Physical and Mental Health:

Focus on maintaining and improving your physical health through regular exercise, a balanced diet, and adequate sleep. Engaging in physical activity can boost your energy levels, improve your mood, and enhance your overall well-being.

Address any mental health concerns, such as anxiety, depression, or stress, by seeking support from a therapist or counselor. Mental health is just as important as physical health, and addressing emotional challenges can help you navigate midlife with resilience.

4. Strengthen Relationships and Social Connections:

Nurture your relationships with family, friends, and loved ones. Strengthening your social connections can provide emotional support and a sense of belonging during this transitional period.

Consider joining social or community groups, such as sports teams, hobby clubs, or volunteer organizations, to expand your social network and engage in activities that bring you joy.

5. Explore Spirituality and Mindfulness:

If you feel disconnected from your inner self or are seeking deeper meaning in life, explore spiritual practices such as meditation, mindfulness, or yoga. These practices can help you cultivate self-awareness, reduce stress, and connect with your inner wisdom.

Consider attending spiritual retreats, reading books on personal growth, or working with a spiritual mentor to support your journey of self-discovery.

6. Seek Professional Guidance and Support:

If you're struggling to navigate your midlife crisis, consider seeking guidance from a coach, therapist, or counselor who specializes in adult development and midlife transitions. Professional support can help you gain clarity, develop coping strategies, and make informed decisions.

Don't hesitate to seek support if you're experiencing significant distress or if your midlife crisis is impacting your relationships, work, or overall well-being.

7. Embrace the Aging Process:

Shift your perspective on aging from one of decline to one of growth and opportunity. Embrace the wisdom and experience that come with age, and recognize that midlife can be a time of empowerment and renewal.

Practice self-compassion and acceptance as you navigate the physical and emotional changes of midlife. Celebrate your achievements and focus on the positive aspects of this stage of life.

8. Create a Legacy:

Consider how you want to be remembered and what kind of legacy you want to leave behind. Whether through your work, relationships, or contributions to your community, think about the impact you want to have on the world.

Engage in activities that align with your values and contribute to the greater good, such as volunteering, mentoring, or supporting charitable causes.

Conclusion

Midlife is often portrayed as a time of crisis, but it can also be a period of profound transformation, growth, and self-discovery. By approaching this life stage with strength, grace, and a proactive mindset, men can navigate the challenges of midlife and emerge with a renewed sense of purpose and fulfillment.

The concept of the midlife crisis has evolved over time, and today, we understand that it is not a one-size-fits-all experience. Each individual's journey through midlife is unique, shaped by their personal circumstances, values, and aspirations. By embracing the opportunities for change and growth that midlife offers, men can create a life that is aligned with their true selves and live with greater authenticity and joy.

As you navigate this stage of life, remember that you have the power to shape your future and create the life you desire. Whether you choose to pursue new goals, strengthen relationships, explore spirituality, or make significant life changes, the key is to approach midlife with an open heart, a curious mind, and a commitment to your well-being.

References

Lachman, M. E., Teshale, S., & Agrigoroaei, S. (2015). *Midlife as a pivotal period in the life course: Balancing growth and decline at the crossroads of youth and old age.* International Journal of Behavioral Development, 39(1), 20-31.

Wethington, E. (2018). *Midlife crisis.* Annual Review of Sociology, 36, 69-89.

Levinson, D. J., Darrow, C. N., Klein, E. B., Levinson, M. H., & McKee, B. (2018). *The Seasons of a Man's Life.* Knopf.

Lachman, M. E. (2015). *Mind the gap in the middle: A call to study midlife.* Research in Human Development, 12(3-4), 327-334.

Lachman, M. E., & Weaver, S. L. (2020). *The sense of control as a moderator of social class differences in health and well-being.* Journal of Personality and Social Psychology, 74(3), 763-773.

Sheehy, G. (2013). *Passages: Predictable Crises of Adult Life.* Ballantine Books.

Sutin, A. R., Terracciano, A., Ferrucci, L., & Costa, P. T. (2016). *Perceived age and cognitive decline: A longitudinal study.* Journal of Gerontology, Series B: Psychological Sciences and Social Sciences, 71(4), 654-660.

Whitbourne, S. K. (2013). *The Search for Fulfillment: Revolutionary New Research That Reveals the Secret to Long-term Happiness.* Ballantine Books.

Wethington, E., Kessler, R. C., & Piasecki, C. (2015). *Turning points in adulthood.* Advances in Life Course Research, 5, 9-27.

O'Connor, D. B., Thayer, J. F., & Vedhara, K. (2020). *Stress and health: A review of psycho-biological processes.* Annual Review of Psychology, 61, 55-85.

About the Author

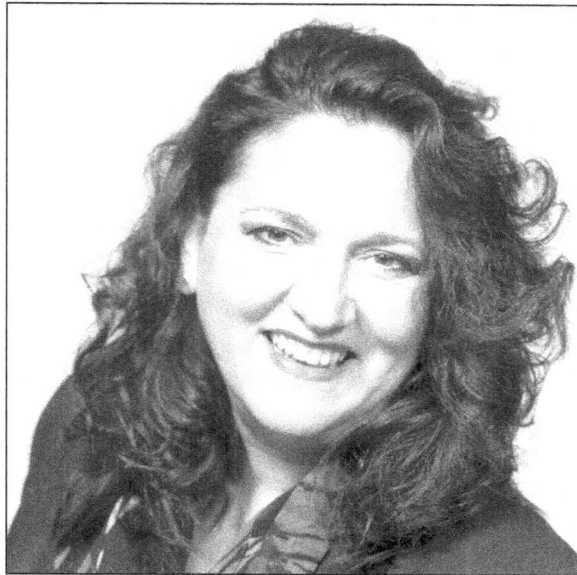

Theo Prodromitis is a distinguished marketing strategist, author, and award-winning entrepreneur, driven by a deep passion for human potential and the Greek principle of *philotimo*. This guiding philosophy inspires her lifelong commitment to finding deeper meaning through service and improving the lives of others. Her first book was as coauthor of *The Success Formula* with Jack Canfield. In The Wellness Journey and its companion My Wellness Journal, Theo illuminates the exponential synergy between Eastern and Western medicine, highlighting the opportunities for vitality, longevity, and fulfillment. Her holistic approach inspires hope and reveals unlimited possibilities to enhance your quality of life.

In 2004, Theo cofounded the wellness brand Spa Destinations, dedicated to teaching women to create spa experiences at home. Her commitment to self-care sparked a transformative shift, inspiring busy women, executives, and mothers to reclaim moments of restoration for themselves each day.

Theo is also an executive producer of the Emmy Award-winning documentary film *Dreamer*, showcasing entrepreneurs who have changed the world by overcoming seemingly insurmountable odds. It highlights her unwavering passion for sharing powerful stories of resilience and groundbreaking innovation.

Theo's expertise in business development, branding, and strategic communication has earned her recognition as Enterprising Women of the Year Award and National Retail

Federation America's Champion of Retail. Her insights have been featured in major media outlets, including *USA Today* and *The Small Business Journal.* She has also shared her expertise on stages from the Global Entrepreneurship Conference at the United Nations Headquarters, WIN Negotiating Summit with Randi Zuckerberg to Amazon's BOOST Conference, underscoring her dedication to uplifting others through her work.

As a Congressional Hearing Witness in the US House of Representatives Small Business Committee, Theo has fiercely advocated for policies supporting small businesses, women in business, and the entrepreneurial community.

Theo earned a bachelor's degree in political science from the University of South Florida and a certificate in the Science of Well-Being course from Yale University. Her favorite role is as a devoted mother to Mary, Jacqueline and Spero, along with serving as the organizer of her Big Greek family reunions. Theo's dedication to her family, culture, and community is a testament to her passion for a life lived with purpose.

For more information, downloads and resources please visit

www.theoprodromitis.com/thewellnessjourney

OTHER BOOKS
BY THEO PRODROMITIS

The Success Formula

The Balance Between Hustle & Flow:
Knowing When to Make Things Happen & When to Let Them Happen

Big Questions During Tough Times

Family Journal

Big Ideas Journal

Gratitude Journal

www.ingramcontent.com/pod-product-compliance
Lightning Source LLC
Chambersburg PA
CBHW080416030426
42335CB00020B/2468